After School

Lives of Manitoba Normalites
(Class of 1950-51)

R. L. Duane Duff

DUFF PUBLISHING .CA
Surrey, British Columbia, Canada

Editor, cover: Sean G. Duff

ISBN 978-0-9810784-4-1
Printed in the United States of America

Duff Publishing
13866 60 Avenue
Surrey, BC V3X 2N1
Canada
www.duffpublishing.ca

To the memory of
the administration, staff, and students of
Manitoba Provincial Normal School
class of 1950–51

A teacher affects eternity;
he can never tell where his influence stops.
—*Henry Brooks Adams*

The object of teaching a child is
to enable him to get along without his teacher.
—*Elbert Hubbard*

Contents

List of Photographs 11
Preface 13
Acknowledgements 17
Introduction 19

Class A 27
1. Ruth Armson 29
2. Harry Backlin 35
3. Joan (Barr) Allison 39
4. Shirley (Bold) Fairbairn 45
5. Edna (Brown) Dreger 59
6. Marie Brownlees 63
7. Frances (Burnett) Dickinson 75
8. Dorothy (Carnegie) Blakeman 81

Class B 85
9. Winnie (Cathcart) Wolfe 87
10. Mary (Dishnick) Chubey 93
11. Audrey (Donald) Henitiuk 103
12. Eugene Doroschuk 111

Class C 115
13. Cecile (Droux) Fisher 117
14. Duane Duff 124
15. Virginia (Eilers) Lyons 133
16. Jacob Enns 137
17. Helen (Finlay) Morrow 145
18. Betty (Forsyth) Sumner 151
19. Abe Friesen 155
20. Peggy (Friesen) Lawrence 159
21. Shirley (Fulmore) McCracken 169

22. Ethel (Galloway) Currie.....175
23. Isla (Gliddon) Lawrie.....179
24. Evelyn (Graham) Jones.....185
25. Joyce (Griffith) Garner.....189

Class D.....197
26. Aileen (Harbottle) Huss-Siedel.....199
27. Wilma (Hedley) Treloar.....205
28. Henriette (Heiget) Leduc.....211
29. Keith Huss-Siedel.....215
30. Emily James.....227
31. Vera (Jones) Skayman.....231
32. Ena (Kandall) Sparrow.....237
33. Peter Peters.....243
34. Dorothy (Twilley) Shewfelt.....251

Class E.....257
35. Sylvia (Lee) Haverstick.....259
36. Jean (McClelland) Tully.....263
37. Irene (McFee) Coleman.....273

Class F.....279
38. Henry Dick.....281
39. Jerry Hildebrand.....287
40. Lois (Leigh) Moore.....293
41. Rose (McColl) McIver.....297
42. Wilma (Miller) Furniss.....307
43. Bernice (Morrow) Lewis.....311
44. Jack Morton.....315
45. Sarah Evaline Muir.....323
46. Isabelle (Neeley) Dowling.....329
47. Delphie (Olson) Norberg.....333
48. Doreen (Olson) Lindquist.....341

Class G.....347
49. Dorothy (Brownridge) Haithwaite.....349
50. Betty (Hughes) Doroschuk.....355

51. Orest Roscoe....359
52. Harry Rudy....365
53. John Ryan....371
54. Gladwyn Scott....381
55. Viola (Sigurdson) Wild....389
56. Elaine (Slimmon) Dale....395

Class H....401
57. George Krahn....403
58. Shirley (Solar) Maurice....407
59. Verna (Spurr) Lavergne....415
60. Steve Stasiuk....419
61. Emily (Szarkowicz) Hilhorst....423
62. Olive (Tarbath) Johnson....427
63. Tina (Thiessen) Hildebrandt....431
64. Roy White....435

Class J....441
65. Carl Braun....443
66. Elaine (Wall) Rex....459
67. Pearl (Young) Langille....465

Appendix....471

List of Photographs

1. WECO Ticket..15
Front, Winnipeg Electric Company (WECO), circa 1950. *[courtesy Manitoba Transit Heritage Association Inc., used with permission]*

2. WECO Ticket..15
Back, Winnipeg Electric Company (WECO), circa 1950. *[courtesy Manitoba Transit Heritage Association Inc., used with permission]*

3. Plaque..16
Near the entrance of the chapel of the former Normal School, now Canadian Mennonite University. *[courtesy Isla Lawrie]*

4. Central Normal School, Winnipeg..........................19
1905. Archives of Manitoba, Winnipeg – Schools – Normal 2 (N3690) *[courtesy Manitoba Provincial Archives, used with permission]*

5. Normal School, Brandon..20
Built in 1912. *[courtesy Queen's Printer for Manitoba, used with permission]*

6. Frontenac Hall Boys..21
Normal School. *[courtesy Mary Chubey]*

7. Strathcona Hall Musicians..22
Normal School. *[courtesy Mary Chubey]*

8. Mr. Moorhead..23
Principal of Manitoba Provincial Normal School. *["Normal Lights", 1951]*

9. Teaching Staff..25
Manitoba Provincial Normal School. *["Normal Lights", 1951]*

10. Class B..86
Normal School. *[courtesy Mary Chubey]*

11. Broadview School..95
Near Morris, Mary (Dishnick) Chubey and her first class in 1951. *[courtesy Mary Chubey]*

12. Class C..116
Fad Day at Normal School. *[courtesy Isla Lawrie]*

13. Denepro School..118
Near Grandview, where Cecile (Droux) Fisher taught. *[courtesy Cecile Fisher]*

14. Cheval School..162
Near Morden, where Peggy (Friesen) Lawrence taught. *[courtesy Peggy Lawrence]*

15. Parkland School Div. #2197....................................170
Near Virden, where Shirley (Fulmore) McCracken taught. *[courtesy Shirley McCracken]*

16. Campaign Poster..221
Over rear entrance for Keith Huss for Student Council President. *[courtesy John Ryan]*

17. McCreary School..227
Where Emily James attended high school. *[courtesy Emily James]*

18. Turtle Plains School...228
Where Emily James first taught. *[courtesy Emily James]*

19. Osprey School...228
Near Neepawa, where Emily James taught. *[courtesy Emily James]*

20. Class E...258
Members at the 1996 reunion. *[courtesy Jean Tully]*

21. Loon Straits...266
An almost finished two-room school where Jean (McClelland) Tully was principal, teaching in the high school. *[courtesy Jean Tully]*

22. Ladies' Hockey Team...274
At the 2001 reunion. *[courtesy Gladwyn Scott]*

23. Bear Creek School..299
#762, near Gladstone, where Rose (McColl) McIver first attended school. *[courtesy Rose McIver]*

24. Class G...348
Members at the 2001 reunion. *[Courtesy Gladwyn Scott]*

25. Portage Avenue Streetcar and Bus..........................351
In Front of Eaton's Store, Winnipeg Electric Company (WECO), circa 1950. *[courtesy Manitoba Transit Heritage Association Inc., used with permission]*

26. Men's Hockey Team...383
At the 2001 reunion. *[courtesy Gladwyn Scott]*

Preface

Everyone has a story. Some have told it; some have not. As one passes through life, there are many experiences—in one's childhood years, in one's teenage years, in one's working years, and in one's senior years. What may be routine or uninteresting for one person may be interesting or educational for another. We all can share with others what we have learned during our lifetime.

Having written two books about specific people in several countries and one about a few Canadian naval veterans, I embarked on one about the experiences of my colleagues of the class of 1950–51 at Manitoba Provincial Normal School in Winnipeg. When I was laying my plans, Gladwyn Scott sent me his copy of the book that was compiled in 2001. That was an ambitious undertaking, one in which the committee is to be commended. Much work went into its production.

With the encouragement of Gladwyn and a few others, I set my plan into motion. More encouragement that came from others after I began sending out letters was much appreciated. Since I have had very little contact with my Normalite colleagues over the years, I wanted to produce this book for them, especially since all of us are up in years. I feel rewarded for the time, cost, and frustrations of producing this book. I would like to thank all for whatever they have done to help to make this book possible. If there be any errors or omissions, please accept my apology.

As the submissions were received and I composed the chapters from them, I felt happy with the successes of various persons, sad with the trials of others, and proud with the determination of many in not being defeated by adversity. Every achievement, no matter how small it may seem to the person, stands out as worthwhile. The lives of the participants took on new meaning for me. I have come to know them as I had never known them before. It was truly an educational experience for me, and I hope that it will be the same for anyone who reads these stories.

When a submission was very short or made a comment that posed a question to me, I contacted the writer by email, postal mail, or telephone to obtain more information. This was successful. As I have compiled stories for about 140 persons with the completion of this book, I have learned about interviewing. This has been an ongoing experience, beginning with an interview with the Mexican Ambassador to Canada as he was driving to work while snow was falling.

If there be a disappointment, it would be that more persons could not have been involved. Several letters were returned because of people having moved. However, about one third of those contacted made submissions, which is good, considering the health of many. Some contacted me via email while others wrote their stories by hand and sent them by postal mail—some with physical difficulty. There was no problem in reading any of them. In a few cases, a telephone interview was used instead, with good results.

Another disappointment is that I could not obtain sufficient information about our teachers to include. However, I have included their photographs that are in the 1951 yearbook. There is also a class list with the names being as listed in the same source.

There are differences in the structure and nature of the context of the various chapters. Those of Carl Braun, Jake Enns, and Jerry Hildebrand were submitted for my book *I Have a Story to Tell, Too* and the one for Gladwyn Scott was submitted for a book which had to be abandoned. These have been edited a bit for this book. I was unable to make contact with more Normalites for those books. The lengths of the submissions varied and a few were virtually in final form.

As many of the submissions came in telling about one-room school experiences, I felt that it might be good to include photos of such schools. Eventually, I contacted a number of persons who had email addresses and received from them the photos which appear in this book. I regret not being able to include photos of rural schools of more of our class who were students or teachers in them.

I was able to obtain photos of public transportation that we used and of the tickets we deposited on entrance into a vehicle. These may bring back memories of our travel in the city.

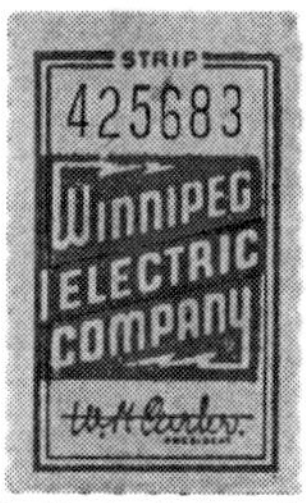

1. Ticket, front

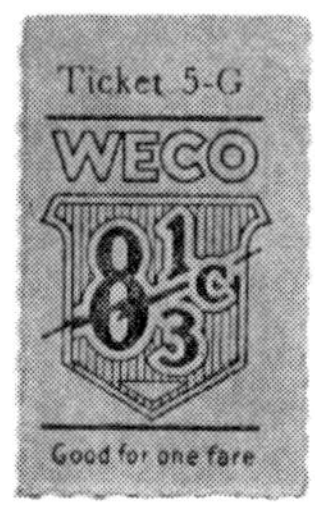

2. Ticket, back

There has been something unique about the students of our year—right from the beginning. That may be why the reunions have continued and comments appear in these stories about having kept contact with friends we made in that Normal School year.

Each person has his/her own skill. If writing your story be not one of them, you can find someone who can do it for you with your help. Your life experiences are important for others—your own descendants or the general public. If you have not already committed your story to print, it is my hope that you will. So many stories will be gone forever if you do not tell them. This encompasses one of my reasons for compiling this and other biographical books.

May you enjoy the stories of our colleagues!

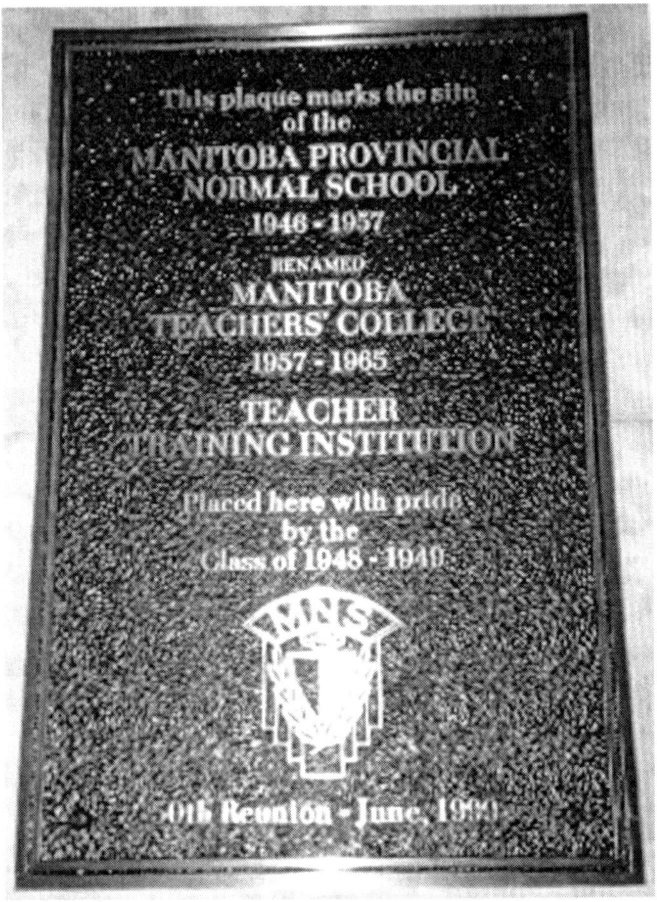
This plaque marks the site
of the
MANITOBA PROVINCIAL
NORMAL SCHOOL
1946 - 1957
RENAMED
MANITOBA
TEACHERS' COLLEGE
1957 - 1965
TEACHER
TRAINING INSTITUTION
Placed here with pride
by the
Class of 1948 -
MNS
Reunion - June,

3. Plaque

Acknowledgements

I would like to thank everyone who sent submissions and who offered encouragement in regard to this book. I would also like to thank the persons listed below for their contributions. All helped to make this book possible.

With the assistance of family members, Christine Moore, Sharron Arksey, and Janet Brunger provided stories for their corresponding mothers, Lois (Leigh) Moore, Viola (Sigurdson) Wild, and Emily (Szarkowicz) Hilhorst, respectively.

Shirley Maurice provided an extensive list of Normalites, with addresses and telephone numbers, as available. Abe Friesen provided his copy of *Normal Lights 1950–51* for use when contacting participants and when receiving submissions.

School photos were provided by Carl Braun, Mary Chubey, Cecile Fisher, Emily James, Peggy Lawrence, Isla Lawrie, Shirley McCracken, Rose McIver, John Ryan, Gladwyn Scott, and Jean Tully.

From the office of Queen's Printer for Manitoba, Jill Bemi sent permission documents and Cindy Stevens gave permission to use photos of the Normal Schools in Brandon and Tuxedo.

Sharon Foley, Manitoba Provincial Archives, provided permission to use the 1906 photo of the Normal School in Winnipeg. Alex Regiec, City of Winnipeg Transit Department, provided photos of public transportation vehicles and tickets.

From Manitoba Education, Citizenship and Youth, John Tooth provided data regarding the Normal School principals, Nessa Herman sent the list of the principals, and Lee-Ila Bothe drafted the letters in response to our requests.

Matea Tuhtar, Manitoba Teachers' Society, provided data regarding former MTS general secretaries. The information on pages 23–24 comes from articles in the February 1957 and September 1975 issues of the *Manitoba Teacher.*

From Canadian Mennonite University, Winnipeg, Paul Friesen, helped in making contact with the appropriate official at the university and John Longhurst provided permission to use the text and two photographs from http://www.cmu.ca/about_founders.html.

Alejandro Duff assisted with the recording of telephone interviews and with touching up photographs. Pam Duff scanned the print photographs and saved them to computer. Sean Duff did the editing, layout, and publishing of the book.

Introduction

Saint John Baptist de La Salle, founder of the Institute of the Brothers of the Christian Schools, founded what is generally considered the first normal school in Reims, France, in 1685. The term "normal school" made its way to North America in the early 19th century from the French *école normale*.

The French concept of a normal school was to provide a model school with model classrooms to teach model teaching practices to its student teachers. Its purpose was to establish teaching standards or norms, hence its name. The children, the teachers of the children, the student teachers, and the teachers of the student teachers were all together in the same building. Although a laboratory school, it was the official school for the children—primary or secondary. Most such schools are now called teachers colleges; however, in some places, the term normal school is still used.

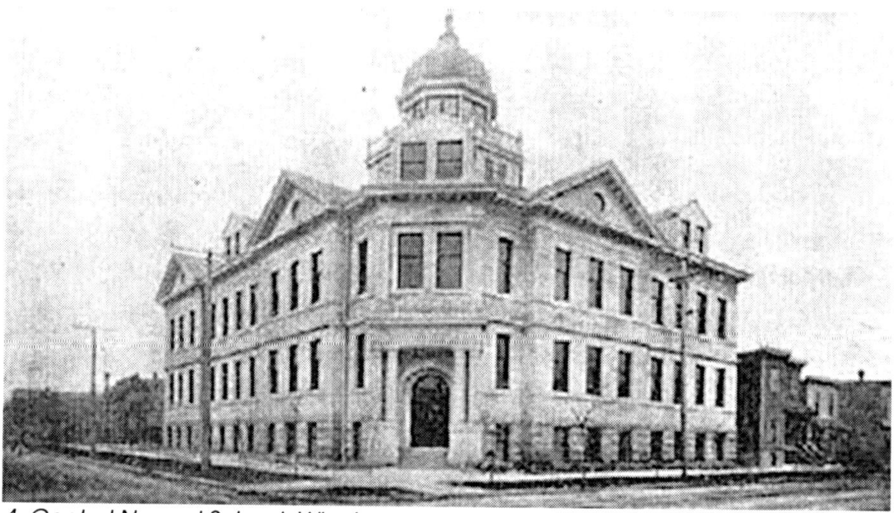

4. Central Normal School, Winnipeg

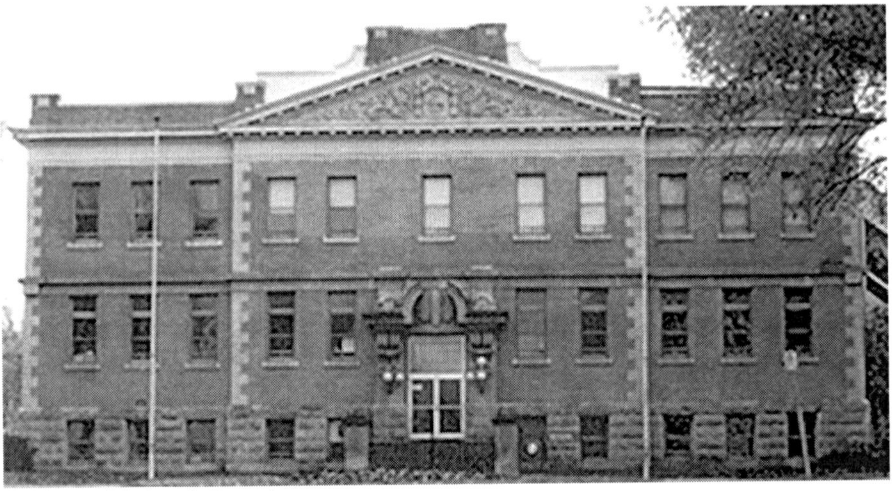

5. Normal School, Brandon

Manitoba Normal Schools were opened in 1882 for Protestant teachers and in 1883 for Catholic teachers in response to such factors as the rapidly growing population through immigration and the subsequent need for trained teachers.

Four Normal Schools were built and opened under the direction of the government of Premier Sir Rodman Palen Roblin: St. Boniface (1903), Manitou (1904), Winnipeg (1905–06), and Brandon (1912–13).

The Normal School building located in Tuxedo has a long tradition of housing education. Constructed in 1921–22 by the provincial government as a custom-built campus for the Manitoba School for the Deaf, the building featured limestone walls, Tudor arches, cove ceilings, gargoyles, spires, and a four-storey tower at the main entrance. Designed by American architect John D. Atchinson, the English collegiate style campus boasted a main instruction building with sixteen small south-facing classrooms, a large auditorium, and vocational instruction in home economics, printing, and carpentry.

Girls lived on the third and fourth floors of the north-south (C) wing, boys on the third floor of the classroom (B) wing, with the dormitories separated by a solid brick wall. Electrical shaker units were attached to each bed to wake students in case of fire, and each dormitory was equipped with emergency strobe lighting. The dining hall had separate entrances for boys and girls at the south and north.

Two decades later, the live-in deaf and hard of hearing students were moved to Saskatoon or Montreal to make room for the war effort.

For the five years between 1941 and 1946, thousands of new recruits to the Royal Canadian Air Force studied radio communications at the new #3 Wireless School. Six H-huts—two dormitory buildings linked by a washroom, forming the letter H—were constructed to the west of the dining hall, and a large hangar-style gymnasium was constructed to the north of the main building. Young airmen from across Canada and the Commonwealth lived and studied at #3 Wireless for an intensive 28 weeks.

After the war, the campus made another change, becoming the Manitoba Provincial Normal School, later Manitoba Teachers' College, for the training of young teachers. Four hundred or more future teachers spent a year studying here, with most living on campus in the military barracks or the main building dormitories.

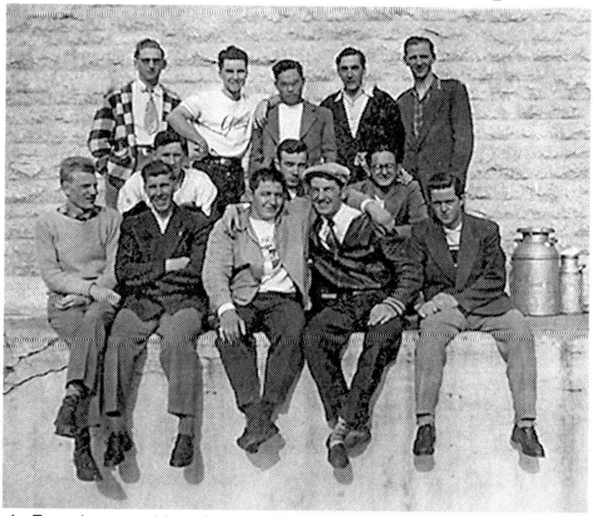

6. Frontenac Hall Boys

For a period, the provincial Normal School in Tuxedo was the only residential Normal School in

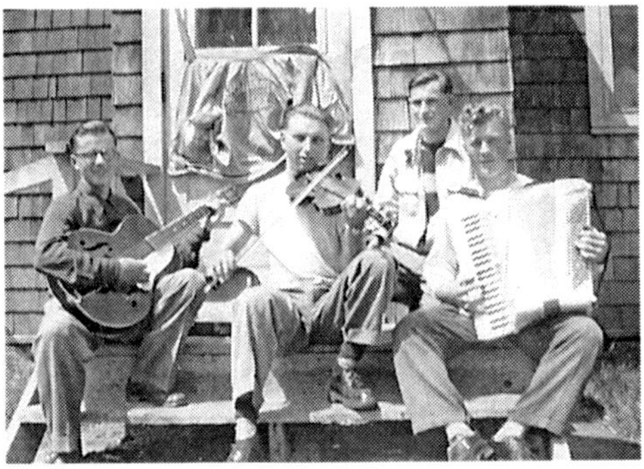
7. Strathcona Hall Musicians

Canada, housing students in eight residences. Former principal, Bruce Moorhead, said of the residences that "almost every racial background is represented here. They have worked together, played together, solved problems together. There is much evidence of an enrichment in living together." During the 1950–51 year, there were five residences for women (La Verendrye, Mackenzie, Radisson, Rupert, Thompson) and two for men (Frontenac, Strathcona).

The Tuxedo campus also boasted a canteen for student gatherings, an 8,500 square-foot (790 m^2) gymnasium, a playing field large enough for three baseball diamonds, as well as volleyball and football areas and a skating rink.

The Normal School in Winnipeg became the only one in Manitoba after the closing of the institution in Brandon in 1942. The enrolment of 307 was the highest for any single teacher training institution in Canada in 1943. The Normal School moved from William Avenue at Gertie Street to the Tuxedo site in 1946.

The barracks at #3 Wireless were converted into emergency housing for low-income Winnipeggers after the war. About four dozen families resided in apartments carved from the H-huts, sharing common washrooms and laundry facilities in the connecting corridor. Children up to grade four attended a small "model" school on campus.

By 1965, teacher education was transferred to the University of Manitoba campus, and the building reverted to its original use as a School for the Deaf.

After a brief period as the administrative centre for the 1999 Pan-American Games, a century-old dream to establish a university in Southwest Winnipeg was finally realized when Canadian Mennonite University purchased the campus in 2000. Extensive renovations transformed dormitory rooms into offices, small classrooms into lounges and seminar rooms, and vocational areas into instructional spaces to accommodate students who now study at CMU.

Designated as a provincial heritage site in 2000, what is now known as Founders Hall at CMU provides an architectural link to the importance past generations placed on formal education.

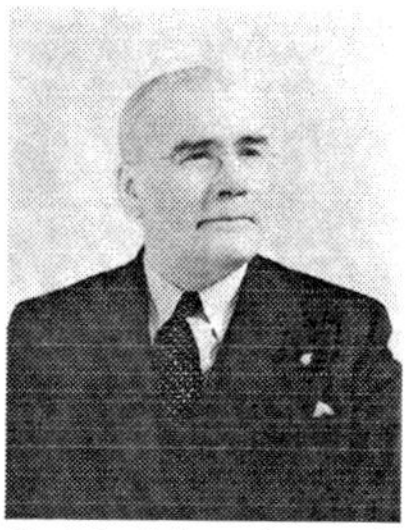
8. Mr. Moorhead

Mr. D. B. Moorhead, principal of the Manitoba Normal School, died September 28, 1951. Mr. R. W. Lightly took over as principal after three months as acting principal during the illness of Mr. Moorhead. He had become assistant principal in 1949. On January 1, 1957, Mr. Lightly became Chief Inspector of Schools for the province and Mr. G. W. F. Brisbin of the inspection staff was named as Mr. Lightly's successor.

Thomas McMaster was General Secretary of the Manitoba Teachers' Society during the year when we attended Normal School. He was born at Clydebank, Scotland and served in the Royal Navy during World War I. After emigrating to Canada in 1921, he attended St. John's College and Normal School. By 1936, he had completed his Bachelor of Arts, Bachelor of Education, and Master of Education degrees and had been teaching in Winnipeg. During World War II, he was in the Canadian Legion Educational Service. Among other responsibilities, he set up educational services for Canadian servicemen at Oxford, Cambridge, and the Sorbonne.

Tom was appointed as General Secretary of the Manitoba Teachers' Society in 1945, serving as a member of the general curriculum committee, the discipline committee of the Department of Education, the teacher recruitment and retention committee, and the Collective Agreement Board. In 1950, he wrote a book entitled *Beyond Collective Bargaining*, which is believed to have been the only guide in North America for teachers on the subject at the time.

He was a member of the Masonic Order, the Manitoba Command of the Canadian Legion, the Winnipeg Chamber of Commerce, and the Winnipeg Rotary Club. He was also a life member of the National Education Association of the United States, and an associate member of the American Institute of Management. Tom died in 1956.

Emerson Arnett was Assistant General Secretary during the year when we attended Normal School. Emerson started his career in education as a teacher in a one-room school at Sulphur Creek, Manitoba, in 1932. Later, he became principal in Headingley and Tuxedo. Finally, he was a member of the staff of a junior high school in Winnipeg. He served on the Provincial Executive of the Manitoba Teachers' Society from 1946 to 1949, after which he was Assistant General Secretary. In 1956, he succeeded Tom McMaster as General Secretary.

When Emerson retired in 1975, he had set a record. He had served on the Society staff longer than any staff member ever employed by the Society. In his years with the Society, he saw the scope of the organization grow from one serving about 4,000 members in 1949 to one serving about 12,000 members in 1974 and having its senior staff increasing from two in 1949 to twelve in 1974. The Emerson L. Arnett Bursary for students continuing their education is named for him. Emerson died in 1975.

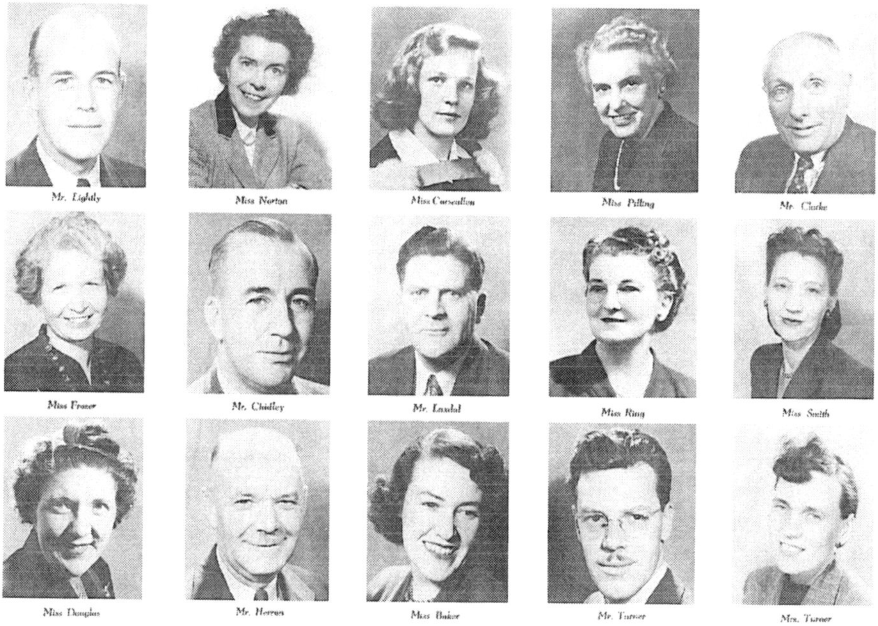

9. Teaching Staff

During our year at Normal School, Mr. Moorhead was the Principal and Mr. Lightly the Vice-Principal. Our teachers were Miss Baker, Childhood Development (Psychology); Miss Carscallen, Physical Education (after September); Mr. Chidley, Mathematics II (Practical); Mr. Clarke, Classroom Management; Miss Douglas, Music; Miss Fraser, Librarian; Mr. Herron, Science; Mr. Laxdal, Mathematics I (Methods); Mr. Lightly, Social Studies; Miss Norton, English I (Methods), Miss Pilling, Art; Miss Ring, Health; Miss Smith, English III (Practical); Miss Stewart, Physical Education (September only); Mr. Turner, English II (Speech); Mrs. Turner, Basic Techniques (Primary Methods).

Other members of the administrative staff included Miss Bain, linen; Mr. Cartwright, chef; Mr. Evans, bursar; Mr. Foster, cleaning; Mr. Fyles, food stores; Mrs. Gardiner Main Building; Miss Gordon, infirmary; Mrs. Owen, housekeeping; Mr. Rousseau, assistant chef; Mrs. Savage dining room; and Mr. Shead, engineering.

CLASS A

Paul Alexiuk
Yvette Allard
Phyllis Anderson
Doris Andres
Ruth Armson
John Atamanchuk
Maxine Atcheson
Harry Backewich
Eileen Barkley
Doreen Baldwin
Joan Barr
Sigrid Bardell
Merle Bech
Dorothy Beisher
Fay Bent
Jake Bergman
Fleurette Bernardin
Ann Berzowecki
Frances Bilanski
Garth Bishop
Doris Boak

Mary Bocek
John Bodnaruk
Manuel Boguski
Shirley Bold
Helen Borthistle
Estelle Boulic
Joan Bowey
Lillian Boyko
Isobel Brabant
Maurice Brabant
Inez Bray
Edna Brown
Marie Brownlees
Nancy Bunting
Frances Burnett
Dorothy Carnegie
Simone Carriere
Ruth McInnis
Leonie Rey
Phyllis Webb

1

Ruth Armson

Are you interested in a different, but fascinating adventure, in Canada? For all of the beauty of the southern parts of Canada, Ruth suggests a breathtaking trip in the autumn up the Dempster Highway. This adventure begins just south of Dawson City in the Yukon, winds its way through mountain ranges, valleys and across the vast Arctic tundra to the lowlands of the Mackenzie Delta in the Northwest Territories. From there it is possible to take a plane to Tuktoyaktuk, an Inuvialuit settlement at the mouth of the Mackenzie Delta on the Arctic Ocean.

The traveller is always surrounded by nature and very, very few people or settlements. The autumn colours are unbelievable! The highway is not paved, except for a bit at the beginning and at the end. Thus, the potential exists for a chipped windshield and flat tires. Will you let this stop you? At Eagle Plains Hotel, about halfway along the highway, tires can be repaired. Since trucks are quite common on the highway, a driver can obtain a ride if there is a car problem. Ruth highly recommends this trip. Is there anyone who will accept the challenge?

Ruth was born in Portage la Prairie and lived on a small farm nearby. The first school that she attended was Beaconsfield School, Rignold District, in Portage.

Normal School, for her, was a wonderful year. She was a young girl, barely seventeen. She had so much fun with the girls in Radisson Hall, loved dancing at the canteen, made so many new friends, and did other activities in her "spare" time.

After Normal School, she obtained a Bachelor of Arts degree and a Bachelor of Education degree.

She had a range of teaching experience in different parts of Canada. The locations were as follows: Euclid School, Portage la Prairie; Addington School, Goodlands: Fort la Reine School, Portage la Prairie; Brandon; Hay River, N.W.T.; Cold Lake Air Force Base, Alta.; Manitouwadge, Ont.; Fort Garry; Whitehorse, Yukon; and Victoria, B.C. She worked in six provinces and territories in Canada because she loved seeing new places. However, she was particularly fascinated with the North.

Outside the teaching profession, she worked for one year in Portage la Prairie as Christian Education Coordinator for Portage United Church.

One of her favourite books as a child was *Girl of the Limberlost*, by Gene Stratton-Porter. As an adult, she enjoyed *Fugitive Pieces*, by Ann Michaels, and reads books by such authors as Paolo Coelho.

Ruth takes time for such hobbies as photography, card making, cross-country skiing, walking, travelling, reading, mentoring, and cooking.

She has been active in numerous organizations: Habitat for Humanity, Yukon Council on Aging, Mentorship Program for Beginning Teachers, Kumon Skills Program, Yukon Retired Teachers Alumni, and Senior Writing Program on Memoirs.

Habitat for Humanity builds houses for people who cannot afford them. It is a new programme in Whitehorse. Ruth was on the Selections Committee when it began. Her group chose the first family to benefit from the programme. The third unit, a multiplex, was started in 2008.

Kumon is an international basic mathematics and reading skills programme for children. Children work on the skills at home outside of school time and go to Kumon to be updated and to get help.

One of the most memorable features in her career has been receiving several awards. These include two Hillroy Fellowship Awards; an Innovations in Teaching Award, which is given by the Yukon Government annually; a National Computer Award for an innovative programme; the Commissioner's Award, which is given for community service in the Yukon; and the Queen's Jubilee Award.

During her lifetime, Ruth has visited over fifty countries. One of her most memorable trips was to Antarctica during the southern summer. The stark beauty, the feeling of being overwhelmed by nature, and the hope that man can cooperate in the last frontier on Earth cannot be forgotten. The fascinating scenery is such that it is difficult to describe. Her numerous incredible photos provide evidence of the mystic beauty of this wonder-world.

She considers this to be the most beautiful scenery on the planet. There are large expanses of glaciers and icebergs, towering mountains, much water, and no people. Many penguins and huge birds, like the albatross, abound.

She arrived there on a refurbished Russian icebreaker across Drake's Passage from Ushuaia, Argentina. The group sailed south of the Antarctic Circle until they met pack ice and then returned by sailing up the Inland Passage. Each day they listened to lectures by the scientists on board, viewed the incredible landscape, and ventured out in inflatable Zodiacs to view wildlife.

One night was spent sleeping in tents on the mainland. The temperature was between 0°C (32°F) and 10°C (50°F)—very comfortable at this latitude. This is another tour that she would recommend.

Another time, she was in a group of about one hundred people who circumnavigated the globe on a chartered 757 jet. The flight was operated by Travel Guild Inc. of Ontario, an offshoot of the Ontario Teachers' Association, in an annual event. The group stayed at 4-star and 5-star hotels en route. Her voyage, which was in 2006, included stops in Japan, Hong Kong, Viet Nam, Cambodia, India, Dubai, Nairobi, Egypt, Prague, and Iceland. She particularly enjoyed the beauty of Viet Nam. An outstanding point was the Taj Mahal, in Agra, India.

In speaking to teenagers, she would tell them to become informed world citizens and, through kindness, hard work, and respect for others, help to make their mark on the world in a positive way. Also, have fun, travel much, respect all cultures, and lend a helping hand to the less fortunate.

For those contemplating her profession, she would tell them that teaching is a profession like no other. It is so rewarding and so much fun. They should love children, be kind, be competent, and make children's lives better by giving them a sense of security, a sense of self-worth, and a sense of accomplishment.

She particularly liked her high school geometry teacher, Mr. Garrett. His subject was one that she loved!

She has a friend of forty years, Peg Hanulik, who has had a positive effect on her life. The Hanulik family has always treated Ruth as a family member. This has grounded her and helped her so much in making Yukon her home. Both Peg and her husband, Tony, are role models, and Ruth loves their children and grandchild.

She has great respect for Stephen Lewis, who has done so much for the underprivileged in other countries and has brought to the general society an awareness of the poverty and injustice in so many countries, including our own.

For her, life is wonderful and each experience helps her to grow in knowledge, wisdom, and caring. She can have fun and, at the same time, work hard at a career that she loves, be kind to others, understand and respect other cultures, and give back to the community that has been so good to her.

On top of all of that, she loves the Yukon, a land of such beauty, such interesting people, and so many opportunities.

2
Harry Backlin

Would you like to try a new adventure in fishing? How about the Douglas Channel, an arm from the Pacific Ocean that reaches inland as far as Kitimat, B.C.? Near this inside port, there is fishing year round. Depending on the time of the year, one can fish for cutthroat, steelhead, chinook salmon, pink salmon, chum, and coho salmon. These waters must be really attractive to Harry because he has been going there whenever possible for twenty-five years. He enjoys seeking out salmon from his thirty-foot (9 m) boat, the *Harry O.* This is also part of the area where the spirit bear, that also likes salmon, makes its habitat.

Harry was born in Oakburn. He received his grades one to eleven in Sandy Lake.

He obtained a Bachelor of Arts degree at University of Winnipeg in 1956 and a Bachelor of Laws degree at Manitoba Law School in 1960.

Before entering Normal School, he taught as a permit teacher in a rural school in Miami. After attending Normal School, he spent two more years in teaching.

His best memory of Normal School was being elected as Student Body President. In our year, there was an elected council for the first term and a different one for the second term. Harry served in the first term.

Mr. Turner, our speech teacher at Normal School, was probably his greatest teacher up to that time. Harry holds him in high esteem.

Harry practised law in Winnipeg following graduation from Law School. In 1969, he moved to Vancouver, B.C., where, from then to 1975, he engaged in life insurance and business consulting. In Prince George, from 1975 until the present, he has been a commercial realtor-developer. At the current time, he is with Coldwell Banker Boardwalk Properties.

The late Judge Hamilton was most instrumental in carving out Harry's legal career, so much so that he benefits from the judge's counsel daily, even though he is now in a different profession.

His favourite reading is "motivational" books, especially by Napoleon Hill. *Think and Grow Rich!* is his choice. The theme was inspired by a suggestion from American billionaire Andrew Carnegie. It was published in 1937, at the end of the Great Depression. It was the biggest seller of Napoleon Hill's books, selling a claimed twenty million copies over the next fifty years.

Harry was a director of the Prince George Hospital Board, chairman of the Prince George Hospital Foundation, and fund-raiser for the Prince George Hospice Society and for the Prince George Community Foundation.

As chairman of the Prince George Hospital Foundation, he was instrumental in assisting in raising $5,000,000 for their first MRI for the hospital. It was a wonderful experience!

The one message that Harry has to all teenagers is to learn to be humble, to show gratitude, and to be able to say, "Thank you," or "I'm sorry". It is indeed a regrettable phase in the formative years of all younger students that they are not taught money management. This is something upon which all parents should act. As for a career choice, the advice which he always gives is that whatever the mind of man can conceive and believe, it can achieve.

A memorable trip which Harry made was one to Moscow, Russia, where he met people from all walks of life. On returning back home, he was able to appreciate all "our freedoms" and "lifestyles" much more than before.

For tourists coming to Canada, and Canadians themselves, the number one place to visit for a few days is Vancouver, B.C. This is one of the finest and top-rated cities of our continent.

Stanley Knowles—one of Canada's most respected politicians—dedicated his life to enhance the health and the education of all Canadians. Many people, including Harry, consider him to be one of the great Canadian leaders.

Harry lives—and has lived—as the one basic philosophy of life: "To care and to share" and be a caring and sharing person.

3
Joan (Barr) Allison

She had returned to her hometown of Flin Flon to attend a basketball reunion. As she and her sister, who was also a player, were walking along a street, they noticed that a store window exhibited a display. What was it? On closer scrutiny, she perceived that about 75% of the display was about her. What a shock it was to see that without any warning! Her sister decided right then to nominate her for the Manitoba Basketball Hall of Fame.

Going back several years, a young girl started playing basketball in high school in Flin Flon, spending four years in the game. She was in a junior league and gained experience by playing against the seniors. After graduation, she became a student at Manitoba Provincial Normal School, in Winnipeg. She played on city teams while she attended Normal School and then when she taught in adjacent St. James.

Her major claim to fame was that every team on which she played won the Manitoba championship—eleven teams in nine years. That was quite a feat! One year her team won the Eastern Canada championship, defeating a Toronto team. In trying to achieve the Western Canada championship, the girls lost twice to a Saskatoon team. Sometimes, this star was team captain; and, sometimes, she was leading scorer. She enjoyed a brilliant career in this sport. Despite her achievements, she does not consider herself as making the difference since everyone worked as part of a team

On a visit to Winnipeg, she and a couple of members of the family visited the Basketball Hall of Fame housed in the downtown Hudson's Bay store. She whooped a shout of excitement as she approached and saw her name. Even the curator hurried over to the display to see who she was. Again, it was a shock to see this recognition. The selectors chose her for induction into the Manitoba Basketball Hall of Fame in 1985.

Joan was born in The Pas, and obtained her schooling in Flin Flon.

Most of her teachers in elementary and high school were remarkable, although a few others stood out because of what she feels were injustices. One time, because she handed in her completed mathematics assignment in the fourth period instead of before nine o'clock as she was supposed to do, her teacher strapped her. Mathematics was her favourite subject. This sad experience remained in her memory all of her life.

On another occasion, her high school physics teacher gave her 46% on a test. When her teacher was checking the papers with the class afterwards, Joan found four more marks. When she told her teacher, he said that he would check into the oversight. The test was worth ninety-five marks with five bonus marks given to all. When he calculated Joan's actual mark as a percent, it was 49.4%. Despite the closeness to passing, he would not pass her. He did not do this to show meanness, but to show her that she did not deserve to pass. Again, this incident stayed with her all of her life. Nevertheless, she enjoyed school, but mainly for social activities and sports.

When she was at Normal School, she had a boyfriend and she played basketball—both off-campus. Since these interests took two or three nights a week and weekends, she was not involved in many on-campus activities. She recalls sneaking into her dormitory after hours on occasion, a common occurrence with numerous students. Overall, she does not recall any negative experiences at Normal School—and no really outstanding positive ones, either.

She performed her teaching in St. James, and in Fort Frances, Ont.

Joan married Bill Allison in 1953. During the year when she was at Normal School, 1950-1951, he was playing hockey for the Brandon Wheat Kings. In 1956, they moved to Fort Frances, Ontario. Bill taught at the high school—majoring in history and economics.

After leaving full-time teaching to raise a family, Joan continued to serve as a supply (substitute) teacher. Since Fort Frances had a demand for such teachers, she was able to teach in every school in the district and from kindergarten to grade 13. She did not want to be a full-time teacher when she had to care for her family. She felt that she could not perform justice to both if she tried to do it.

Both as a child and as an adult, she has read so many books that she is unable to say that any one stands out as being the one that she can classify as her favourite.

She and her family had the opportunity to live in Wales for one year and found it to be a good learning experience. Bill was participating in a teacher exchange programme. They lived in a three-bedroom house that did not have central heating, but had small coal fireplaces in each room. As the fires would go out during the night, it was necessary for Bill to rise early to rekindle the fires. During the day, Joan would carry a small electric heater from room to room as she performed her household work.

During their stay, they travelled to other parts of the British Isles and to Europe.

Teenagers are at the stage when they have interest in acquiring various possessions. Joan would advise them that amassing things never brings happiness. There is more in life that is needed. For those considering the teaching profession, they should think carefully about it. She considers it to be the most important job, besides parenthood, that a person will ever do.

She would recommend that visitors to Canada see the Fort Frances area of Ontario, especially because of the clean lakes.

She feels that Pierre Trudeau made a great impact on Canada, being forward-thinking and epitomizing the philosophy "live and let live".

She has always tried to keep busy. As a hobby, she participates in fund-raising. Doing census work for election campaigns has been enjoyable. She has also worked for most campaigns in helping her party in the Rainy River Constituency.

For the past eleven years, she has been a member of the local Riverside Hospital Foundation Board, most recently chairing the Special Events Committee. In the past, she has served on the Housing Board and the Hospital Board. She has found her activities rewarding and all-consuming.

So many people have had a positive influence on her that she hesitates to name any one person as having done more than the others.

Bill and Joan had four children—two girls and two boys. The girls attended Mohawk College in Hamilton, Ontario, and the University of Winnipeg. Currently, they reside in Fort Frances raising their families. The boys went to play hockey, giving their parents many wonderful places to visit.

David played in the American Hockey League with teams in Halifax, N.S.; Sherbrooke, Que.; and Newmarket, Ont., and then coached in the AHL with teams in Prince Edward Island and Iowa. For a time, he coached the Ottawa Senators in the National Hockey League. He has also coached at other levels of hockey. As this is being written, he is coaching junior hockey in Des Moines, Iowa.

Michael played eleven years in the NHL—six with New York Rangers, two with Toronto Maple Leafs, and three with Los Angeles Kings. He was inducted into the Northwest Ontario Hall of Fame in 2003. After hockey, he completed his Bachelor of Arts degree, but, after one year of teaching, he decided it was not for him.

Her husband Bill spent the last three years of his life in a personal care home, suffering from Alzheimer's, and passed away in 2007.

Joan's philosophy of life is to try to live in the moment. She still lives in her family home. Three of her children reside in Fort Frances, too. Life is good!

4
Shirley (Bold) Fairbairn

A brother can be so embarrassing to his sister, especially if they are in the same grade. This was the case with Billy and Shirley. During her school years, they were in the same grade since grade two. He was always the "class clown", which made the situation worse. Involving Miss Lawson, their grade eight teacher and one of her favourites, increased the embarrassment.

This was one of those days when Billy chose to act the clown. The teacher always dismissed her class by saying, "Class, pass out." Billy took her literally. Down he fell, flat on his face! He had passed out as she had told him. No, it was not a real faint, but one of his antics.

Every day, he had the class in stitches over some incident; and Miss Lawson would always say to him, "Billy, I will see you after school." Poor Miss Lawson! His sister was always so embarrassed. Shirley felt so sorry for Miss Lawson. She was such a patient and good-natured teacher, a kind and gentle soul who was loved by all her students—even Billy.

Shirley was born in Minnedosa. She attended school from Class A (no kindergarten in those days) until she graduated from Minnedosa High School in 1950.

It was after her first day of school in grade one that her parents asked her how her first day was. She announced that she was going to be a teacher—and she cannot remember ever changing her mind. She can sincerely say it has been the most satisfying endeavour of her life.

Probably her favourite teacher of her school days before Normal School was her grade one teacher, Miss Jackson. She had such a profound affect on Shirley regarding her life's vocation. If ever there were a teacher who personified a teacher, it was the one in artist Norman Rockwell's painting "The School Teacher". That figure so resembled Miss Jackson. She was tall and thin and had been teaching for many years. Even her attire was similar —a grey flannel skirt, a white tailored blouse, and black-laced oxfords with a Cuban heel. Also, her body language that one could feel from the portrait matched. Shirley truly thought her teacher must have been a very clever person in order to teach all the girls and boys in her class how to read, do arithmetic, print, and write stories. She was so fascinated with her teacher. She even had a solution on how to tell the set of identical twins in her class apart. She had Barbara wear blue laces in her sneakers and Betty wear red laces in hers.

Her days at Normal School were quite predictable after she had settled into her daily routines. Every day there were our classes and three times a day, our treks outdoors to the dining hall building to see what surprises the chefs and cooks had prepared for the daily anticipated mobs who descended to their assigned tables.

One of her favourite aunts, who lived and worked in Winnipeg, always seemed to arrive at the dining hall on her days off work. The students at Shirley's table always honoured her by having her sit at the head of the table. They all affectionately called her Auntie Rene. Everyone enjoyed her friendly and upbeat personality and she enjoyed the young people as much as they enjoyed her.

This was a ritual that occurred at least two or three times a month.

There were so many times when the students of the fourth floor of MacKenzie, her dormitory, were up to some sort of fun and high-jinks, not always what they should have been doing. On Saturdays, there was usually a group of the girls who would walk through Assiniboine Park out to a Portage Avenue trolley to go downtown to shop.

Shirley still remembers being so impressed by the big bronze statue of Timothy Eaton, sitting in his huge bronze chair on the first floor of Eaton's store. Having come from a small town, she was not used to seeing something like this statue, as he looked larger than life.

It seemed that, with their limited amounts of money, their shopping excursions were quite limited in buying power. They all loved to window shop and stop for lunch at the food floor. There was so much from which to choose. In the winter months, they had to be aware of the time as the days were shorter and darkness came earlier. It was necessary for them to catch the trolley and be able to walk through the park before darkness set in. Being at Normal School was a time of enjoyment, with so many changes in her life.

When she had completed Normal School in 1950–51, a group from MacKenzie Floor decided that they would attend Summer School at Gimli, in July and August 1952. Was this ever some reunion! Of course, they had lectures, but *wow*, what a good time they all had at those parties on the adjacent Lake Winnipeg beach. She completed the requirements for her Manitoba Permanent Teaching Certificate in Winnipeg the following year.

She feels that Mr. Clarke left an impression on the students in our Normalite year, 1950–51. He approached Shirley one day in the spring session, a time when all were wondering where they would teach in the 1951–52 year.

He was well-known and very fond of the school districts in southern Manitoba around Boissevain, between Brandon and the southern border of Manitoba, having been a superintendent of schools in that area. He had placed the previous teacher at Fairburn School District #61, south of Boissevain. Because of a tragic snow storm, or a white-out, as the local people referred to it, the teacher perished in the extreme weather conditions. Mr. Clarke, on this particular day, asked her if she would accept the position of classroom teacher, with grades one to eight, in the 1951–52 school year.

Shirley was really overwhelmed and felt honoured to have been hand-picked by Mr. Clarke to succeed this particular teacher. She did not hesitate and said that she would welcome the honour which she truly felt that he had bestowed upon her. This was a typical country school —grades one to eight—her first appearance in such a school. It was a very enlightening experience for her.

That year of many "firsts" for her was a rewarding teaching experience. One day they were singing "God Save the Queen" at their closing exercises and had reached the line, "Long may she reign over us." A cute little curly red-headed, six-year-old Garry, who was in grade one, loudly announced, "And it is, too." As all looked out the windows, they saw that, indeed, it was raining.

There was a boy in grade eight who would arrive early to light the fire in the winter months so that the warmth from the heater was welcomed and appreciated by all. He did take his duties seriously and would stoke the heater throughout the winter days, to make sure that everyone would be very comfortable and cosy throughout the many snowy and windy days.

About the third day of the Spring Teachers' Convention in Winnipeg, she met Mr. Clarke, who had sought her from the crowd. They had numerous discussions in which he would refer by name to the school board members where she was teaching. He knew them all personally. Eventually, he asked her what her immediate plans were for the next school term. She told him that she was interested in furthering her education and completing the requirements for her Permanent Manitoba Certificate and that she would like to teach in Winnipeg for the following year. When he heard that, he immediately took her over to meet the superintendent of the Winnipeg School District. He and Mr. Clarke had been friends for many years.

The next thing that she knew was that she was presented with an application and asked to fill it out. With that being done and with her sincere appreciation to Mr. Clarke, her plans were to come to fruition—to be able to teach in Winnipeg. This happened with such speed that she realized that she would have to be in touch with her present school district. She was returning to Boissevain the next day when she received a phone call from the secretary-treasurer. Shirley found herself embarrassed but did explain her actions with Mr. Clarke. She had prepared her letter of resignation the evening before and explained to him the reasons why she would be going to Winnipeg.

Even to this day, she realizes what influence Mr. Clarke had, and she will be eternally grateful to him for what he had done for her in her early placements of her teaching career. He was the type of person no one ever forgets.

The following year, she went to teach in Winnipeg, again as a classroom teacher, but with only one class. She taught in Winnipeg until she married in 1954. It was during the time that followed when she taught in military base schools, as she and her husband now had a little daughter born in 1955, in Moose Jaw, Sask., and a son born in 1959, in Halifax, N.S. She and her husband have lived in Manitoba, Saskatchewan, Quebec, Nova Scotia, and British Columbia; and she taught in each province.

It was when her husband was sent to Cold Lake, Alta., to take his pilot training on T-33 jets that she and the children returned to her home province of Manitoba. It was during the next fifteen years that she proclaimed that being married to a military husband was a series of ups and downs. During those fifteen years, they had moved seventeen times—up with the curtains and down with the curtains.

During this transitional time, her husband transferred from the Royal Canadian Air Force to the Royal Canadian Navy to acquire his wings when he flew T-birds on the aircraft carrier, HMCS *Bonaventure*, and trackers on both the east and west coasts. She was asked to teach at the base schools and then at Dartmouth, N.S.

In 1967, the family was transferred to the west coast to HMCS *Esquimalt* and the airbase HMCS *Pat Bay*, near Sydney, B.C., on Vancouver Island.

At this time, both the children were in school and Shirley returned to teaching at Victoria School District #61 as a classroom teacher. She taught for twenty-seven years, seventeen of them at Willows School in Victoria in grade one and was affectionately referred to by her principal as "Mrs. Willows", named after her school.

When they were in Victoria, Shirley resumed her education at the University of Victoria in 1967. After seven summers and winters, she graduated with honours, including majors in language arts and early childhood education and received her Bachelor of Education degree. After completing three courses toward her master's degree, she had back surgery which left her with permanent damage and other health problems. To her dismay, she was not able to continue her education. After teaching for twenty-seven years with the Greater Victoria School District #61, she retired from teaching because her health continued to deteriorate.

Miss Jackson, her grade one teacher, will never know the personal satisfaction, the joy, and the happiness that Shirley felt teaching the children throughout her career. She sincerely believes that this is a profession that she found most rewarding. It never ceases to amaze her when she encounters a former grade one student from twenty or thirty years earlier. She has even taught the children of her former grade one students. It is then that she realizes that the years are passing her by. However, when they say, “You haven’t changed a bit,” she does feel really elated. She thinks that this may be vanity. In what other profession can one feel the same sense of satisfaction and the rewards one feels when completing a profession started so long ago?

Her only other profession was that of being a mother. This was full-time before the children started to school. She found this to be so rewarding, having their two children and being the wife of a military man. She did, however, take part as a Primary Supervisor at her church, the Oak Bay United Church, during the years of raising her family.

When she was a child, she was exposed to the book *Charlotte’s Web*, by E. B. White. This really left an entertaining and positive impression on her, so much so that when she had a mature grade one class, she would read to them a chapter a day after spring break. The children would anxiously await the following day’s activities of Charlotte. One youngster, Hugh, upon looking throughout the book, seriously announced to her, "This must be a very old book, Mrs. Fairbairn."

When she asked why he said this, he matter-of-factly announced, "It's all black and white."

Oh, the effect coloured television had upon their young impressionable lives! This was in the late 1960s, thus it seemed very logical to him.

There have been many books which she has enjoyed reading as an adult; but now being a grandmother, she has enjoyed the *Harry Potter* series with her grandchildren. She has enjoyed not only his adventures but also has truly found it uplifting to share in each book the suspense one shares with the grandchildren in each volume. When they were young, Ryan, Laura, and Brett anxiously could hardly withhold the suspense, awaiting the next volume.

In regard to hobbies, her health and their living now in a condominium prevent her from taking part in her passion of gardening activities. Nevertheless, she still enjoys her plants. She has tried container gardening—with some success—but their sun room is really too hot for some plants. She plans on resuming her knitting as long as her hands can do it.

She would like to share her efforts with the Ladies' Auxiliary at their local hospital, the Royal Jubilee Hospital, where their daughter took her RN training. Her daughter has since pursued her educational endeavours in California, where she now lives and works. She has obtained her Masters in Health Administration degree and is a director for the Kaiser Health Foundation in Los Angeles.

Because of her health and family obligations, she has not participated in any service clubs or community organizations this past year, but continues her interests in the clubs and organizations in which she was active in before this past year.

It was during her first year of teaching in Winnipeg that she met her husband-to-be. During her first years as a young family, they took many trips to such hot spots as Hawaii, Mexico, southern California, and Arizona. When they were in Mazatlán, they purchased a new penthouse time-share condominium which was still under construction. This time-share gave the family various locations from which to choose. Even with having a young family, the choices were many.

It was, however, their tour to the United Kingdom that was most memorable to the family. The children were in grades eight and four. Often the trips included Grandma, Shirley's mother. They visited such tourist attractions in London as Buckingham Palace, changing of the guards, touring around London in a double-decker bus, the Tower Bridge, many beautiful parks, many museums, and other attractions. They travelled throughout England, Scotland, Ireland, and Wales. Included in the tour were many chapels and castles, as their tour guide was a very experienced and knowledgeable person. In Edinburgh, they attended a *Ceiladh,* where the practice is to pipe in the whole pig (cooked, with an apple in his mouth). They even sampled haggis and all the trimmings.

They travelled by bus to the most northerly point of Inverness. The countryside was so impressive with waterfalls and hills which were covered with flowering purple heather. In Wales, they walked behind people, just to listen to them speak. They have such a lyrical lilt to their speech and a very rich resonance, especially the men's choirs. Here they saw the Irish step-dancers performing wherever they went. They soaked up the local customs, song, dance, military tattoos, and relished in such foods as Welsh scones, Devonshire cream, and fresh strawberry jam. The whole time was so enjoyable.

As they travelled from coast to coast, they enjoyed all situations as they arose and had many experiences and observed so much throughout Canada. However, one place was the most beautiful and inspiring of all. This was in the province of Quebec, as they were travelling through the Saguenay Valley on their way to a posting at HMCS *Bagotville*, near the city of Chicoutimi. At the time, it was in the fall season. The trees on the hillsides on both sides of the highway were like a rich-coloured patchwork quilt of the most vivid golds, reds, oranges, greens, and browns—truly a magnificent display of the autumn colours that left a lasting memory with Shirley.

In Bagotville, her neighbour said to her, "You know, your daughter, she swears in French." Their daughter Dawn was only two and one-half years old and had picked up the French language—even words her parents did not know. She had become bilingual while playing with the French neighbours' children.

Although she had never addressed a group of teenagers during her teaching career, she was a parent to two teenagers as they passed through the various phases in their development during these years. Being there for them was most important to her as their father was away for long periods of time in his vocation.

There is another age group that she found to be most important and impressionable to a child's development. That was a most positive time for a child as he/she began formal learning development as a six-year-old in grade one. Shirley had much experience in this area. Being able to make this transition as smoothly and positively for the child's academic development throughout his/her life is of vital importance.

It is along this line of thought and reasoning that has expressed how she felt, and from experience, to many of her student-teachers. She tried not only to express her feeling but also to show the importance of the child's meeting success and having a positive feeling towards himself/herself and his/her abilities towards success in the early academic and social development in life. Primary teachers have a wonderful opportunity to give each child this positive experience to the best of their abilities.

The person who had the greatest positive effect in moulding Shirley's life was very near and dear to her—her mother, Mrs. Florence Bold. Most people should be able to say the same, but how many have exhibited the strength while afflicted with extreme hardship? It was a teaching lesson well-learned by Shirley.

When she was twelve years old, her father passed away, leaving her mother a widow at thirty-one years of age with seven children from ages thirteen years to one and one-half years old. Shirley was the oldest girl in the family. It was at this stage that she and her mother became inseparable, going off to work after school to earn money to help raise this family which included seven children and their mother. They would scrub floors, clean medical offices, and wash and dry dishes at the local café in their small town of Minnedosa. By the time that she was fourteen years old, she started waiting on tables. This was a promotion as she was not only earning twenty-five cents per hour, but she also received gratuities. She knew all of the people in town and in the surrounding area as she still went to school. These activities occurred after school and on weekends. It was during high school that she was crowned carnival queen and was given the option of taking a cash prize—two hundred dollars.

Her mother continued washing dishes and peeling potatoes to be made into potato chips. Shirley continued working on the weekends and in the summer holidays. By grade eleven, she was working in the drug store on Saturdays and during the summer holidays. By the time that she had completed grade twelve, she had saved enough money to go to Normal School. What an achievement she accomplished!

Despite her having jobs, she was on the honour roll throughout her high school days. It truly was from her mother that she had learned her work ethic and, therefore, was able to fulfill her desire to become a school teacher. Her mother has always been an inspiration to her. In 2001, she passed away. The whole family really does miss her. She was an exceptional person; one about whom Shirley can say, "I was always very proud of her. Yes! My mother."

When she thinks of someone who has contributed to the well-being of people—not only in Canada, but throughout the world—it results from an incident that occurred in her own family. Her niece was twelve years old when she was diagnosed with juvenile diabetes. Each day, she would have to test her blood sugar level and then would inject insulin according to the requirements she needed at that time. She would repeat this routine several times in a day. She did this for over thirty years and certainly had her ups and downs during those years. Two Canadian doctors, who were co-workers, Sir Frederick Banting, a scientist, and Dr. Charles Best, a physiologist, discovered insulin in 1897. They have changed the lives of many diabetics around the world. Shirley's family is justly proud of these two prominent Canadian doctors.

In 2005, her niece received a kidney transplant, a perfect match from an RCMP officer. Then, her niece received a pancreas transplant, another perfect match, in

Vancouver. Both transplants were successful and are functioning properly. She is now injection-free of her insulin shots. How wonderful this is! Ironically, her great-grandmother, Mrs. O'Reilly, was one of the first diabetics to receive an insulin injection in the first year of availability. Shirley has a sincere appreciation to not only her nephew, the kidney donor, but to all organ transplant donors.

Explaining her philosophy of life is difficult because she feels that actions speak louder than words. She has tried to live her life accordingly. There have been many incidents throughout her life in which she, like others, has been called upon to make many decisions which would affect others. What we do and say can have a lasting effect upon both the giver and the receiver. If we all do the very best that we can do and seek a positive consequence. One cannot ask for more.

As of 2008, Shirley and her husband are in their fifty-fifth year of married life. This year is proving to be one of change for their immediate family. Her husband has been tested and diagnosed with the beginning stages of Alzheimer's disease. With Shirley being the primary caregiver, she knows that she needs to be strong to meet the challenges of every day. She prays that she will be able to meet all the changes.

There is a wonderful support group in Victoria which has a large proportion of elderly senior citizens. With their help and your prayers, she hopes that she can meet each new experience and challenge. She will do her very best to meet these needs. The only constant in life is change, and she and her husband will go on from there on this final stage in their journey in life.

5
Edna (Brown) Dreger

A crime had been committed in the coal shed which was attached to the school! Who was the guilty person? This was the mystery facing the teacher of the school where Edna spent her first ten years. A broom had been broken and no one would admit guilt. What was the teacher to do now?

Since someone was obviously hiding the truth, everyone would be sentenced to a strapping. That still did not evoke a confession. The teacher recognized her predicament and decided to exonerate the grade one class. That was a relief for Edna as she was in grade one. Then the teacher felt pity for all the girls and excluded them from punishment. That left the boys. However, she based her conclusion on a faulty premise. The boys had often played "swords" with the laths in the coal shed. The broom was housed there. The boys must be guilty. Therefore, by strapping all of them, she would punish the guilty person.

Edna felt sorry for her brother as he exited the school and put on his leather mittens. That must have hurt him! Stories came back from children of the trustees that a group of men had attended a drinking party in the shed. One of those men was the actual culprit. The moral of this story is that one should be absolutely sure of the facts in any situation before taking action lest an innocent person become a victim.

Edna was born in Winnipeg, and commenced her schooling at Union Point. When the time came for her to prepare for higher education, the Minister of Education, Dr. Miller, advised her dad that she should attend Normal School before teaching because she was so young. That gave her another year to mature. As a result, she picked up many useful pointers prior to embarking on her career.

Miss Ring, our health teacher, helped Edna with some health problems by referring her to a doctor. She seemed truly concerned about the welfare of her students. Mr. Lightly, our vice-principal and social studies teacher, also impressed her. He towered above everyone and was so positive. He told Edna that she would be successful, no matter where she taught. That comment gave her confidence for her future.

Dormitory life could be eventful. One night, she awoke suddenly from a very sound sleep. She heard doors banging and water running. She must have overslept! She grabbed her towel and ran for her shower in the Mackenzie Hall bathroom. She was almost dressed for the day when she realized that something was wrong. These girls were not brushing their teeth to go for breakfast or to class, but to go to bed. They had just returned from their dates! Edna sheepishly returned to her bed.

In addition to Normal School training, her post-secondary education included the earning of a Bachelor of Arts degree and a Bachelor and Master of Education degrees. This was accomplished in the period from 1970 to 1983, during which she worked full time and raised six children. Her husband and her children helped her considerably so that she could fulfill her goals.

She spent her teaching career at Armour School in the Municipality of Morris, at King Edward Primary

School in Winnipeg, and at Morris Kindergarten in the Town of Morris. When she was in Morris, she drove to Rosenort during the noon hour to teach kindergarten there in the afternoon. She also drove to the Lowe Farm to teach kindergarten for a year.

As a child, she enjoyed the *Katydid* series, by Susan Coolidge, and now likes to read books by Pearl Buck.

Ann Huch, from Netley Lake, was Edna's grade seven and eight history teacher. This teacher's mode of dress etched its way into the young student's mind as it was a novelty in this area of the province. She dressed prettily, wore cute shoes, and polished her nails.

One day many years later, one of Edna's kindergarten students brought a tape to school for the class to enjoy. At the end of the day, the mothers were at the school collecting their young children to take home. Edna was horrified! That tape was right on her desk a moment ago. Now, it was gone! Immediately, she notified the owner—a mother with the proverbial red hair disposition. Like a flash, she stormed out of the school in hot pursuit of someone. She suspected who had taken it —and she was right. She caught the thief pulling away from the school. What a relief that was for Edna!

Teenagers, in considering your future, do what you really want to do and stay with it. Be honest and ask for help when you need it. If your interest be in a teaching career, it is advisable that you obtain the necessary training and then teach at the level which you like best. Never be afraid to admit to your students when you have made a mistake, but point out to them how you have learned from that mistake.

Over the years, Edna has been involved in such community affairs as Women's Institute of Morris, Morris Museum Board, United Church of Canada, and in serving meals for Parkside Villa. With these activities, her career, and her family, she still has time to enjoy scrapbooking, gardening, reading, sewing, and crafts as hobbies.

For anyone paying a visit to Manitoba, she would recommend spending time at St. Malo Beach, about one-half hour from her home—but definitely in the summer.

Edna is not partisan-oriented when she affirms that Conservative Prime Minister Diefenbaker and Liberal Prime Minister Pearson were leaders who made substantial contributions to Canada. The former finally provided a voice for the West after many years. The latter led the way in establishing a distinctive Canadian flag and, in general, followed good policies.

Her trip to Costa Rica in March 2008 was a dynamic learning experience. It was a cultural trip in which she and those who accompanied her learned how the Ticos—the name by which residents of that country are commonly known—live, work, and play. Jorge Avila, the very environmentally conscious guide, told the group about every bird, animal, or flower which he spotted.

Their bus stopped frequently so that the visitors could obtain a close-up of a hanging sloth, or a slithering snake, or other creatures. The group clambered up dormant volcanoes, trudged through dense rain forests, experimented in cooking delicious Costa Rican food, bathed in soothing hot springs, visited the local indigenous community, and so much more. Life is good!

It was an experience of a lifetime, one that she will never forget. Her follow-up was the completing of a scrapbook of all their experiences, which was like making the trip all over again.

Her personal philosophy of life is to smell the roses as she works hard. Life is too short to do nothing but work. She also feels that if one wants to accomplish something, just go ahead and do it. Well begun is half done!

6
Marie Brownlees

Amazing events can occur in a high school science laboratory. Two girls, in their spare periods, and two or three boys, when they preferred not to attend scheduled classes, would, at times, meet in the "lab". Usually, they talked or exchanged stories. It was those other times that could be unpredictable.

As the supplies and equipment were not locked from amateur scientists seeking to make an astounding discovery, these students decided to find out their capabilities. Normally, they followed textbook directions and had no problems.

Then, the abnormal burst forth! They decided to become a little more inventive. Unlike true chemists, they neglected to record ingredients and quantities. They had been mixing their invention in a very large flask when, to their amazement, the liquid thickened and became frothy. Then, it rose higher and higher in the flask. Soon it overflowed, running down its sides onto the acid-proof, fire-proof counter.

Gradually, it stopped expanding. Then, the students learned that the counter top was not acid proof. What should they do? When the concoction had eaten its way through the counter top, the students decided to disappear from the room.

Their memories, their eyes, and their ears erased all records of the event. They wondered if they might have helped shorten World War II if they had known how to repeat the effect and if the timing had been a couple of years earlier.

Marie was born in Selkirk. She began her education in Windsor School, St. Vital. She had lived in six homes by the time that she entered school.

During grade one, she suffered through numerous illnesses. Her most lasting impression of that grade came from her teacher on the last day of school.

There were fifty-four students in the class. When the teacher called out the names of the children who passed at the end of the year, she called them from highest to lowest. Marie was determined not to let her fear show as each name—but not hers—was called. She clenched her teeth and closed her eyes to hold back the tears. She tried to console herself by repeating to herself "I don't care if I don't pass, I was only here twenty days" as each name was called. Finally, her name was called. "Marie Brownlees—passed on trial." How awesome those words sounded as they rang in her ears!

Had this not happened, she would not have known what it felt to be last as, from then on, she was always at the top. Later, she learned that her new mother and her teacher had decided that, with help over the summer, Marie probably would be all right. As a result of this experience, she became a better teacher than she may have been had it not occurred.

She has always recognized the call for help from a student who does not care. She never failed a child without both the child and the parents knowing ahead of time the positive aspects—that "repeating" was not "failing". She has always made sure the children at the low end of the scale knew ahead of time that they were passing, and if "on trial", what they could do.

Marie has not remembered the name of that teacher, but she certainly has remembered what that teacher did for her. As a result, she allowed each child in her classrooms to be a winner by making "improvement", not an "A", the goal.

Marie's high school mathematics class participated in a provincial test. She scored 99% while another student, better known as a long distance runner, scored in the high teens. The teacher, Mr. Wyatt, congratulated the poorer student for having raised his grade. Then, he turned to Marie and told her how disappointed he was that she had not scored 100%. She should have checked her work. She was quite upset until she examined her work and found a simple subtraction error that should not have occurred if she had taken more care.

As a teacher, she used this story frequently to instil in her students the importance of checking their work. Mr. Wyatt always stood out as an example of a person who knew when to build up a student and when to "prick his/her balloon". Over time, he interjected much good advice without preaching.

While attending senior high school, she was in an accelerated class, taking grades ten, eleven, and twelve in two years. Somehow, she and a friend had three or four spare periods per week. In addition, they seem to have been left often on our own.

Much of the time, they would sit at the back of Mr. Wyatt's business arithmetic class, where they tried to beat him when he was proving the answer to a long involved question. They would look for errors as they were being made, then smugly wait until the lengthy question was completed—incorrectly, of course. Then, like self-reliant Girl Guides, they would come to the rescue by pointing out the error, which was usually in the second or third line.

Mr. Moorhead, our Normal School principal, would often confuse the identities of her and Isla Gliddon. He would spot the girls together and accuse Marie of too many late nights. She would object and assure him of her innocence. He would look a little confused and apologize for his error. At other times, he would stop them and accuse Isla of skipping too many classes. She, too, would declare her innocence, and again, poor Mr. Moorhead would apologize. Marie does not think that he ever learned to identify the girls correctly.

One day, on entering a friend's room in La Verendrye Hall, she discovered a huge wasp nest—obviously a specimen for science class. As she was about to leave, she noticed movement near it. Since the nest was located on a bed, Marie felt that it should be removed. Where should she take it? She decided that a temporary location would be the porch at the entrance of the building. Since the time was winter, this place would serve as a freezer unit until Mary, who had collected it, returned to her room.

Later, a young man offered to store it in the rumble seat of his car until a method could be formulated to kill the wasps and save the nest. The science teacher suggested that they enlist the assistance of the maintenance crew to enclose the nest and to use a gas-emitting motor.

On obtaining the motor, the crew placed the nest and the motor inside a huge carton, covered it with blankets, and plugged in the motor. When they returned later, they discovered that the box was alive with the sound of hundreds of angry wasps. The plan had not worked. At that point, no "man" wanted to be a part of the project.

Marie recalls pulling on the cord to the motor to try to free it. After the motor had cooled, and it appeared safe, she and her friends dragged the branch with the soggy nest toward the outdoor rink. Then, they rushed through the cold to their rooms.

After graduating from Normal School, she taught grades one to nine in Wilson Glen School District, Treherne. (There was only one school in the district.) Then, she moved to Maple Ridge, B.C., where she taught grades two to seven for thirty-four years in School District #42. She retired and completed her career by teaching art in grades three to ten in Meadowridge Independent School for six years.

Marie and Hazel, another teacher, were producing a musical, *Tom Sawyer*. All of the children from grades four to seven—140 in all—were involved. Classes were held in the old Haney Central School, while the musical was to be held in the new Eric Langton School.

After about four months of practice in the classrooms and hallways, it was time to practise where the musical was to be performed. Since the gym was new, they placed newspapers along the back wall. When the children made their 7:30 a.m. entrance, they would remove their shoes and put them, their coats, their homework, and their lunches on the papers. After that, practice would begin.

One very wet miserable day, just after 9:00 a.m., the fire alarm sounded. While Hazel escorted the children out, Marie proceeded to find out what was happening. As she started down the hall the secretary spotted her, and exclaimed, “He didn't tell you?”

“Tell me what?” Marie replied, realizing that the secretary was referring to their new, young head teacher, Danny.

As the secretary went to notify Hazel to bring the children into the school, Marie proceeded down the hall to Danny's classroom. She saw through the window that his grade seven class was standing in a line outside in the pouring rain. Danny was sitting on the railing at the top of the steps, slowly and deliberately calling the roll. On seeing Marie, he gasped, "I forgot about your practice."

Then, he quickly explained why there had been a fire drill. It was April Fool's Day and one of the students in his class had poured water on his chair. He sat in it. Not to be outdone, he said to himself, "They like water, I'll give them water."

He went to each classroom, but not to the gymnasium, and told all of the teachers to ignore the fire alarm. When Marie returned to the gym, the dripping, wet children and Hazel, too, put wet feet into dry shoes, dressed, and returned to Haney Central.

Oh, what a joyous day that was! Wet clothes were drying everywhere and children in gym strip, with wet hair and bare feet, were sitting in their rows of seats. The stench of wet shoes and socks drying on the radiators was overwhelming. Danny was left to ponder about "Pay Back Day".

Marie's trip to Russia, Mongolia, China, and Hong Kong was a learning experience both before and during the trip. She was part of a tour group consisting mainly of professionals. Since the three countries were Communistic, the group received information—including how to eat with chop sticks—prior to leaving Canada. The trip took place a couple of years before the Tiananmen Square incident in China and before everything became highly geared for tourism.

The Soviet Union had historic buildings and exquisite art and crafts. Communism was not quite as hard-lined as it had been. For the most part, there were few restrictions and even those were extremely easy to obey. The guides were knowledgeable and friendly. Wherever the group went, people offered "big bucks", mainly for their jeans, cameras, and tape recorders.

The accommodations were modern and well run. However, the food left much to be desired. The Soviets were used to catering to Americans and, as a result, steak and fries played a prominent role.

There appeared to be a shortage of fresh fruit and vegetables. No matter where they were, from Moscow to Siberia, these tourists barely had a taste of true Russian food. The stores had little variety of such everyday items as clothes and toys. However, there were excellent places where they could buy crafts.

Part of the trip was travelling on the Trans-Siberian Railway to Ulan Bator, capital of Mongolia, another Communistic country. Mongolia is a large country with a small population. The government chose to ally with the Soviet Union and promptly set about trying to prove what great Communists they were. There was military everywhere. The tourists were detoured into the Gobi Desert so that they would not be able to see a parade that was slated to be a show of military strength.

Marie entered a small bookstore and purchased a book about Ulan Bator and a large map of Mongolia. When her friends entered the store about ten minutes later, there were no books, maps, or similar items available.

In Ulan Bator, the accommodations were modern. The food was based mostly on what Americans might expect. They did, however, have some Mongolian foods when they were living in *gers* (yurts) in the Gobi desert. Again, there was a lack of fresh fruit and vegetables in their meals. The *gers* were quite comfortable—much like camping in large, well-furnished tents. The guide's main object was to limit their travel to avoid contact with anyone other than selected individuals and to attempt to confuse the tourists as to the true location of many of their destinations.

Because the Mongolians had not allied themselves with China, they had a tendency to do whatever they could to delay tours going to China. If a tour were late reaching its Chinese destination, it made it difficult for the Chinese to bring the tours back on track. The group heard horror stories about this from the time that they entered Mongolia.

In order for them to leave on time, the American, Chinese, and British ambassadors were involved. Even the Russian ambassador was contacted. It was also made difficult to make outside contacts. They did not know, until the time to board the train, whether they would be allowed to leave. In order to ensure their safe departure, all of the ambassadors were at the station. It helped that the engineer of their train was Chinese because he was told by the Chinese ambassador not to move the train unless a car were added for the Canadians. (That day 158 tourists and a Swedish tour leader were detained.)

Entering China was like waking up on a bright sunny day. The accommodations were exceptionally good. The food was delicious and almost entirely Chinese, except for breakfast, which was influenced by the Americans. Generally, fresh fruit and vegetables were abundant and definitely available to the Chinese people.

The guides were open and eager to learn about Canada. They had survived the Cultural Revolution and were eagerly looking forward to a bright future. The tourists visited all types of life—farms, factories, homes, universities, communes, and historic locations—and were able to watch varied artisans at work.

China was the most open of the three countries. For the most part, they were very hard working, optimistic people. The "one child, one family" rule was probably one of the hardest, if not the hardest, rule with which they had to live. Even the poorest were anticipating a better, brighter future.

They could spot a tourist in a crowd and would go out of their way and politely make contact—not to buy items like the Russians—but to "practise" their English and learn about Canada. Most places had not yet become tourist traps.

Hong Kong was British, waiting to be turned over to China. The tourists were told not to go out alone at night. There were handicapped beggars, often sleeping in doorways on the streets. Even in Russia and Mongolia, it was safe to walk alone; and, in China, one felt totally safe walking through the night streets. As she flew home, she wondered if things would be better in Hong Kong with the Chinese in control.

When she was a child, Marie read books by Lucy Maude Montgomery and Rudyard Kipling. In addition, she enjoyed reading Nancy Drew mysteries and children's poetry. As an adult, she has read both children's stories and adult books. Those which stand out are *Owls in the Family*, by Farley Mowat; *The Secret World of Og*, by Pierre Berton; and *Winnie the Pooh*, by A. A. Milne. She also enjoyed Agatha Christie mysteries, westerns, biographies, autobiographies, and other non-fiction titles. She states that she cannot restrict herself to one book at either level. From age eight until she became blind, she did not just read books, she "devoured" them.

Before she lost her sight, in about 1999, she dabbled in a bit of everything. Her hobbies included the following: painting (mostly acrylics), photography, copper tooling, pottery, silver smithing, lapidary work, stained glass, etching, sewing, silk screening, bird watching, back packing, hiking, and travelling.

Now, she is limited. She does some writing, using her computer. It is a Macintosh with a built-in magnification programme that allows her to use the internet with its virtual library of information. The computer reads text aloud to her, allowing her to enjoy "hearing" from people through e-mails. She scans pictures or articles, using Adobe PhotoShop to edit her photos for making various types of greeting cards. She can import questions from study books, answer them, and read her answers in class.

Marie has worked in numerous groups, some of which are the following: Maple Ridge Teachers' Association, Rebekahs, Ladies Encampment Auxiliary, Ladies Auxiliary to the Patriarchs Militant, guiding (Brownies and Guides), Maple Ridge Lapidary Club, Maple Ridge Astronomers' Club, Maple Ridge Photography Club, Meadow Highlands Ceramics Club, MacWest Computer Society, Alcoholics Anonymous, St. George's Anglican Church organizations, and White Cane Club.

She met Hazel—not the teacher in the fire drill episode—many years ago when Hazel's daughter joined Marie's Brownie pack. Hazel became the pack's Tawney Owl and also became the sister whom Marie had never had. Later, the two friends organized a guide company. They attended the same church and study sessions. Hazel did volunteer work in Marie's classroom and on field trips. Her nursing background was most helpful. She taught Marie what it was to have a friend and how to be a friend. She could instantly spot a child who was hurting physically or mentally.

Hazel believed in her as a teacher and as a person. As a result, everything that Marie did was better than it would have been if her friend had not been there to appreciate her efforts.

Now neither can drive and, unfortunately, Hazel does not use a computer. Marie once wrote a poem when she was going through a rough time, "There's God and You and the Telephone". In 2008, Hazel fell and badly bruised her hip and received a mild concussion. She is unable to go for walks without help. Since she has trouble with her eyes, she cannot read and has trouble seeing the television. She was always a vibrant person. This was evident, even over the telephone. The two friends still talk at least once a day.

Of the many places that she could suggest for visiting, Marie feels that Quatsino, B.C., at the northern end of Vancouver Island, is a unique spot to see. It is a very tiny town, with a population just under 100. It can be reached only by plane, boat, or water taxi. The community has a remarkable history, beautiful scenery, good fishing, good kayaking, fabulous birding, and roads that go nowhere. This is a location where a person can relax and forget the problems of the outside world. It has one of the last one-room schools in the province.

Her advice to teenagers is to cease loafing and to forget the idea that the world owes them a living, as it does not. They should learn how to find work, do it well, and be proud of what they do. In short, they should create a life which they can truly call their own.

A Canadian, who has left his mark, not only on Canada, but also on the world, is Terry Fox. Years after his death, his legacy has continued to grow.

If you do not love children, if you do not have a great sense of humour, if you are short on patience, if you do not want to work overtime for no pay, if you do not want to spend even more time keeping up-to-date, you should not become a teacher. That would not be fair to yourself and would be a disservice to each and every child you would teach. That is her advice for anyone considering teaching as a profession.

Marie did not obtain a university degree. At the time when she needed only two more courses, she taught with several persons who had masters degrees. Noting that they were not the best examples of teachers, she decided that a piece of paper does not necessarily make a good teacher. She knew full well it would affect her future pension. However, having received it regularly for over thirty-three years and looking forward to many more, she is not complaining about what she has received since retiring.

She feels that she is only a work in progress with whom God is not finished. No matter how "old" she becomes, she has much to learn, and hopefully much to give and even more to enjoy. Now that she has lived long enough to be able to look objectively over her life, she feels that, in spite of what has happened from her birth until the present moment, God has most assuredly watched over her.

7

Frances (Burnett) Dickinson

What draws the attention of many people in Canada and other countries in early October? It is the Fall Classic, otherwise known as the World Series of baseball. This is an event that crosses the barriers of age. How many high school students would rather be watching or listening to the games than be in a classroom working on their studies? The high school at Medora, experienced the magnetism once many years ago.

The principal noted the depleted classroom and confronted his wayward students on their return, “Where have you been?”

“We have been listening to the World Series on the radio.”

The students were surprised to hear his response. “Do not let it happen again.”

There was something about the way in which he said it that struck a nerve in their guilty consciences. They had expected a greater repercussion. The unauthorized absence from class did not happen again.

Frances was born in Medora. She commenced her schooling at Purple Hill, a country school northeast of Medora.

One of her favourite teachers was her grades one and two teacher, Aileen Casselman, from Lauder. She taught her pupils to print and write in the first year, so that they would not still be printing all their work in the higher grades as pupils do today! This grand lady is still alive and alert at age 97 (as of 2008), living in Deloraine. Frances recently had a good visit with her.

She remembers Miss Smith, our Normal School practical English teacher, for her emphasis of the fact that, in the Lord's Prayer, it is "forgive THEM that trespass" *not* "forgive THEY". Since then, Frances has always said the word "them". Until recently, when a minister at a church service said it when repeating the Lord's Prayer, she had never heard anyone else use the word "them". Finally, someone is on the same wave-length as Miss Smith and Frances!

She recalls how living in Rupert Hall, on the second floor of the main building, made it easy to rush to the balcony for assembly and classes. Back then, she thought that the chapel was huge.

In 1951–52, she taught grades one to eight at Thirlstane School, northwest of Deloraine. Her dad's sister many years earlier had taught at this school and had boarded in the same house that Frances had. In 1952–53, she taught grade four and part of grade five at Deloraine. In 1953–54, she taught grades one and two at Waskada.

Accepting a position at Waskada School frequently resulted in a time of stress. What caused it? It was initiation day for new teachers. They had no idea what was going to happen to them. High school students set up the torture chamber in a room completely devoid of light. In walked the victims for what they knew not. It was the fear of the unknown that worked in the students' favour. When the session had been completed, the new teachers had to admit that it was not really bad after all.

The next profession on which she embarked commenced in July 1954 when she became a farmer's wife, partner, go "for", and chief cook and bottle washer on a farm west of Waskada.

Teenagers should work hard, putting effort into all that they do. They should be depended on to do their best. They should also be aware that they will reap from life what they have put into it.

Frances advises young people to become more involved in what is offered and be better prepared for their life's work. When she was young, she was naïve and felt somewhat out of place. Those who had taught on permit were far ahead of her.

Anyone entering the teaching profession should be aware that all children are different and, thus, have different needs. Work hard to bring the best from each one. Attend the functions in which they are involved to show that you care and observe how they interact on the community grounds.

Often Frances needed the suggestion for a speaker or information on a topic which she was responsible for presenting. She considers Marlene Baskerville, who was known as the "Home Economist" many years ago, to be a "walking dictionary" because she could always be counted on to have an answer for what Frances needed. If she did not, she would find a source that could provide an answer.

Adelaide Hoodless was a young Ontario housewife who had lost her eighteen-month-old son as a result of the use of impure milk. She decided that she would do everything in her power to help other women gain the education necessary to prevent similar tragedies. She was responsible for a group of women meeting in 1897. These women decided to organize a Department of Domestic Economy in affiliation with the Farmers' Institute. It later became known as the Stoney Creek Women's Institute. The purpose of the first Institute was to raise the standard of homemaking.

This organization carries on today in all provinces of Canada, focusing on personal development, family, agriculture, rural development, and community action—locally and globally. In 2008, environment was added. The Women's Institute presents resolutions to the government. One resolution presented that came to be an actuality was the "stop arm" on school buses.

It is an organization that continues to work for the good of all, regardless of religious belief, political affiliation, or ethnic background. We owe the contributions of this organization to Adelaide Hoodless, by whose speaking out to women provided the means to improve the standard of homemaking.

An affiliate group is the Manitoba Women's Institute. The provincial body will celebrate 100 years in 2010. Frances is her region's representative on the provincial board.

She has worked in a Neighbour's Goodwill Club, which consists of folks from two former school districts. The club assists with the needs of the bereaved, the sick, and the shut-ins and looks after bridal showers, special anniversaries, and any other community needs.

She is also active with church attendance, church board, Sunday school, and church-related mid-week groups. She is on the local library board and a member of the Southwest Farm Women's Network.

She has been a 4-H leader for many years and then the 4-H programme assistant in her Agricultural Representative's area until the government phased out that part of the organization. Working with 4-H members has been the most rewarding of all her volunteering. It was wonderful to see these members develop organizational, speaking, and communication skills which they will always need when they go out into the world.

A very educational trip was one which she and her husband took to Holland. Her husband's cousins, who live near Amsterdam, met them at the airport. Amsterdam's name comes from the fact that it was built on a river that was dammed. There is a saying that "God made the world, but the Dutch made Amsterdam."

Downtown Amsterdam has tall shops because the owners are allowed only a small street frontage. Many have cranes on top to hoist up their wares and furniture. Most of the houses are joined, but the gables are often different. At a flower auction, they saw thousands of flowers being bid on to go to many destinations. They drove through a tunnel under the water to reach the house of another cousin.

They drove to Zeeland to see the Delta Dam where the North Sea is on one side and the inland water is on the other side. The regular inspection of the dams in the area is a must. They also drove across the "Enclosing Dike"—twenty miles (32 km). This water was known as the Zeider Zee before the dam was constructed. They walked through patches of heather, saw the windmills, and learned much history about the war damage.

For Canada, she recommends visiting the International Peace Garden, nestled in the Turtle Mountains on the Manitoba and North Dakota border. The best time is late summer when the flowers are at full bloom or early fall when the trees are turning colour. There is also much history to learn here.

Her favourite childhood book was *Anne of Green Gables*, by Lucy Maud Montgomery. In her adult life, there has been no special favourite, but she does enjoy mysteries and Zane Grey's western books.

Her hobbies include reading, knitting, playing board games, camping, and square dancing. For several years lately, she and her husband have driven sixty miles (97 km) once a week to participate in this dancing. No fools like old fools the saying goes, according to her. She also solves crosswords to try to keep her mind from slipping too much!

Her philosophy of life is to live life to the fullest, work hard, laugh considerably, have compassion for all people, and be a doer instead of a whiner.

8

Dorothy (Carnegie) Blakeman

A trip to England, Wales, and Scotland can be very memorable to someone who lives in North America. Such was the case for Dorothy. She rented a car in London and drove to Lye Regis and then to Wales. She and those with her visited friends in both places. From there, they headed north to Scotland. After that, they drove down the east coast back to London.

There is so much history everywhere that she would love to go back and spend more time. It was so thrilling to visit many places about which she had been hearing and reading from her school days and later.

Sometimes, there seems to be a moment in lifc that stays in one's memory. It is not always in a very important place; but, for some reason, it seems meaningful. Such an instance occurred for her one bright, clear morning as they were driving along a country road in Scotland. They approached a man strolling by the side of the road, carrying his fishing rod and the biggest, most attractive salmon that she had ever seen. It struck Dorothy as being so typical Scottish scenery, and it remained in her memory as if it were yesterday. For her, it typified the simple, but pleasant, country life. Too often, people are not observant of their surroundings and, thus, miss the beauty in simplicity.

Dorothy was born in Cypress River. She attended school from grade one through grade twelve in this town.

Her favourite teacher, although not always at any given time, was Kae Owens, who later married and was known as Kae Anderson. She was totally dedicated to seeing that all children who passed through her classroom learned as much as she could teach them

Dorothy received a teaching certificate from Manitoba Provincial Normal School in 1951. It seems so long ago when she was at Normal School. She remembers the year at Normal School as having been a good experience. Nevertheless, she also was very much looking forward to graduating and returning to teaching.

However, she does remember how the girls on her floor would gather in her room in the evenings. Joan Barr and Yvonne Ver Wilgen were her wonderful roommates. The three girls occupied one of the larger rooms. Therefore, it was the place to go and talk and try to solve the problems of the world.

She particularly remembers Miss Ring, our health teacher. Her classes were interesting and she was always very pleasant.

Her teaching career began in 1947–48, when she was a permit teacher at Gordon Union School, in Rathwell. For the following year, 1949–50, she again was a permit teacher, this time at Mafeking School, in Mafeking. From 1951 to 1954, she taught grades one and two at Woodhaven School, in St. James, a part of Winnipeg. Then, in 1954–55, she was a substitute teacher at Kapuskasing School, in Kapuskasing, Ont.

Her husband, who graduated as a mechanical engineer from University of Manitoba, obtained a position at the New York *Times*—a great newspaper—in 1962. They moved to the New York area and have enjoyed their lives there since then. They had thought that, perhaps when they retired, they would return to Canada; but, by then, their children were both married and settled in the United States.

From 1970 to 1980, she taught adult education classes at Northern Valley High School, in Demarest, N.J., and in Fort Lee High School, Fort Lee, N.J. One of those classes consisted of mostly Japanese women who spoke very little English. She incorporated graphics into her lessons to the students to help them to comprehend. This experience was very rewarding for her.

In 1980, she began the position of service contracts administrator in the computer division of Hewlett Packard Company. Her job was being a liaison between the software engineers and the customers. The customers with whom she worked were located in Manhattan and required trips throughout New York City to review their software requirements. Her office was the penthouse at One Penn Plaza in that city. This position provided her with many opportunities to become familiar with midtown Manhattan. She remained with the company until 1991.

Since 1992, she has been actively involved with the Meals on Wheels programme as a deliverer of food and as a member of thc board.

As a child, she enjoyed reading *Heidi*, by Johanna Spyri, because the setting in the Alps was so different from the rolling hills of Manitoba where Dorothy lived. She has read and enjoyed so many books as an adult that it is difficult to name only one, but *The Return of the Native*, by Thomas Hardy, will always be a favourite.

Sometimes, a childhood memory is not pleasant. One day, some boys in grade seven put a dead garter snake into the desk of a girl classmate. There seemed to be a high population of garter snakes in Manitoba that year. As it happened, the girl whose desk was involved reported it to the teacher quite calmly, who, in turn, requested one boy to return it outside the building. That was the end of the matter. Dorothy was glad that it had not been placed into her desk. Since she had a snake phobia, she would have most likely shrieked loudly and made a scene. That would have caused the boys to be in trouble. However, cooler heads prevailed—much to Dorothy's satisfaction.

Once she read an article in the New York *Times* telling of how the garter snakes in northern Manitoba would emerge in great numbers from the caves in the spring. Her sister, who lives in The Pas, has told her that, in the spring up there, the highways are blanketed with dead garter snakes that have been run over by the cars.

Dr. Ron Stegall was a friend and minister who had an influence on her because he was a good listener and because he was able to give sound counsel.

She would suggest that, for a unique experience, tourists visit a northern Canadian town in the dead of winter to experience the northern lights. What an amazing sight it can be as the sky becomes a glow of colour!

She would advise a young person to visit other countries and travel and spend time in them. This should be done as much as possible while they are young. It would be a very valuable learning experience.

She would tell anyone contemplating the teaching profession as a career the same as she told her daughter, who became a teacher. Teaching is a wonderful profession. You have an opportunity to make a positive difference in the life of a child.

Her hobbies now are playing bridge, needlework, crossword puzzles, tennis, and, of course, reading. Her philosophy of life is to treat each day as a gift and enjoy it.

Class B

Ernest Braun
John Carrol
May Cathcart
Winnifred Cathcart
Florence Chambers
Alice Chanin
Roberta Chapman
Sophie Chatwell
Ardythe Chisholm
Stanley Cholka
Roberta Clark
Ethel Clarke
Yolande Combot
Robert Connolly
Charlotte Cooper
Pricille Cormier
Ann Couch
Frieda Couling
Margaret Coutts
Fred Daciw

Donnella Darling
Loretta Darling
Denise Davison
Ada Dawson
Joyce Demchuk
Edward Demkiw
Natalie Demkiw
Gloria Dick
Clarice Dickenson
Joan Dickson
Mary Dishnick
John Doerkson
Audrey Donald
Eugene Doroschuk
Ivy Douglas
Pansy Douglas
Marion Dracass
Sister Edith Marie
Sister Gerard
Sister St. Rose

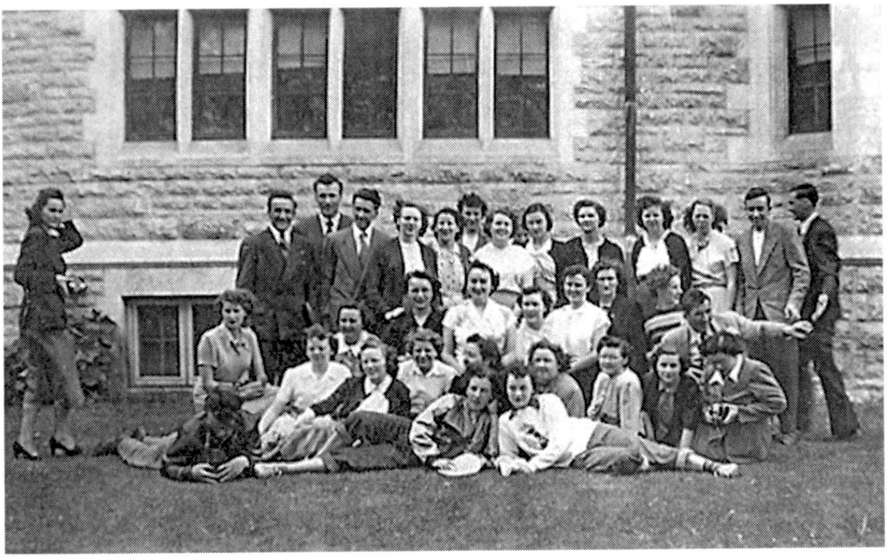

10. Class B

9

Winnie (Cathcart) Wolfe

One year when she was attending Southfield School, there was no snow on the ground until after Christmas. She commenced the year going the five miles (8 km) from home with a team of horses and a buggy. When the ground became frozen, the buggy wheels wore out. Thus, it was necessary for her to switch her means of transportation. She then rode horseback until the snow covered the ground. Now, she drove the team hitched to a sleigh.

One day, disaster struck! The horses ran away, leaving her and the sleigh behind. What would she do? She need not worry because help was on the way. Neighbours were hauling hay on that road. Seeing the plight of the girl, they dropped what they were doing and chased the horses until the team was under control. They returned the horses to the sleigh and hitched them to it. Since there was nothing broken on the harness, the girl assumed that she had not hooked the harness properly to the sleigh. You can be sure that she checked very carefully in the future to avoid such an experience again. As may be expected, she was teased about that incident for a long time.

Winnie was born in MacGregor. Currently, she lives in the Rural Municipality of Daly.

She attended three schools in receiving her grades one to ten education: Pratt, Great Carlton, and Southfield. These schools were close to Pratt. She took grades one to six at Pratt School; and then, because there were so few students, she moved to Great Carlton for grades seven, eight, and nine. She next moved to Southfield to take grade ten by correspondence, after which she attended MacGregor School for grades eleven and twelve. Because it was fifteen miles (24 km) from her home at Pratt, she boarded in MacGregor.

Miss Francis taught her all subjects, including music and art, from grade one to grade six in the one-room school at Pratt. At noon hour and recess, this teacher went out to the schoolyard and taught the children numerous games. Miss Francis made much use of the blackboard and often announced short tests. Her method of teaching stayed with Winnie to her own teaching days.

She remembers Miss Smith, who taught English grammar at Normal School. She had a manner of teaching verbs, nouns, and other parts of speech that made grammar an interesting subject to study.

Winnie was one of the girls who prepared the tables at Normal School before the other students came in to eat. The meals were served buffet style, but the girls served the dessert. She remembers that, when a raisin pie slice was served, the students usually wanted a second slice. There was only so much for everyone, but the waitresses managed to give an extra one to some of the students. This job at meal times made it quite rushed for the girls, but they enjoyed doing it. The fifty cents a day that they were paid helped. After the students left the dining room, the girls cleaned the tables so that they would be ready for the next meal. Since the meals were not mentioned in the yearbook, Winnie decided to tell how all of us managed to be fed.

She was a permit teacher at Hermfield School, which was five miles (8 km) south of Waskada. After Normal School, she taught for three years at Spring Valley School, which was about ten miles (16 km) north of Alexander. That was the extent of her teaching career.

When she was teaching at Spring Valley, there was always a Christmas concert to prepare with a tree, gifts for everyone, and Santa to hand out the gifts. One time, when Santa entered the room, Winnie walked down the aisle to meet him. She kissed him. The audience was aghast! Was she not being a little forward in kissing Santa, her future husband? Little did they know. However, she knew by the friendly "Ho, Ho, Ho" that Santa was actually her father. He and her mother had come to see the concert and take her home to Pratt for the holidays. She was really thrilled with her dad's surprise.

After teaching, she married a farmer and has been a farmer's wife ever since. To pass the long winter evenings on the farm, she crocheted; but since doilies have long gone out of vogue, she has not crocheted for a few years. Now, she passes the time doing crossword puzzles. In the summer, she is usually in the garden or going for walks.

She was an avid reader of books about animals when she was young. One was *The Call of the Wild*, by Jack London, which she read several times. She remembers a book called *Heather*, which was about a pony in Scotland. As an adult, she is reading less. However, she has read Margaret Atwood's books *The Blind Assassin*, *The Robber Bride*, and *Alias Grace*. Now, she prefers to read books written by Catherine Cookson.

She was secretary for United Church Women for nineteen years until it folded because of the closing of the church. Her most interesting service was being director of the Harding Fair at Harding. She began as director of the school work; but after five years, she was transferred to being director of the cooking. She spent over thirty years in this role. When she reached seventy-five years of age, she relinquished the director position because she felt that someone younger would have new ideas. Nevertheless, the current directors still ask her to help out if they have need.

If visitors were to go to Manitoba for a day, she would suggest they go to the Harding Fair. It is always held on the third Friday of July. There is a little bit of everything there, including cattle, light horses, and heavy horses. In 2008, there were five six-horse teams in the ring at the same time. There is baking, sewing, and garden produce to see. It is small compared to the big well-known fairs, but it is friendly and there is plenty to eat and drink. Winnie invites everyone to visit this fair next year.

One time, she and her daughter Arlene travelled to North and South Dakota. The first day, they reached Belle Fourche, a twelve-hour drive. The next day, they continued to Spearfish Canyon. At Deadwood, they saw the gravesites of Wild Bill Hickok and Calamity Jane in Mount Moriah Cemetery. On the way to Custer, they saw the Crazy Horse Memorial. Near Custer, they toured Jewel Cave. At Custer State Park, they followed the wildlife loop and saw buffalo, deer, goats, and bears. Next, they drove on Needles Highway and saw gorgeous rocks and mountains. The next day, they visited Mount Rushmore National Memorial, and then went to Wall, home of the famous Wall Drug tourist attraction, for the night. The following morning, they drove to Badlands National Park and roamed the hills. They continued on to Pierre, South Dakota state capital, where they spent the night. They left

Pierre the next morning for the drive home. It was a very pleasant and informative tour.

She has not addressed a group of teenagers since she last taught school. Life for the young now is much different from what it was back then. Her advice to teenagers and anyone in general is to be very careful with whom they associate. There is so much more about which to worry, with drugs and alcohol so prevalent. She would advise young people to find a good job which they enjoy instead of spending their time loafing. A person can receive so much satisfaction from a day's work. Then, when one has earned money, one must not waste it by gambling, but spend it wisely or save it for a rainy day.

The teaching profession is one which can be very rewarding if you like to work with people. You can start as a substitute teacher and then become a teacher of a single room. After a few years of teaching, you can become a principal. A later goal could be to become a superintendent. When you feel like retiring, you can reverse the procedure until you are again a substitute teacher. It is up to the individual what route he/she will take, but such possibilities as the one stated here are available.

10
Mary (Dishnick) Chubey

Count on a child to say something amusing while trying to be serious. Mary was substituting in a grade one classroom after she retired. As it is a good idea to tell little children one's name, she did. She introduced herself as Mrs. Chubey at the beginning of the first day. In case that this name might be unfamiliar, she informed them that her name would be easy to remember if they thought of her as being chubby.

All went well until the next day. As young children love to do, they crowded around her desk at noon, each one trying to tell her something. This was too much for one little boy who could not say his piece before someone else did. Becoming impatient in waiting for his turn, he tugged at his teacher's sleeve, calling, "Mrs. Skinny! Mrs. Skinny!" That set off a roar of laughter from his classmates. As this hurt his feelings, he started to cry. Mary understood. She placed an arm around him and gave him a big hug. She assured him that he had made only a little mistake, but that he had just made her day. That did it. He was all smiles then. However, he forgot what he was trying to tell her.

Mary was born on a farm near Arnaud on a very cold and stormy day with a midwife present. She is an only child.

She attended North Star School, one and one-half miles (2.4 km) away from home, from grade one to grade eight. She usually walked to school, unless it was very stormy. Later, her parents purchased a bicycle for her and she rode to school on it in the warm months.

For grade nine and grade ten, she boarded in Arnaud and attended Arnaud School. For grades eleven and twelve, she attended St. John's Technical High School in Winnipeg. In July, after she had completed grade ten, her parents gave her money for a train ticket to Winnipeg. In answer to an advertisement in the *Free Press* wanting a student to help at home in return for board and room and an opportunity to attend school in Winnipeg, she walked from the Canadian Pacific Railway station to the address given—and was hired.

She stayed there for the two years and found it very interesting. She lived with a Jewish family and learned about their culture. At the same time, she looked after two young boys and helped the mother with some housework. The disadvantage was that Mary could not participate in any extracurricular activities because she had to be at home soon after school. She could not start studying until the boys were in bed. She was not paid, but she was able to go to the movies with the children every Saturday. On Sundays, she could visit with her friends.

She obtained her teacher's certificate after her year in Normal School, and then went on to take summer school courses to obtain her Permanent Teacher's Certificate. Later on, her school inspector, Mr. Gerard, advised her that she should attend university to acquire her Bachelor of Arts degree. She achieved it by taking five correspondence courses and the other five through summer courses and night school courses in winter. This was carried on while she was teaching and being a mother and housewife. She graduated in 1975, but she continued to attend summer school classes to help her teach the Ukrainian bilingual programme in school.

She gives much credit to her husband for helping her obtain her university degree. In summer, she drove to Winnipeg by herself; but, in winter, he drove her to her classes. He would wash dishes and do some housework and garden work so that she could study.

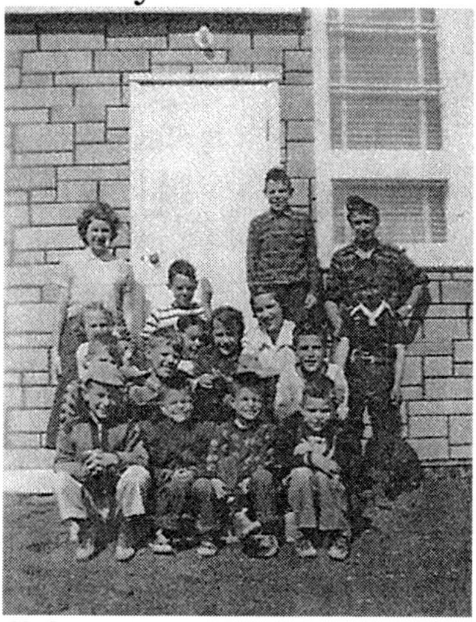

11. Broadview School

She began her teaching career in Broadview School, grades one to eight, near Morris. After her marriage and in between having her family, she taught in the local schools: Baskerville School, Senkiw School, Plankey Plains School, and River Ranch School. All were grades one to eight. When the schools amalgamated, she taught grades one to three in Plankey Plains School for two years. Then she was moved to Shevchenko School in Vita, where she taught grades two or three, depending on the year. She retired from teaching in 1988 after thirty-one years in the classroom.

The only other professions which she had were being a farmer's wife, a homemaker, and a mother.

As a child, she enjoyed reading the book *Heidi*, by Johanna Spyri. As an only child, Mary found her life fascinating. As an adult, she read many books; but there was none that stood out as much as the Bible.

A sad experience occurred when she was a teenager going to school in Arnaud. She became friends with a Japanese girl, Hatsue, who had come from a family that was displaced from British Columbia and relocated in the

Arnaud area during World War II. When Mary's parents found out, they told her that she could not be her friend because that girl was an enemy. Both girls were hurt by this attitude. Unfortunately, this attitude was expressed in regard to both Japanese and Germans living in Canada at that time.

Her hobbies are vegetable and flower gardening, writing Ukrainian Easter eggs, reading, crotchet work, wheat weaving, doing puzzles, and exchanging email with friends.

Mary has been an active member of the Rosa, Olha Kobylanska Branch of the Ukrainian Women's Association of Canada, for many years. In 2007, she was honoured with an Award of Excellence plaque from the Ukrainian Self-Reliance League of Canada. She has been a member of the Vita Horticultural Society, on the board of the Vita and District Resource Council, a member of the local Good Neighbors Club, and a 4-H judge many times.

A very memorable trip that she and her husband Harry took was to Ukraine in the fall of 1988 after Mary had retired. They flew from Toronto to Austria, where they transferred to a plane to the Ukraine. On disembarking from the first plane, they saw armed soldiers telling the guide where to go to board the next plane. What an uncomfortable feeling that gave the visitors!

Everything went according to schedule until they arrived in Lviv. Members of Mary's side of the family were waiting at the hotel, as had been previously arranged. As this was their first meeting, it was exciting for everyone. Mary had no other relatives in Canada besides her parents. Since they had passed away, her side of the family consists of only her children, grandchildren, and great-grandchildren. It is very fortunate for her that Harry had come from a big family. Thus, Mary inherited many in-laws.

Her family wanted them to visit with them. The tour guide said that they could, but they were not to tell anyone. Someone from the family could come and take them if they would not go further than twenty miles (32 km) away. They had to be in the hotel by 11:00 p.m.

The husband of one of Mary's cousins was a taxi driver. Therefore, he came for them and drove them to the villages in which her relatives lived—more than twenty miles (32 km) away. That fact was kept a secret from the tour guide. Since Mary's family was aware of the situation, those who lived further away came to visit in the villages that were closer to Lviv.

When they arrived in Ukraine and visited with their relatives, Mary noticed that the people had milk pails upside down on fence posts as her mother did when Mary was a child. They lived in a village, yet each one of them had a cow and some chickens, turkeys, ducks, or geese in the yard, just as her parents had when she was little. Each family had a garden and all seemed to have to work hard to survive.

In every home where they went, they were served a meal which consisted of several courses. While one course was served, the next one was being prepared. This meant that it took a long time to finish a meal. The first course was probably digested by the time the last course arrived!

There was a special store where tourists could shop, but the local people were not permitted to shop there unless they were with the tourists. Mary and Harry could go out in the city of Lviv on their own, but there were soldiers everywhere. They were very friendly, though.

One day, the couple, wanting to see a Ukrainian store, set out to find one. They were successful. It was like an outdoor farmer's market. What amazed Mary was seeing freshly killed chickens hung up for sale. When they realized that they were lost, they asked a soldier for directions. He was very friendly and helped them find their way back to their motel. She felt that they were constantly being watched. There seemed to be eyes everywhere! She did not feel free throughout the time that they were there. A fear that they might do something wrong lingered over them.

Being able to speak the language certainly helped. A stranger asked her from what part of Ukraine had she come. When she told him that she was from Canada, he found it hard to believe, noting that she spoke with an accent like those near Lviv. She had learned that accent from her parents because that was the way in which they spoke.

In the city, the public bathrooms amazed her. There were stalls, but in each stall was an open hole in the floor with running water in it—not very inviting. Here you did what you had to do. The hotels had much better bathrooms. In one motel, the bathroom consisted of a sink and a shower head with a hole in the floor for the water to escape. There was no hot water because the system had broken down.

Many of the married children lived with their parents; and, while the children went to work, the parents looked after the animals. Someone had to take the cow out to where there was grass so that she could graze. In 2006, Mary received a letter from her cousin's daughter saying that they had to sell their cow because the father was sick and could no longer take it to graze or make hay for it.

What really amazed her was the people's approach to work. One of her cousins told her about her first job. She was working in a factory doing piece work. She worked hard to complete as many pieces as she could, thinking she would be paid well. When payday came, she discovered that she was docked money because she had done too much. She said that from then on she never did more than she was required to do.

Mary and her cousin were very upset because they both felt that the youth in Ukraine would have no concept of the work ethic that the older generation still had. She and Harry tried to explain to them their way of life. They told them that they had beef cattle and purchased their milk. It was unbelievable to these people that, in Canada, a farmer could have cows and not milk them.

Despite their way of life, they seemed to accept their situation very well. Mary remembers her parents talking about their life back home in Ukraine. To her, it sounded like the feudal system. There was a lord in the village. Her parents were allotted strips of land that they purchased. They still had to work for him in return for special privileges.

When they were leaving Ukraine, they were asked by the officials about what they were taking back. These Canadians told them exactly what they had. However, there were others on the tour who were questioned and whose luggage was searched. Tourists were certainly not free to come and go as they pleased. Mary and Harry felt very relieved to pass through customs and be on their way home.

As a result of this trip, Mary learned to appreciate Canada deeply as her home country for the freedom which we have here. At that time, she felt that their way of life was forty years behind ours.

Their son and grandson went to the Ukraine in 2006 with a group of dancers and said that there is much more freedom now. They were not restricted as the others had been. Everything was more modern now.

She would suggest to visitors in Canada from another country to attend Folklorama in Winnipeg at the beginning of August. In two weeks, they would have the opportunity to see the pavilions of many different countries, taste their food, and learn about their culture.

If she were to address a group of teenagers, Mary would emphasize the fact that they should not be swayed by peer pressure, but put much thought into their actions so that they would not regret in the future what they had done. They should pay attention to their teachers and parents for good advice. She would stress honesty, good manners, and sincerity in all they do. They should also develop a good sense of humour.

She has a few questions that she would ask anyone contemplating entering the teaching profession. Are you sure that you like children and are prepared to accept teaching children with different abilities? Are you ready to spend much time in preparation for the classroom? Do you realize that extracurricular activities with the children are also important? Have you thought about the talents which you have and how you can use them in the teaching profession?

Reverend Wasyliw had a positive influence on Mary's life. At the time that he was the priest for their parish, her sons were teenagers. He was able to involve them in Sumk (a youth club), and that helped their parents guide the boys through their teens.

Nellie McClung made a great contribution to Canada. She was instrumental in bringing women's issues forward. In 1916, because of her efforts, the Liberal party gave the Manitoba women the right to vote.

Mary believes in accepting life as it happens. Have a strong belief in God and let him guide you through life. Also have a good sense of humour!

Miss Douglas, our music teacher at Normal School, always seemed to be happy and spontaneous in all that she did. Mary and her husband have always had a love for music. He played an accordion and was active in musical bands. It seems that they passed on their love for music to their grandchildren. One plays guitar and sings in band called *Sloohai*. (In English, the word means "listen".) The youngest one takes part in Ukrainian dancing and has travelled to many parts of the world. Youth now have so many opportunities that their parents did not have.

Her year at Normal School was very special to her. She enjoyed the classes as they seemed to have real meaning for her future profession. The assignments were easy and fun to do. By being in residence, she had time to make many new friends and to have fun. She is still in contact with a number of them. Like other former Normalites, she regrets that many are no longer with us.

Mary lives on a farm near Carlowrie. This used to be a little village with a store, post office, dance hall, and several households; but now there are only a few homes and mailboxes. She has lived there since 1953, not long after she and Harry Chubey were married.

They had two sons, Taras and Tom. Both live in Winnipeg. Taras taught school in Winnipeg and retired in 2008. Tom was a Winnipeg transit driver and has also retired. Mary became a widow in 1996. She has five grandchildren and four great-grandchildren.

She still enjoys her vegetable and flower gardens which she tends—with little outside help. She is blessed with a grandson Glen and his wife Holly and two great-grandchildren (Owen fourteen months old and Lucas two months old) living nearby. Thus, help is not far away if it should be needed.

11

Audrey (Donald) Henitiuk

In her first year of teaching, her rural school had thirty-seven students from grades one to nine. She loved every minute of it, although she had her challenges. She even reveled in those. Two brothers, ages ten and eleven, provided much of that challenge—even some amusing moments. They were consistent in creating trouble for themselves and their teacher. She felt that she was prepared for them because she was told when she arrived that they had been shooting the insulators off the telephone poles and that the police had to investigate.

Most of the time, they went hunting gophers with their dad's .22 rifle instead of attending school. Their dad worked away from home, and thus was not available to supervise often. They took advantage of this in order to talk their mother into many things. However, Audrey had been raised with six brothers and thought that she knew how to handle any shenanigans.

One day, she isolated the older boy in the girls' cloakroom after school to let him think about his behaviour that day. When she went to retrieve him to deal with the problem, he had outwitted her. He was gone! Not desiring to be imprisoned there, he climbed out the window and went home! So much for that. She thought it was hilarious at the time.

Another time, the same boy had to be reprimanded and, thus, she kept him in after school. As he sat at the back of the room, she could hear some grumbling. He was saying, "Why don't you strap me and get it over with?" However, Audrey did not believe in that kind of punishment. Therefore, after an appropriate lecture, she sent him home. That seemed to end her troubles with them. Could it have been, instead, that it was because they moved to another district?

Audrey was born in Treherne. She began her schooling at Louise School, in a farming community six miles (10 km) north of Treherne. Her school days certainly were in another era and were a long time ago. There were the usual strange things that happened along the way—playground teasing and being taunted about wearing red knee socks that her aunt in Winnipeg had sent to her because they were different, coming from the big city.

She remembers going to school in midwinter, skiing across the snowdrifts as she followed her brother the mile (1.6 km) to school. Sometimes, if the weather was particularly stormy, her dad would take the children with the horse and cutter. She says that makes her feel *oooold*!

She taught on a permit in 1949–50 and after two years received her permanent Manitoba teaching certificate. Later, over a period of years, she obtained a Bachelor of Education degree from University of Alberta, grade ten piano from the Toronto Conservatory of Music, third year Certified General Accountant from Grant MacEwan Community College and Northern Alberta Institute of Technology—both in Edmonton, Alberta.

She attended the University of Alberta when she could as she and her husband raised their family of four. Their daughter Valerie obtained her Ph.D. degree there as well and is now Associate Director of Literary Translation at the University of East Anglia in Norwich, England.

Miss Smith, our language arts teacher at Normal School, taught her the grammar which she had somehow missed up to that time. This experience helped her for many years afterwards. Miss Douglas, our music teacher, fulfilled the need in her life for music.

Life at Normal School revolved around the dormitory where she could associate with, help or receive help, and console or be consoled by other girls. Mackenzie Hall was a place of fun. Coming into the building through the tunnels after the doors had been locked at night was an experience. If she could do it all again, she would have more fun instead of doing so much work.

She has taught in the following schools: Springbrook in Austin; Allendale in Rossendale District; Burnside, near Portage la Prairie; Victoria Elementary in Portage la Prairie; Manning Elementary in Manning, Alta.; and Robert Rundle Elementary in St. Albert, Alta. She has also taught as a substitute teacher in various schools in Spruce Grove and Stony Plain, Alta.

While she was teaching school, she was also a piano teacher after hours in Manitoba rural schools from 1951 to 1955. She worked out of her home with her piano classes in the towns of Manning, Alta.; Whitehorse, Yukon; St. Albert, Alta.; and Spruce Grove, Alta., from 1955 to 2006. She has been a public accountant since 1980 in St. Albert and Spruce Grove.

Girl of the Limberlost, by Gene Stratton-Porter, was her favourite book when she was a child. *The Stone Angel*, by Margaret Laurence, was her favourite in her adult years. For pastimes, she plays piano, violin, and organ; sings in a choir; dabbles in oil painting; and gardens.

In Alberta communities, she has been a member of the Royal Purple. She also has been Manning United Church organist, St. Albert United Church Sunday school teacher and superintendent, Winterburn United Church organist and choir director, and choir member of St. Andrew's United Church in Spruce Grove.

She had an enjoyable visit in Dijon, France, where her daughter taught for a year. She met Valerie in Paris. This city is always an interesting place with all the museums, ornate churches, tiny shops, the Eiffel Tower, and such other sights as artists' wares along the Seine River. From there, they travelled by train toward Dijon. The French countryside is always green and beautiful.

They arrived at Valerie's apartment, which was ideally situated in the university area where Valerie worked. After Valerie headed out to work, Audrey would go for a walk, sketching the street layout in the area so that she would not be turned around and hopelessly lost. The apartment was easy to locate, with its spoke-like system of streets around a town square, as long as she took the correct street.

Medieval half-timbered houses lined the streets in the oldest parts of the city. A century-old fountain was topped by a bronze statue of a nude grape-stomping winemaker. She would sit on a stone bench to rest and watch the people go by or browse the tiny shops until it was time to hurry back to meet Valerie when she would return home after work. There were many international students in the city.

As Audrey and her daughter walked through the narrow cobble-stoned streets of the old town, she imagined the clatter of history of others on foot, on horseback, and in carriages, who had gone over the same stones and worn them smooth since at least the 12th century.

They visited the 150-foot (46 m) Tower of Philip the Good—built as a lookout by the duke. They climbed the 316 worn stone steps in a tightly spiralling staircase. From the top, they could see a panorama of the countryside. What a majestic view that was!

Walking along the narrow stone streets between the houses, they espied a good luck charm built into one corner. The charm had been worn very smooth with the touching of hands over the centuries. Also along the route were many Gothic churches and other buildings with beautiful architecture.

Then, they travelled by train to Lyon to visit a friend who lived there. Michelle and Audrey had been pen pals since they were in high school, fifty-two years earlier. This was their third get-together, twice in Lyon and once in Spruce Grove, Alta. While her mother visited here for two weeks, Valerie returned to her work.

Michelle and her husband Marcel had a car and spent many days showing their guest the sights. He sped along the roads and as a car would cut in front of him or come too close, he would shake his fist and blurt a stream of *le français* that Audrey could only guess the meaning.

They saw the remains of an old Roman amphitheatre and amazing Roman stone roads, the wine district where they stopped at a friend's winery, and visited many shops and winery caves in quaint villages. Audrey discovered that her high school French was not good preparation for total French immersion. She could read the language fairly well and understand what her friends were saying, but putting timely sentences together was a struggle. Eventually, her conversation skills improved.

When Mother's Day arrived, there was a family gathering for the weekend at a very "ancient" mountain cabin. The back half of the building had been the original dwelling with space for animals, a large fireplace for heating and cooking, and a dirt floor. The walls were made of stones two feet thick. The structure must have been in existence for centuries. The part added on was fairly modern. The large gathering room had a big table and many chairs. Obviously, this close-knit family had spent much time there over the years. Too soon, she and Valerie boarded the train back to Paris to commence her flight home. It had been such a wonderful holiday!

On another occasion, she and her friend Phyllis enjoyed a bus tour of England, Ireland, Wales, and Scotland. After a busy tax season, they packed their bags and headed for London. The trip was well organized by Globus Tours. Thus, they had little planning to do. Usually, one or two nights were spent in a place. Then, early in the morning, they were on the bus heading toward another place. On the way, the guide would point out the historic sites.

The first stop was at Hampton Court, built in 1514 along the River Thames. This was King Henry VIII's favourite summer home. They toured the wide halls and enormous dining areas. The kitchens had a massive fireplace for cooking the venison or other meat. There were reportedly the ghosts of two of his wives still haunting the rooms. It must have been very cold in this home in winter weather.

They visited Stonehenge, which seemed so small, but those stones, which probably had been at this place for 5,000 years, were massive. As much of the stone is buried in the ground as appears above the surface. What an engineering feat it was to have transported those rocks!

After a visit to Bath with all its statues, they passed through southern Wales, where they took a ferry across the Irish Sea to Ireland. Her dad was from Scotland and had a wonderful tenor voice. She can remember, as a child, hearing his clear, strong voice singing many Irish and Scottish ballads as he worked around the farm. The songs kept coming back to her head as they stopped at such places as Galway Bay, Tipperary, and Dublin.

Beautiful green country with rolling hills, quaint homes, remnants of fortresses, and misty rain seen here have appeared in many novels. One overnight stop was in an old country manor house—now a hotel. A family was still living in it, but most of the building was roped off for tours. She was impressed by the stately rooms with high ceilings and ornate trims, carved fireplaces, and fabulous wall hangings.

Trinity College, in Dublin, displayed millions of books on shelf after shelf that filled the enormous high-ceilinged building. The Book of Kells was displayed under glass. Its pages richly decorated and the embellished script certainly told of another time.

In the northern part of Wales, thousands of sheep covering the hillsides and many waterfalls and streams made the country very picturesque. A short visit to Edinburgh followed. Edinburgh Castle loomed overhead in the mists. Here, they walked the Royal Mile and braved the windy ramparts of the castle. Later, as they stopped to view the remnants of Hadrian's Wall, they were amazed that it is still standing in many places. The spires of Oxford appeared as they headed south. Back in London, a short tour of Windsor Castle ended their holiday.

For a tourist in Canada, Audrey recommends a visit to the Okanagan Valley of southern British Columbia in the spring. The blossoms of the fruit trees with a backdrop of mountains and lakes exhibit amazing scenery. In addition, there are numerous interesting places in the area to see.

Her advice to teenagers is to stay at school and obtain the most out of every day. Each day goes by anyway, so you may as well accomplish something in that time. Aim for the best; you just might reach your lofty goal.

For anyone contemplating teaching as a career, she has this exhortation. Be sure you enjoy the students and subject matter. Be kind. Try to find the fun in your work.

Beth Garnett was her grade seven teacher in a rural school. She taught all subjects. Audrey liked the way her teacher mixed handicrafts with the daily work and took a personal interest in each of her students. How excited the students were when her boyfriend pulled up on a motorbike to visit her! She stayed in the community after marrying and kept in contact with Audrey.

Her mother's first cousin had a big influence on Audrey's life. She and her husband Bill lived in Winnipeg, had no children of their own, and gave her the opportunity to live with them and go to high school at St. James Collegiate. She introduced Audrey to the world of classical music; helped her to see the importance of doing well with each endeavour; showed her how to help in the community, schools, and churches; and instructed her on a myriad of things the big city had to offer.

Audrey had been raised on a farm and her mother—the strongest influence in her life—had sent her there to acquire an education and become a teacher that had been her own lifelong desire.

Many of the women who were ahead of their time showed what can be done with their lives. One of those was Dr. Mary Percy Jackson. She came from a well-to-do family—mostly teachers—in England and became a doctor. Her first posting was in the Peace River area of northern Alberta in 1929. Here she married, raised a family, and provided medical services to the ever-expanding community, overcoming insurmountable difficulties. She received the Order of Canada and other notable acclaims during her lifetime of ninety-six years.

Aim to be the best you can be and to attempt things that may seem impossible. You never know where it might take you. This is her philosophy of life. She presents a saying along this line: "Even a fool knows you can't reach the stars, but that doesn't stop a wise man from trying."

12
Eugene Doroschuk

He was playing second base on his elementary school team. A little fly ball drifted toward him. He reached out to grab it. The ball missed his hands, but it made a direct hit on his right eye. Ow! That hurt.

He received an opportunity to redeem himself when another little fly ball floated toward him. Up went his hands again. This time, there was a direct hit on the left eye. That was too much! Two black eyes convinced his father that his son was extremely short-sighted and needed glasses. However, he did say, "Anyway, you certainly kept your eye on the ball." That was not funny, Dad!

Eugene was born at SW cor SE ¼ sec 3-33-20W, near Pulp River. This address actually appears on both his birth certificate and his passport. For anyone who has never lived on the Canadian Prairies, that is an official farm location. When his dad went to register him at birth, he was told that the community he stated did not exist. Therefore, he gave the school cottage location where the birth occurred. This address remains.

He commenced his schooling at Loon Lake School District, a rural school about thirty miles (48 km) north of Dauphin. The person who was his favourite teacher was his father, who taught him in grades one to eight and supervised his grade nine correspondence. Beyond that, he gave Eugene a love for music, learning, and sports.

Eugene was a permit teacher at Fryer School District at Silver. Following Normal School, he was an assistant principal at Balmoral; a principal at Belmont; and a teacher and principal at Chateauguay, Que.

He had a great respect for Mr. Moorhead, our principal. As house captain, Eugene was one of a group who had a meeting with him every morning before class. His calmness and commanding presence were very impressive.

Because of his responsibilities in Frontenac Hall, Eugene was closely involved with all the "comings and goings" of the house members. Running the election campaign for Harry Backlin and organizing the election rally concert were among the many memorable experiences at Normal School.

Eugene obtained a Bachelor of Physical Education degree at University of British Columbia, a Master of Science degree and a Doctor of Philosophy degree at University of Illinois.

The person who had a great effect on his life was Dr. T. K. Cureton, his mentor at the University of Illinois. He lived his theories of physical fitness.

Eugene held several positions in the field of physical fitness. He was the director of physical fitness laboratories at the University of Montreal and Laval University. Then, he was physical fitness consultant in Montreal, Ottawa, and Quebec City, where he worked on Centennial fitness awards, CAPHER fitness for children, fitness for adults, fitness of the Canadian ski team, and fitness of championship athletes at the Olympic Games and the Pan-American Games.

He and a few colleagues from University of Illinois began work in Canada. The CAPHER Fitness Testing

Programme, which they developed, was adopted for Canada. They found Canadians at the time to be in very poor physical shape. He has seen little improvement over the years. There is now much obesity.

He checked athletes who came to the Montreal area, including some local professional hockey and football players. One of the tests would be to measure for fat thickness in their bodies. He tested various athletes competing in the Olympics and Pan-American Games in the 1960s and 1970s. He had the occasion to perform a fitness test on Bruce Kidd, a member of Canada's track team, before the 1964 Summer Olympics in Tokyo. He stressed good diet, but did not go into specifics regarding nutritional choices.

Eugene feels that physical education programmes in schools go only part way in regard to physical fitness. Sports alone are not enough. When he worked with young children in school, he would make rules for their playing basketball and volleyball so that everyone would be involved. He did not want a small player or girls being overlooked by other players on the court.

He was becoming disenchanted with the progress of physical fitness in Canada since people did not take the matter seriously. He mentioned to someone that he would work with anyone who would listen. The opportunity came when a neighbour asked him to work with his race horse. Although this was unusual, he accepted the challenge and was so successful that the horse became a winner. He showed what can be done.

With the passing of time, he focused his attention on the music field where his wife Betty was excelling. Together, they formed an opera company in Montreal. He has been President of Ballet Victoria and accordionist in the Victoria Balalaika Orchestra, which played at various seniors' homes and community centres. The orchestra, having an average age of about seventy-five, folded in 2008 because of lack of young members. He also leads sing-a-longs at four or five seniors' homes. He has really enjoyed working with a Down's syndrome group, which has grown considerably in numbers. Again, he has shown what can be done with those who try.

Two books by Ernest Thompson Seton, *Wahb: The Biography of a Grizzly* and *Rolf in the Woods,* were favourites in his childhood. Later in life, he enjoyed *The Cossacks*, by Leo Tolstoy, and a Tolstoy short story, "How Much Land Does a Man Need?"

He and Betty took a trip to Soviet Union at the time of the Summer Olympics in Moscow in 1980. He enjoyed that visit very much. A trip to Cuba revealed to him how American propaganda distorts the advances which Cubans have made in their country. The people live better and are happier than what is being publicized. He and Betty had a very pleasant time there.

For those who like to see large cities, he recommends Montreal as an ideal place to visit at any time of the year.

His advice to any age group and for those contemplating the teaching profession that they acquire as much education as they can, never stop learning, and question everything around them.

His hobbies include reading, cooking, playing the accordion, and racehorse training. He lives by the philosophy, "Be nice and do good!" He is very pleased with the achievements of their sons with their singing group, *Men Without Hats*. He sees great potential with his granddaughter in the field of opera.

Over the years, he has always been thankful for the first annual reunion of our class. It was there where he and Betty began their close friendship that culminated in their marriage. They have remained happily together since that time.

Class C

Cecile Droux
Margaret Drozd
Duane Duff
Lois Dureau
Joyce Dyck
Thelma Dyck
Bill Eastcott
Margaret Eastman
Virginia Eilers
Donalda English
Jake Enns
Pat Enns
Art Fast
Peter Fast
Helen Finlay
Joyce Flatt
Muriel Forfar
Betty Forsyth
Lucille Freynet
Abe Friesen
Abram Friesen
Rowena Friesen
Shirley Fulmore
Ethel Galloway
Elsie Genik
Gwen Georgison
Marjorie Gilman
Isla Gliddon
Helen Goertzen
Margaret Gorowski
Evelyn Graham
Joyce Griffith
Joyce Griffiths
Genevieve Grudeski
Rose-Ann Guagliardo
Theresa Guimond
Donna Gustafson
Mary Gwozd
Sister Alfred
Sister Augustine
Sister Raymond

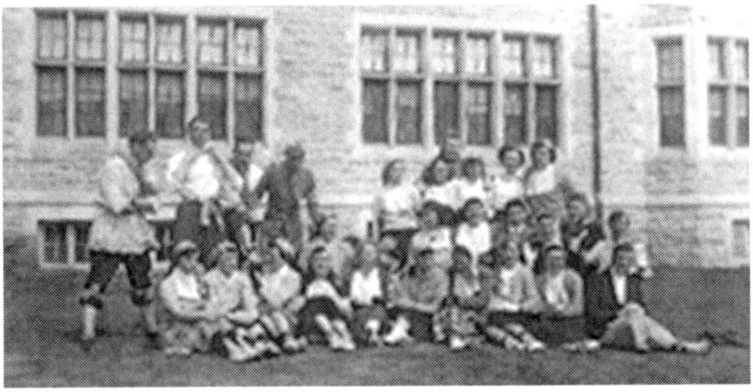

12. Class C

13
Cecile (Droux) Fisher

Oh, what a stench it was! Upon entering her classroom one morning, she could hardly breathe. It reeked of garlic! How had this happened? She quickly learned that one of her students had kindly shared his supply of garlic with the whole class.

It did not take long to determine who the generous supplier was. It was not amusing at all. As a punishment, she required him write twenty lines: "I will not give my classmates any more garlic!"

Knock, knock! was immediately heard at the classroom door. Then, to the young teacher's horror, there stood the inspector. "Oh, no! My job is in jeopardy," was the thought that raced through her mind. To her amazement, he laughed and dismissed the class to go outside and play ball. He, too, had been munching on garlic. What a relief that was! Now, her heartbeat could retreat to normal speed.

Cecile was born in Manitou. She acquired her grades one to eleven in Manitou and her grade twelve in St. Jean Baptiste.

In addition to her Permanent Teaching Certificate, she has taken numerous university courses, only two short from attaining a degree for a professional librarian.

When she was in grade eleven, her physics teacher shocked her with an impromptu assignment. He asked her to teach the lesson on the electric bell to the class. Taking up the challenge despite her extreme nervousness, she accomplished her mission successfully. Then, she discovered one positive side effect of the ordeal. She wanted to become a teacher! Since this teacher frequently asked her for help in preparing his lesson, Cecile's desire to become a teacher increased. One can see why he was her favourite teacher.

Normal School meant much to Cecile. Since she had a desire to teach, she did everything that she could possibly do to achieve good marks—studying diligently and attending class to learn to be a very good teacher. Her motto is, "Whatever you do—do well!" Take on any challenges and you can do anything that you set your mind to do, and work at your utmost potential. This she did and was thankful for attending Normal School.

Mr. Lightly, our vice-principal and social studies teacher, caused her to like the subject, in general, as he explained the lesson so well.

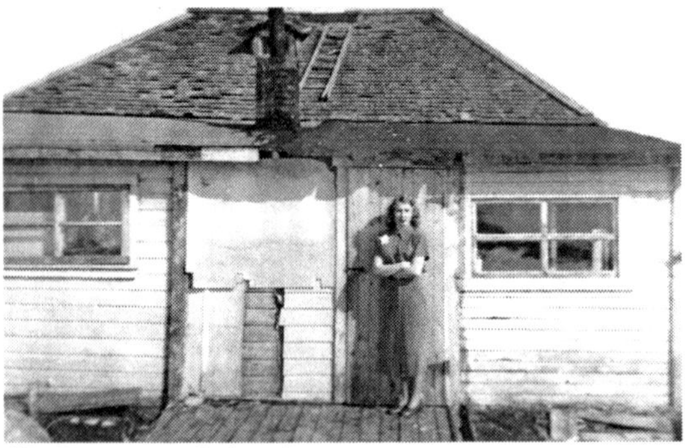
13. Denepro School

Prior to attending Normal School, she taught on permit in Grandview and in Manitou. Later, she taught at Denepro (near Grandview), Roblin Elementary in Roblin, Oak Lake, and Elkhorn.

Since the existing country school, where she taught on permit, was too small for the large enrolment, the trustees and community gutted an old house and transformed it into a classroom. It had a large room, an unheated cloakroom, a porch, but no indoor toilets. It was used for three years until an addition was built on the school. Creating the temporary structure proves that you can make use of anything available. Cecile feels that it is highly unlikely that the building would pass today's standards.

This was such a wonderful community, even to the point that she met her husband Tom here. The year 2009 marks their anniversary of fifty-four years of marriage—and they are still counting.

Besides teaching, she has worked in other areas. At Marr's Leisure Products, in Dauphin, she was a sewing inspector for recreational campers. At ARC Industries (Adult Rehabilitation Centre), also in Dauphin, she was a sewing instructor for the handicapped. She taught several phases of sewing, for example, quilting, crocheting, knitting, cross-stitch, candle wicking, and rug-making. She assisted with ceramics and woodworking for eight and one-half years. After that, she opened her own body-toning studio in Dauphin. Finally, in 1988, it was time for her to stay at home.

When Cecile was a child, two of her favourite books were *Silver Chief to the Rescue* and *Silver Chief, Dog of the North*, by Jack O'Brien. In later years, she located all of Jack O'Brien's books about Silver Chief at her library and followed the route on a map of Alaska. This was a very interesting project. In addition, she has also read many books on the experiences of teachers.

There are numerous hobbies that she enjoys very much, including sewing, knitting, crocheting, embroidery work, Crewel embroidery, quilting, beadwork, and any type of crafts. As this book is being written, she is collecting men's ties to make a "tie" quilt and other crafts using ties.

A neighbour lady was a seamstress who made so many beautiful articles that Cecile developed a keen desire to learn to sew. The lady helped her to make her first pyjamas and a white blouse on which Cecile embroidered. Her high school teacher taught her to crochet. Since then, she has purchased many craft books and ventured on her own.

Playing cards is another one of her delights. She convenes the cards events for Elkhorn Leisure Centre in the Westman area and also tends to the cards played in the centre every Monday night. If those interests do not keep her occupied, she partakes of such outdoor activities as hunting and fishing.

In her community, she works with SAIL (Seniors Access to Independent Living), which offers much assistance to the elderly, Meals on Wheels, and trips to shop or medical appointments, and musical outings. However, she eventually had to cut back on these activities for health reasons.

It was such a delightful trip to New Zealand to meet Tom's relatives whom they had never met, although some had visited Tom and Cecile in Canada. They were able to tour both of the main islands. How beautiful they are! She would recommend this trip to anyone who is able to go there.

For visitors to Canada, she would suggest that they tour the whole country as it is beautiful. Manitoba has such scenic spots for sight-seeing, hunting, and fishing as Lake of the Prairies, Roblin, Childs Lake, Lake Manitoba, and Riding Mountain National Park. In Ontario, Elora and Elmira are also places of interest. The countryside in this region is lovely! These are only a few places that she can suggest.

Cecile would tell young people to explore the outdoors in every avenue of life—hunting, fishing, curling, skating, and all types of sports—and to enjoy the beauties of Canada. She feels that there is too much reliance on our computers for information that libraries are being neglected by many people for reading and research.

For those interested in teaching as a career, Cecile would recommend that they do enter the teaching profession and become involved with various kinds of more constructive activities.

She does not consider that she has any favourites as great Canadians. Some have performed well for our country and some have performed badly.

We really do not know what we have until we lose it. The most important things in life one cannot buy. Be careful with our resources, as you cannot buy them back. Look for the good aspects in life—not the bad aspects. Life is what you make it—this is a system for guiding you in life.

Cecile and her husband Tom have a lovely family of three daughters, six grandchildren—three girls and three boys—and five great-grandchildren.

14
Duane Duff

Tossing a ringer is the desired goal of any horseshoe player. However, on one occasion, it was not.

When he was in grade eight, the boys played horseshoes at the side of the school. There were two girls who did not want to play, but tried to disrupt the boys in their activities. Their contribution was to pull out one or both of the pegs. After their being successful a few times, the boys decided to stop the girls.

Now, as two pairs were throwing horseshoes on the only pitch, the two boys sitting out would fend off the girls. It was the turn of Duane and his partner to be guards for the boys who were playing. They held the girls against the nearby wall of the school.

Suddenly, he was knocked backwards with his head hitting the ground a few inches in front of the post. The thrown horseshoe was on its way! It scored a direct hit on his face. Blood appeared from a cut in his left eyebrow. Anxiously, the other boys escorted him to the washroom where one boy donated his coloured handkerchief to help stop the bleeding. Another boy ran for the principal.

On his arrival, the principal removed the handkerchief, took his injured student to the staffroom-library, and had him lie on the chesterfield. He washed out the wound with a white cloth that had been soaked in alcohol. How that stung! He left the student there for the rest of the afternoon. When class resumed, Duane could hear the principal scolding the girls. At the end of the day, he walked the mile (1.6 km) home by himself. His parents could not take him to a doctor. For many years, there was a small scar in his eyebrow, so close to the eye.

Duane was born near Corinth, Ont., about 15 miles (24 km) north of Lake Erie. He obtained his grades one to eight at the two-room Corinth Public School. For grades nine to twelve, he went to Brownsville Continuation School, in the community of Brownsville, three miles (5 km) north of Corinth. He attended Aylmer High School, in the nearby town of Aylmer, for grade thirteen.

He holds a Bachelor of Education degree from University of Alberta, including courses toward that degree from the Universities of Saskatchewan, Calgary, British Columbia, and Washington. He also holds a Diploma in Advanced Accounting from La Salle Extension University.

He remembers the two evenings of the class presentations at Normal School, one for our teachers to grade, and one for teachers of Winnipeg. He did not have the skills to be a director, a writer, a singer, a backdrop artist, a clothes designer, a dancer, or an actor. What was left for him to do? Since Class C was presenting a story of an African-American slave uprising on a Kentucky cotton plantation, lighting was an important factor. Thus, Duane was given the responsibility of manipulating the lighting from a huge panel of switches on the wall at the side of the stage. He performed his duty successfully—and really enjoyed it. The whole class performed admirably. In fact, all of the classes performed magnificently during both evenings.

Although something positive can be said about all the teachers, it is Mr. Chidley, one of two mathematics teachers, who stood out. He taught in a subject area that Duane liked. He had a quiet, friendly air when speaking with his students. This teacher was his overseer during practice teaching and arranged for him to observe and teach in two schools—one upper elementary and one junior high.

His career took him to three Canadian provinces and one U.S. state. He taught at Holmfield, as a permit teacher; and a teacher at Langruth; Minnedosa; Harlowe, Ont., also principal; Union, Ont., also principal; Caroline, Alta.; Condor, Alta.; Vauxhall, Alta.; and Atherton, Mo., a private school.

At Dallas, Tex., he was a volunteer tour guide for school classes and the outreach coordinator at a railroad museum, taking a presentation to children in schools and public libraries. For twenty-four years in Alberta, he was a school librarian. As a member of the School Library Council, he was provincial treasurer for two years, and president of the Central Alberta and Southern Alberta Regional Councils. For a broader account of his memories of his schools as a student and as a teacher, visit http://www.innvista.com/society/education/schools.

Field trips can be so much fun—at times. When he was at David Thompson High School, Duane and a student teacher were assigned to accompany the grades seven and eight students on two consecutive Saturdays, one grade each day, late in the school year to Edmonton, Alta. It was a 6:00 a.m. start each day from their school, located beside the highway between Red Deer and Rocky Mountain House, Alta. The visits were to Edmonton International Airport, Queen Elizabeth Planetarium, the Legislative Building, and Al Oeming's Game Farm. The first trip proceeded well all the way. They arrived back at the school after supper, which they had at the Juniper Lodge Restaurant, along the new freeway near Lacombe.

The second trip proceeded well until the bus was about forty miles (64 km) south of Edmonton on this freeway on the way back to the school. Then, the driver sensed a problem on a wheel. He stopped the bus, checked the wheels, but could find nothing amiss. Shortly after resuming the trip, a tire blew. The driver had difficulty in holding the bus from swerving or upsetting, but he was successful in bringing the vehicle to a safe stop. He then tried to remove the wheel to replace it with another. However, the lug nuts were so tight that they would not budge. There was now a problem.

The accompanying car had gone ahead to the Juniper Lodge Restaurant where all were going to stop for supper. That was another thirty miles (48 km) farther from this spot. A pickup truck from Alaska stopped and offered to take Duane to the restaurant. When he arrived, he phoned his wife Pamela to alert parents who would be waiting at the school. Then, he phoned a service station in the nearby town of Lacombe. The person who answered suggested it might be better if Duane contact a repair shop in the town of Ponoka, which was closer to where the bus was. His colleague then drove him there.

A repairman accompanied them in his tow truck to the site of the breakdown. Since the bus had a flat front, the repairman did not want to tow the bus for fear that the winch would break through the windshield. Therefore, after having the bus removed from the road, he took the wheel and the bus driver back to his shop to make repairs. Again, everyone waited patiently. Eventually, they returned and placed the wheel back onto the bus, which now could be driven back to the school.

Although the group did not see a police car, they later learned that the police knew about the bus, as they received some anxious telephone calls. The bus arrived back at the school at 2:00 a.m. the next morning. It had been a long day!

Duane left the teaching profession briefly in 1953, spending about four months in the Royal Canadian Navy in Toronto, Ont.; Cornwallis, N.S.; and Halifax, N.S. His short term was the result of a medical discharge.

As a child, one of his favourite books was *Hoot Owl*, by Mabel Guinnip La Rue. In about 2003, he was able to obtain a copy of the book on interlibrary loan from Wayne State College, in Wayne, Neb., and to read it again.

For having been a school librarian and having volunteered in school and public libraries after retiring, he was not an avid reader. He did enjoy reading books about railroad history and had a collection of about eighty books.

When his family lived in Vauxhall, Alta., he served as treasurer of his church's district and of the local agricultural society. He was on the board of the community library and was chairman for two years. He also chaired the local police advisory committee and served as a board member with the farmers' market. In Dallas, Tex., he was on the board of the Southwest Railroad Historical Society. In Surrey, B.C., he has been a volunteer for a Canada Revenue Agency programme working on tax returns for low income persons and also has served as treasurer for the Green Timbers Heritage Society.

The most impressive trip that he took was in 2000 when he and his wife Pam transported his collection of Bible versions—which he donated to Tyndale House Library—to Cambridge, England. While in this college city, they visited nine of over seventy college libraries and one public library branch. They were given an apartment for two weeks as well as guided tours of the huge Cambridge University main library, the British Bible

Society library, the new Jesus College library, and the King's College library. Duane took time to do some research in four libraries for his website. It was a thrill to their eyes to see original works by A. A. Milne and Sir Isaac Newton, books dating back as far as 800 C.E., and the largest Bible known.

In of nearby town of Ely, they participated in a tour of a huge cathedral whose construction commenced in 1083, a stop at a local tea house, and a quick tour of the former home of Oliver Cromwell. For anyone interested in British history, old and new books, Bibles, Old World architecture, and left-side driving on the highway in a beautiful countryside, this is a paradise.

His philosophy of life is to be honest and fair in all your dealings with others. Develop a personal spirituality —which is rarely the same as being religious.

Prepare yourselves well for the vocation of your choice, and then work at it to the best of your ability. Do not expect that it will be without difficulty from time to time. Be honest in all that you do. Consider the rights of others. Make healthy choices about the food and drink that you consume. Exercise sufficiently. Continue learning for the rest of your life. This would be his advice to a teenager about life in general.

If you like working with children and are willing to put effort into preparation and teaching, by all means follow the profession of teaching. If you are an impatient person and your sole purpose is obtaining a pay cheque, choose something else. The profession can be very frustrating or very rewarding, depending upon you and the environment around you. This would be his advice to anyone considering teaching as a career.

Miss Kirk was one of Duane's teachers in grades nine to twelve and principal for the last three of those years. Early in his grade ten year, Duane became ill with rheumatic fever for most of the autumn. Miss Kirk encouraged him to return to school as soon as he was well enough to do so. When the winter snow and road blockage appeared in January, Duane gave up hope of returning for that school year. However, his principal had not. She finally prevailed upon him to return immediately after Easter. She and her assistant teacher, Miss Van Luven, set up classes so that he could salvage his year. Latin and agriculture were dropped until the next year. He passed his grade.

In grade eleven, he picked up those subjects and carried the regular grade eleven agriculture course. He completed grade twelve Latin when he was in grade thirteen. When he developed ulcers in grade eleven, Miss Kirk was most cooperative. Immediately after his Normal School year, he had to make a quick trip back to Ontario. Miss Kirk lent him the money for train fare. Even many years after, she would ask his mother how he was doing. From her concern for him, he has ever since had a respect for the plight of students, not only for those with medical concerns, but also for the others, including those who gave him difficulty.

Mr. Halpenny, the principal who left administration after many years for a classroom position, taught algebra, analytical geometry, and trigonometry and statics in grade thirteen. Duane liked mathematics and usually did quite well in these three subjects. Mr. Halpenny helped Duane set up his schedule as he had just transferred to Aylmer High School. After Duane went to Manitoba to teach, he followed his teacher's methods in mathematics classes. They were in contact in person or by letter with each other for a few years after Duane's graduation from high school.

A Canadian leader who has contributed both in Canada and abroad is Lieutenant-General Roméo

Dallaire, a senator. In 1994, he commanded the United Nations Assistance Mission for Rwanda. Since his retirement from the military, Senator Dallaire has worked to bring an understanding of post-traumatic stress disorder to the general public. He is a member of the Senate Standing Committee on Human Rights and the Senate Standing Committee on Aboriginal Peoples. He has been outspoken in his stand on the genocide which took place in Rwanda and how more could have been done at the time and since.

Having been in Victoria, on the west coast, and Halifax, on the east coast, and points in between, but regrettably not in the far north, Duane can name a number of beautiful places to visit. However, for someone who enjoys the beauty of maple trees with their leaves of red, green, and yellow, a tour of southern Ontario in the early autumn is highly recommended.

Before moving to Surrey, B.C., Duane and his family had the opportunity of living in Mexico for just over five years, most of which was in the southern state of Chiapas. This is highland Mayan country with two seasons—wet and dry. During wet season, there would be a raging mountain stream a few feet from their house each afternoon. Because of an improper outlet, their street would be a river for a while. By the next morning, there would be a dry creek bed. Leaves would fall from the trees in late February, during the dry season.

On one occasion, Duane had a medical appointment in Tuxtla Gutiérrez, the state capital, fifty miles (80 km) from San Cristóbal, where the family lived. For the first thirty miles (60 km), the highway has 365 curves—one for each day of the year—and dropped in elevation from about 7,200 ft (2,195 m) to about 1,800 ft. (550 m). As the bus was fifteen minutes late in leaving San Cristóbal, the driver wanted to make up time.

Duane's tendency to acquire motion sickness soon took hold. He staggered to the washroom at the back of the zigzagging bus and promptly lost his breakfast. Since toilet tissue is not issued in public places and vehicles, he left the cleanup job to the company. On leaving the washroom, he promptly plopped into the lap of a passenger as the driver negotiated another turn. He managed to return to his seat where he and Pam, who also was feeling the effects, fought to survive for the rest of the ordeal. It was a relief to leave that bus! Incidentally, the bus arrived on time.

The Duff family became friends of a missionary couple working for the Presbyterian Church. They attended church services with them, even though they could not understand the native language. Duane sometimes accompanied the husband when the latter's wife could not go. One feature was that women sat on one side of the church, and the men on the other. They were always treated well by Mayan people.

The people of each village had their own distinctive colour design for their clothes. Despite the media reports about the Zapatista atrocities, the family felt safer there than in such American cities as Kansas City, Mo., and Dallas, Tex., where they also had lived. From their living in Mexico, they learned to appreciate anything that they have, particularly water, and to take nothing for granted.

One afternoon in October 2007, as Duane was walking home to the apartment in Surrey, B.C., he noticed that police were blocking the street in front of the property. On turning off the sidewalk to go to the apartment complex, he saw police cars in the driveway and police speaking with the managers. On leaving the complex later to walk his wife Pam home from work, he was blocked by a police ribbon and had to take an alternate route. There was a police presence for many days. Twice a detective came to their apartment, and to other apartments, to find out if he could obtain any information. The underground parking and garbage room were closed for nearly two weeks while the investigation took place.

There had been a multiple homicide with four young men shot intentionally and two others because they were in the wrong place at the wrong time. Duane and Pam had lived in that tower for six years and were at the time living in the nearby court. News of the event spread across Canada and even into the United States. The guilty men were apprehended and charged in April 2009.

While he and his family lived in Texas and in Mexico, he built up a collection of about ninety versions of the Bible in English and about twenty in several other languages. These were donated to a Bible research library in Cambridge, England. Then, along with other family members, he built a website of about 4,100 pages on various subject areas, http://www.innvista.com. Following that, his interest turned to writing books, mainly about the experiences of people, which he now does. This pastime also keeps his son Sean busy in formatting and publishing. With all these activities, Duane lives the notion that a teacher never really retires.

15
Virginia (Eilers) Lyons

One evening, a few Normalite girls planned on going off-campus to experience a change from studies and dormitory life. One of them decided to take a bath first. Her room was only two doors away from the bathroom—a little too far on this occasion. On arrival, she decided to turn on the tap so that the water could fill the tub while she would return to her room to bring her slippers. That seemed simple enough—even though risky.

However, what should have been a few seconds turned into minutes. Distractions tend to happen at the most inopportune times, this being one of those unexpected times. What was that noise? Why was there water flooding the hallway? Suddenly, she remembered! She rushed to turn off the tap. Then, the cleanup job began, thus ending the night out. There were some unhappy girls and one very unpopular one in that dormitory as a result.

Virginia was born in Tilston, and started her education in that community. Prior to attending Normal School, she was a permit teacher at Mayville School, near Scarth.

As a child, one of her most memorable thrills came when she saw King George VI and Queen Elizabeth when they toured Canada in 1939, even if it were for only a moment. When the train stopped briefly in Elkhorn, the royal couple appeared before the cheering crowd of citizens to give them a brief wave. Little Virginia and her family had travelled from their home in Tilston to Elkhorn by motorcar, quite an undertaking in those days.

A teacher whom Virginia especially remembers is Miss Edith Moody, who taught her grade twelve English. This teacher had a special way of making her students listen and understand. Although she rarely smiled, her students knew that she cared about their achieving to the best of their abilities.

An embarrassing incident occurred in her grade twelve year. Virginia had been permit teaching the year before, after grade eleven. It was a spare period for her and her friends, and they were chasing each other in the room instead of quietly studying. Little did the girls realize that Miss Moody was in the adjacent room until she appeared in the doorway and firmly said, "Virginia—you are an ex-teacher!" That was enough to turn Virginia's face red and for her to sit down quickly.

The teacher at Normal School whom she remembers most was Miss Pilling, who taught art. Virginia loved participating in art work, but her roommates did not like it at all. As a result, she would create the drawings and they would pass them in as their own—a supposedly innocent act. In one class, Miss Pilling held up a piece of art work; and, after giving the class a scolding, she said to her students, "Why can't you do something creative like this?" Virginia realized that the work was one of her own art pieces which one of her roommates had handed in. Afterwards, the girls had a hearty laugh about that.

Following her year at Normal School, she taught at the school in Arrow River for two years. From there, she moved to Virden Junior High School, in Virden, where she spent thirteen years. Then, she taught in Opasquia

School, at The Pas, for nine years. During the course of her career, she obtained a Bachelor of General Studies degree.

What stands out in her teaching years as one of the most stressful was a certain day when she was supervising lunch hour in the junior high school at Virden. All of the students were seated in the long hallway and her responsibility was to make sure everything progressed without incident. Suddenly, a young boy rose and ran to the washroom! Another student yelled, "He's choking!"

Virginia raced to bring help. Would someone arrive in time? The boy was turning blue as the principal carried him to a car to take him to the hospital. Realizing that he could not arrive in time, he quickly grabbed the child, bent him over, and slapped him on the back. Out popped a huge piece of cheese sandwich—just in time. The boy did go to the hospital, but he was dismissed a little later. What a stressful day it had been!

Although Virginia confesses that she is not an avid reader of books, she is a reader of short stories and newspapers.

She has turned her hobby of sewing into a full-time local business. She does custom sewing for weddings and other events; and also almost all types of repairs, alterations, mending, and making various types of clothes.

In her community activities, she has been a faithful volunteer for forty years with the Catholic Women's League. Her main involvement was helping to cater to all types of dinners. With the money which the League earned, they aided the crisis centre, the needy, unwed mothers, and many other worthy causes.

A memorable trip that she took was to Disney World, in Orlando, Fla., travelling there by automobile. During the tour, she met numerous very interesting people.

For tourists in Canada, she suggests that they visit the Maritime Provinces in early fall. The colours are beautiful.

She would tell young people always to think highly of themselves and always do the right thing in any situation. They should try to discover the good in everyone whom they meet and never do anything to hurt others.

For those considering the teaching profession as a career, she would tell them to "go for it". They should be sure that they care for their fellow man. It is a wonderful profession and one that can be very rewarding.

Virginia's philosophy of life is to do unto others as you would have them do unto you.

16
Jacob Enns

What a racket the loud, blaring amplifiers made! Welcome to Kingston, Jamaica! Jake (as Jacob is commonly known) and his colleagues from Canada were beginning their first day of a week-long mission in this Caribbean city. Their task was building a new facility for Youth for Christ.

This was their first trip—a working trip—to Jamaica. Jake knew a little bit of the history and, of course, was most interested in seeing the country and the people. Kingston is a city with quite a diversity of people. As in many places, there are the very wealthy and the very poor. As a rule, they found the people friendly, but they were warned that there are some very rough parts in that city. Those places were gladly avoided. The market places were in open air. One feature was that the meat for sale was displayed so that flies were busy marinating the food. It certainly did not appeal to the tastes of the group.

Some of the local men were also involved in the building project. Jake is not sure if they were paid or were volunteers. He feels that Jamaicans are very laid back and never very quick on their feet. Their favourite expression was "no problem", one which was very quickly adopted by the Canadians.

The volunteers who had come from Canada had taken several days away for a little break. During that time, the local men who were involved had kept working and were very proud of their achievements, even though they had not accomplished much

The Canadians attended a church service in which the majority of the congregation was black. They were impressed with how charismatic the people were. They did have mixed feelings about their trip and their involvement, but they were happy for the learning experience. Culture shock is a good educator!

Jake was born about eight miles (13 km) from Carnduff, Sask., a community near the Manitoba border to the east and the North Dakota border to the south. His parents named him Jacob, but many people know him as Jake. The name Jake even occurs on some of his documents, for example, his driver's permit.

He began his education at Webster School, in a rural setting approximately seven miles (11 km) southwest of Fannystelle, a community not far from Winnipeg. After high school, he was able to obtain a Bachelor of Arts degree and a Bachelor of Education degree at University of Manitoba.

The first language which he learned was German, both Low and High German. However, he would call English his main language at the present time, although he still can speak German quite well.

Jake has for many years served in various positions in the church where he is a member. He taught Sunday school for a number of years, served in the church council board, and has been involved with the leadership in a senior group. These were all voluntary positions.

Jake has been involved in the teaching profession for thirty-seven years. He taught in rural schools for three years, in a town school for two years, and in a private

Mennonite school for four years. For some of the years in which he taught, his students were classified as slow learners. At the time, various techniques were tried and tested. Junior High was the area in which he was involved for most of his teaching career.

He began teaching after taking the short summer course immediately following graduation from high school. Teachers who did as Jake did were known as Permit teachers and were allowed to teach for one year at an annual salary of $1,100. Jake's assignment was at Herriott School, not far from the village of Waldersee, north of Gladstone.

He decided to attend Normal School the following year. For the two years after graduating from there, he taught in a rural school, Prefontaine School, just south of Iles des Chenes, which is adjacent to Winnipeg. In 1953, he joined the staff in Gretna Public School, a border town south of Winnipeg, to teach grades six, seven, and eight.

Then, he moved to Mennonite Brethren Collegiate Institute, in Winnipeg, where he was assigned to initiate the grades seven and eight programme. After four years which he considers to have been the hardest in his teaching career, he applied for a position with the Winnipeg School Division. He taught at Hugh John Macdonald Junior High School for fifteen years. The principal devised a number of innovative programmes to cope with students who were not achieving the desired results. From that school, he was transferred to Cecil Rhodes School, where he ended his teaching career after thirteen years—eight in junior high and five in elementary grades. He says that he enjoyed his last five years best.

In September 2007, Jake and his wife Nettie visited Turkey. For them, this was a very enlightening experience. Travelling by bus, they toured many places where there were excavations from almost 2,000 years ago when the Romans ruled the country. They explored along the routes of the journeys of the Apostle Paul and visited the seven churches to which the Apostle John wrote in the book of Revelations.

One of the most interesting places was Cappadocia, a community where people in past times had constructed homes in the face of the rocks. Here they tried to find refuge in times of war and persecution. The underground cities with many rooms and passageways also were hiding places during such times.

Turkey is a beautiful and rich country. Even though Jake and Nettie found the journey very tiresome at times, especially because the heat was often almost unbearable, they did enjoy it very much.

As a hobby, Jake enjoys taking pictures. He feels that he is not a very good photographer and needs to learn how to take better photos. Nevertheless, he always finds that pictures bring back memories. Both Jake and Nettie enjoy golfing. It affords some exercise, and they find that they are able to enjoy each other's company and also have friends join them for a round. He also enjoys walking, an activity which he hopes to continue for a long time to come.

Memorable experiences in his life's work have been in connection with people whom he came to know in the course of his activities as a teacher. When he accepted the position of a grade five teacher after teaching grades seven, eight, and nine for so many years, he found it a challenge to orient himself to younger students and different subject material. Fortunately, becausc of the graciousness of fellow teachers, he was able to receive much valuable assistance. The entire staff in the elementary school worked together, thus creating a friendly and understanding rapport among the teachers.

He feels certain that there might be other experiences that he could mention.

In considering where he could have been more successful, he states that he has often regretted the fact that his relationship with students was not as pleasant as he would have wanted it to be. His main goal always was to keep order in the classroom, and he fears that his strictness very often hampered any positive relationships that could have been developed. There probably are numerous other retired teachers who can recall similar feelings.

As he grew up, Jake was taught to do the best that he could and to retain a healthy conscience, which meant being honest and kind and treating others fairly. His parental home was Christian, which meant that the Bible was read and regarded as the Word of God.

His philosophy of life is closely related to his relationship with God. In the New Testament of the Bible, Jesus said, "I am the Way, the Truth, and the Life; no man comes to the Father but by me." Jake has committed his life to Jesus; and, as a result, the way in which he lives should reflect that he believes what He has said. Jake is a follower of Jesus. God should come first. As a result, his home, his conduct, and his vocation must reflect the faith that he has.

Although many experiences have faded from his memory of his Normal School year, he does remember some. One in particular was that he and Duane Duff lived in Frontenac Hall. As he looks back at that, he thinks that place was like a refuge for him. He realized that fact when he heard about all the upheavals that went on in some of the other boys' dormitories. Here, he was close to the classrooms and to the dining hall.

He also worked in the dining room or kitchen for a while, but he has few memories about that experience. He also remembers when one of the fellows from across the hall brought a garter snake from home after spending a weekend there. It slithered into his room in the evening. Jake, for one, did not know what to make of it. He does not remember what eventually happened to that little reptile.

He recalls that they slept in bunk beds, with him on the bottom bunk and Duane on the top bunk. He regrets that they did not know each other better at the time. Neither one was really outgoing. They did not learn about each other's backgrounds or of their future hopes.

Another memory he has is of the chapel where we met every morning. At one of the reunions, probably in 1996, as part of the get-together, those who attended met at the school—which was then the School for the Deaf—and sat in the chapel for a meeting. It appeared much smaller to all in attendance than when we attended there many years earlier.

However, the memory that has remained with Jake is the Christmas programme that was put on. He was chosen to be one of the kings who visited the Child in the Manger. Each of the Wise Men from the East came down the aisle and sang one of the stanzas of the carol "We Three Kings".

Of the teachers who instructed us, he recalls Mr. Clarke, whose subject was classroom management, especially when it came to completing the registers in the rural schools in June. Jake could have wished the job on him. He did use some of the songs that Miss Douglas taught her students.

However, the person from whom he learned most was Miss Smith, who taught grammar, including how to parse sentences. He believes that he may have forgotten most of that by now. Nevertheless, he really did love what Miss Smith taught. He had not known any of the grammar structure before he was in that class. He found that Normal School was really a year of fun, as was the summer school at Gimli, another requirement for certification. It was a fairly easy way to earn a teacher's certificate.

Jake honestly can say that there was not any one person who stands out for having had a very positive effect on his work. He must give credit to quite a few of his colleagues who have been good examples for him. They taught him to be more patient, understanding, and helpful. It has been his privilege to hear many good lectures, which have been excellent in theory, but difficult to put into practice. He has had the good fortune of knowing a number of people whose lives have been a tremendous example to him.

Currently Jake and Nettie live in an apartment suite located in North Kildonan, in the northeastern part of Winnipeg. They enjoy living there as they are very comfortable.

17

Helen (Finlay) Morrow

What a cold and lonely winter it was in that little one-room school on the prairie near Angusville! She was a permit teacher in her first school and faced the challenge of teaching fourteen children in seven grades—and she with so little training.

The spring, with its muddy roads, was not much better. It was so far from her family's home in Birtle—but not in miles. She boarded with a farm family who had children in her class. It was a long walk to reach the school each morning and to arrive back at the farm in the late afternoon. On arrival at school, there was no assurance that it would be warm. Sometimes, it took all morning for a fire in the woodstove to create sufficient heat so that the teacher and her students could remove their coats and mitts. It must have been difficult trying to write! When she finally was able to visit her family for a weekend after the long winter, it was necessary for her dad to transport her back to Boyle School on his tractor—which, to her, was less than dignified. At least, she was able to return to her job.

Her next position, after attending Normal School, was at Linwood School, in St. James, a suburb of Winnipeg—a much better location. This is a school that, still to this day more than fifty-five years later, appears much the same and can be viewed from the sixth floor of the condominium building where she now lives.

Helen was born in a house on a rented farm at Broomhill, in southwestern Manitoba near Melita. Her first and only elementary and high schooling were in the town of Birtle.

She feels that her mother may have been somewhat old-fashioned for the times because she had her daughters wear long stockings, even when the weather became pleasant in April or May. However, as soon as they arrived at school, they would roll their stockings down to their ankles so that the girls could be more like their town peers, who were allowed to wear short socks and have bare legs in March.

Probably, the most memorable experience for Helen occurred when she was working at Great-West Life and took a lunch hour break with a few others at the Child's Restaurant on the first day that alcoholic drinks could be served in restaurants. They ordered a martini each, not really knowing what it was other than it had an interesting name.

The late Robert Lightly influenced her when he was the school inspector during her high school days at Birtle. It always amused the students how short the teachers appeared beside his towering frame. He exerted his influence so that she could obtain a bursary to attend Normal School. When she was attending Normal School, Mr. and Mrs. Lightly used her as a baby sitter, thus providing her with some pocket money. He also encouraged her to work in the kitchen at Normal School, as many of the students did to pay their way.

At this school, Miss Smith taught English, with emphasis on grammar. That was a subject which Helen loved—and still does. She feels that she was not well taught in elementary and high school in this subject area.

She did not involve herself very much in the social aspect of Normal School. Outside interests were more important. She remembers rushing to finish her final exams in the gymnasium as the questions seemed too easy.

Helen did stay with teaching long enough—three years—to obtain her Permanent Teachers' Certificate. She has taken a number of courses; however, probably the only diploma that she earned was an Activity Workers' Diploma.

Soon after she had married, she left teaching for a wonderful clerical job at Great-West Life Assurance Company, in Winnipeg. How could one receive a salary for working in a position that was so easy and to her liking without the added burden of homework at night or class preparation? There she remained until Mother Nature called and reminded her of her purpose in life to add to the population. Therefore, she became a mother and homemaker for several years until she felt that the children were able to be without her during the day.

She had the urge to operate a car in conducting a courier business. This proved to be the ideal job for her, working diligently and being financially rewarded accordingly. After spending nine years of road running, in which she became armed with a working knowledge of city streets, she worked as a Cancer Society employee, dispatching volunteer drivers.

Reading was never a pastime for Helen. She feels that it was not stressed in her home, giving her the idea that people who were reading were not doing anything since she was raised with a strong work ethic. She does not read fiction; but rather, she enjoys self-improvement and psychology books, some biographies, and cook books.

Her hobbies are exercising—walking, line dancing, and an exercise called strength and resistance. She enjoys working Sudoku puzzles, various word puzzles excluding crosswords, and using her computer.

Helen and her husband embarked on a month-long trip to England, Scotland, and a bus tour of Europe. They took a flight to Denmark, where she met three first cousins for the first time. She was surprised to learn that the countries in Europe are so much smaller than Canada, that London restaurants have rats, that dogs are allowed into restaurants in Paris, and that wine flows freely in Venice.

Life is so precious and it goes by quickly. What appears to be old age now is not old by the time a person reaches it. She urges all young people to enjoy their youth, remember to respect others, and be aware that they do not know as much as they think that they do. There is so much to learn within their lifetime.

She would counsel everyone not to stop learning or exercising and to volunteer wherever one can—and keep interested. She laments that it is too bad that young people have to make career choices and other choices when they have had limited life experience. Although teaching was not a good choice for Helen, she admires those who choose to pursue a teaching career.

Miss McArthur was her French teacher in high school. She appreciated the fact that some were paying attention—and did well. She was so pleased when Helen scored a good grade.

Duff Roblin, when he was premier of the Manitoba, led the way in the building of "Duff's Ditch", which is the floodway to help Winnipeg avoid having another flood like the one that devastated parts of the city in 1950. For this leadership, Helen credits him as a great Canadian.

As a volunteer at Winnipeg Airport, she is constantly defending her city and her province. She would strongly recommend Manitoba as somewhere for visitors in

Canada to enjoy wonderful motor trips. There are so many places within the province that are scenic and exciting.

Currently, she is the envelope secretary for her church, a member of her Seniors' Centre, and is a member of the board of her condominium. For several years, she was a member of ITC (formerly Toastmistress), and a member of the Manitoba Association of Parliamentarians.

She lives each day as it comes, paying little attention to weather forecasting and trying not to worry since that is a waste of time and effort.

18

Betty (Forsyth) Sumner

Of what do you think first when someone says soup and spelling? Your first impulse may be to say, "Alphabet soup." However, that would not apply in a certain rural Manitoba school in the late 1930s. Picture a high pot-bellied stove at the front of the classroom. Place a large kettle on top of the stove. Set a chair beside the stove. Then, have the teacher stand on the chair.

Now, place into one hand of the teacher a large spoon, and have her stirring the contents of the kettle—whether it be soup or beans that a mother had sent to school for the teacher to prepare for everyone's hot lunch. Place into the teacher's other hand a speller and have her dictate words for her students to write correctly in their notebooks. If, at any time during the day, the fire should begin to wane, there would be a time-out for the teacher or a student to toss into the stove a chunk of wood or use a long poker to stir the burning fuel.

This was a common sight of the day here, but which would be highly unlikely in today's modern schools. Such a unique way it was for a teacher to carry out two functions in the classroom at one time!

Betty was born in Virden. She attended a one-room rural school in obtaining her grades one to nine. Then, she went to Virden for her high school education.

Normal School was a happy year when a group of high school kids "grew up" to become ambitious teachers ready to take on the world.

She felt that Mr. Lightly really enjoyed his teaching and had a keen interest in local history. He expressed an interest in Betty's local history one day when she showed him that she knew the background history of her grandparents. He had a personable way with students and made each feel important. Specifically, she discovered that he was an excellent listener to her concerns about her inadequacies.

After receiving her teaching certificate through attending Normal School, she upgraded her qualifications over the years by summer schools and evening classes.

She commenced her career as a classroom teacher in Millan School, a rural one-room school located north of the town of Souris. After two years, she moved to the primary room in Oakwood School, in Oak Lake, and then into Brandon.

Millan School was relatively modern for that day, having indoor washrooms, a piano, and good electrical lighting. The sports equipment included a softball, a bat, and a skipping rope. However, there were no telephone, no radio, and no record player. Since there was no well, parents brought water to school each day. The school was heated by a furnace that used wood or coal and had to be stoked by the teacher during the day.

About half of the children travelled to and from school by horseback or horse-drawn carts. Thus, there was a barn to shelter the animals through the day. At noon, the children tended to the needs of their horses.

The children often played soccer in the yard, using logs of wood as goal posts. One day, a boy fell onto one of them and severely cut his head. There was no telephone in the school and the little first-aid kit was useless.

What could Betty do to help her student? She grabbed some tea towels and wrapped the boy's head with them. There was a handy supply of the towels since the school was also used as a community centre. Then, she gently placed the boy into her arms and, as quickly as her legs could travel, carried the boy to the nearest farmhouse, where she received help. Quick thinking and action on her part probably saved the boy from a more serious situation.

Mr. Heapy, who was the first principal under whom Betty taught, had been principal of Oakwood School for twenty-one years. He had a positive influence on her method of teaching as she observed his skill in handing children and in organizing the activities of the school.

Her only other profession was motherhood! She enjoyed a wonderful maternity leave for thirteen years as Betty and her husband raised their three children. When the youngest entered school, Betty returned to the classroom. Then for seventeen happy years, she was the kindergarten teacher in Valleyview School, in Brandon.

There were not many books available when she was a child, as this was the depression years of the 1930s. However, she did read *Heidi*, by Johanna Spyri, many times. Recently, she has read *The Last Lecture*, by Randy Pausch. It is a gripping book, one that makes an imprint on its readers. Within its pages, she has found good advice for living and recommends it as containing sound counsel for all ages.

She and her husband are not travellers; but, as avid curlers, they took a trip to a world curling event in Oberstdorf, a ski resort town in southern Germany. They enjoyed the event and loved that part of the country.

Betty is one of a group of senior ladies of her community who enjoy curling. The quality of curling may not be high, but that of the socializing over coffee after their games have been completed is. Despite the extent of her curling, she has claimed no trophies. However, it provides much fun and exercise. Besides that, it helps to pass the cold Manitoba winters.

In addition to being involved with curling, she volunteers for causes which she deems to be useful. These include Save the Children organization, her church, Habitat for Humanity, the YMCA, and Street Love. One of the programmes carried out by Street Love is the knitting of mitts for local less fortunate citizens.

Every Wednesday afternoon, she joins a seniors' group for oil painting. Her many pictures are packed neatly in a cupboard under the stairs. She muses that they will be recognized as masterpieces in about five hundred years, but she really holds no expectations about their potential value. Is she unaware that many treasures have been discovered packed away in attics or other storage places?

Betty would recommend a visit to Riding Mountain National Park, north of Brandon. Within it is a gorgeous, pristine lake called Clear Lake, which is pollution-free. Near it is a lovely resort area. For those who enjoy bird and animal watching and walking on trails, the park is an ideal place. Since this is a national park, the wildlife is protected. It is an oasis on the prairie, having been formed by glacial action.

To those who consider entering the teaching profession, she has this advice: "Be patient, kind, and genuinely interested in the potential of each and every child. In a very short time, the children will be the adults in our society and you will be richer for having had them touch your life."

For her philosophy of life, she has felt that honesty, loyalty, and her faith have been very important in guiding her.

19
Abe Friesen

Beekeeping can be fascinating—or dangerous—or a bit of both. Those who love it will take the danger risk in stride. For many people, a sting is an annoyance; but, for others, it can be life-threatening.

One day, some bees did not like the presence of a certain beekeeper, and promptly attacked him with a vengeance. This precipitated a hasty trip to the local hospital. As he mounted the steps of this sanctuary for the sick, he began to wonder if he would ever reach the door. He did—and the reception desk, too.

On realizing the extent of the attack, the staff hurriedly placed the man into a wheel chair and rushed him into the presence of the closest doctor. Using the patient's arm like a pincushion, the medical practitioner administered an antidote to the bee venom. Then came the task of withdrawing the abandoned stingers. When the ordeal had subsided, the doctor calmly said to his patient, "You could have died."

That was an understatement for the patient who had realized that sentiment as he approached the door of the hospital. Would he continue his career after surviving this near-death experience? Yes, he would—and he did!

Abe was born in Plum Coulee and started school at Stuartburn.

When he was in grade six, a few older boys egged on a smaller boy to pick a fight with him. Not being willing to be pummelled, he defended himself. That encouraged the instigators as they wanted to see a fight.

Suddenly, the teacher appeared from the rear, passed judgement on the event, and laid the strap to Abe. This was his only experience in being punished in this way. He could never figure why the teacher did not investigate and did not strap the other boy. Abe could see no evidence of justice being administered. To this day, he cannot reconcile the action of that teacher.

Eventually, when he was in grade eight, he found a teacher whom he could call a favourite. Vernon Toews was so friendly compared to his previous teachers.

Abe found Normal School to be “a ball”. However, since he had no background in grammar, the class taught by Miss Smith was quite difficult; but other courses were “a snap”. He did not like attending physical education classes, but he managed to survive them. He liked most of the teachers, but seemed to have a very good rapport with Mr. Clarke, our classroom management teacher.

After graduating from Normal School, he also obtained Bachelor degrees in Arts and Education. He taught in Manitoba in Winnipeg, Vita, and Riverton—being principal in the last place. He also spent two years teaching in Australia.

In the first year on the southern continent, it was a semi-rural school in the State of Victoria, one which Abe felt was poorly administered. There were some very good teachers on the staff, but there were others who should not have been allowed into the profession.

In the second year, he taught in a city school in Brisbane, Queensland, one which was strictly run. Among the students were some who had great ability and showed signs of a successful future, while there were others who would not benefit from the available education. In fact, there was a group of girls who were highly antagonistic to the educational system. The facilities in rural areas were not as good as he had seen in similar areas in Manitoba. However, they were very good in Brisbane.

Abe took the long and slow way home from Australia. After a visit in Kathmandu, the capital of Nepal, he travelled to London, England, by bus, passing through numerous countries that would have been closed to his travel at other times. It was an enjoyable journey, although sickness was a problem when travelling through India and Pakistan. Throughout the trip, he had problems with the food.

When he was a child, Abe read any kind of book that was available. He read so much in school because he was bored in his classes, a practice which sometimes placed him into trouble. In grade five, he was reading books by Charles Dickens and other classical authors. However, he had no particular favourite which stood out. Recently, Abe read *John A.: The Man Who Made Us*, by Richard Gwyn, and thoroughly enjoyed it.

His nomination for a great leader of Canada would be John A. Macdonald. Abe takes the view that Canada would be American today without this man's efforts. It was during his two terms in office that the construction of the Canadian Pacific Railway was commenced and completed in order to prevent that from happening.

As a hobby, he likes to do all types of woodworking and does whatever needs to be done, including furniture. He has had good teaching and experience all his life because his dad was a carpenter by trade. Abe took on the task of doing the finish work on a house which he had framed in Steinbach. The installation of the electrical and plumbing facilities was accomplished by licenced personnel. His dad helped in whatever way he could, including the building of the kitchen cabinets.

In 1993, Abe organized in Halbstadt a reunion of his branch of the Friesen family. More than 300 people attended. In 1994, he produced a Friesen family book with stories and photos of the many descendants of Peter Friesen and Mary Rempel, who emigrated to Canada in 1875.

For visitors coming to Canada, there are so many fascinating places with no one place really better than another. However, for those who do not like cold weather and who are visiting in the winter, he would suggest Vancouver Island, which normally has mild winters. He mentions Halifax as a place that has much history. Personally, he, who grew up in Manitoba, enjoyed being in Victoria and missing the cold weather of winter.

He urges teenagers to go to school and acquire an education.

For those anticipating a teaching career, he would advise them to prepare well and to obtain as much education as possible. Even after becoming teachers, they should continue to read and to improve their qualifications. It is also necessary to have the skill of being a good disciplinarian. If these standards cannot be met, there is likely to be little fun in teaching.

Abe's philosophy of life is to do the best that one can in all endeavours.

20
Peggy (Friesen) Lawrence

A memorable—and highly successful—experience was in teaching her class of thirty-five to thirty-eight pupils, whose ages ranged from seven to nine, to learn to read by abandoning the authorized *Dick and Jane* readers. Instead, she used the children's own stories, which she printed on chart paper, as the reading lesson material.

By using this language experience approach, the youngsters, who lived in the most deprived area of Winnipeg, could learn to decode the strange squiggles that are used in the printed English language without having to struggle with such totally unfamiliar concepts as living on "Pleasant Street" or "Daddy going to work wearing a suit and carrying a briefcase". How observant and ingenious this teacher was in meeting the reading needs of these young children within their own understanding!

The eight staff members supplied food and collected clothing from schools in affluent areas for distribution to the pupils of this inner city school, as needed. Peggy is certain that she taught one frail little boy how to read by giving him a spoonful of cod liver oil each school day. She also hugged her pupils whenever appropriate. How times have changed! Teaching included basic needs, not simply a subject skill.

Peggy was born in Horndean in the middle of a January blizzard. Dr. C. W. Wiebe—who lived to be 106 years old—travelled the eleven miles (18 km) from Winkler to the family's rented home, which was located right beside the railway tracks in Horndean. He started off in a car, then changed to a horse and sleigh, and then travelled the last few miles on a hand-powered railway jigger! A storm was not going to stop him. After assisting in the baby's birth, the fourth of five healthy children all born at home, the doctor spent the night on the living room couch!

Before Normal School, Peggy attended classes in Horndean in a three-room school where her dad was the principal for seventeen years. She continued in Ottawa, Ont., where the family lived for two years during World War II so that her dad could work as a censor of German POW mail, and the family could have the experience of living in a city. After the war was over, the family returned to their home in Horndean.

Mr. Victor Peters was her grades nine, ten, and eleven teacher of all subjects in the Horndean High School of seventeen pupils. He made learning come alive with tales of his life. He made his students feel valued as worthwhile people—and they sang every morning! He and his wife, Elizabeth Peters, brought their own classical records to school and all stayed after classes and received the gift of a lifetime, the appreciation of music from these two loving teachers.

She recalls a Horndean school trip to Winnipeg in which all the pupils, ages fourteen to sixteen, *stood* in the back of a ten-ton truck for the whole two-hour trip, each way. They visited the Canada Packers Meat Packing Plant, where they witnessed cattle being slaughtered and cut up. Afterwards, when they visited Christies Biscuits, the guide gave the students sample cookies to eat. Next, they drove past the Legislative Building and on to the zoo.

Peggy completed her high school education in Winkler, where she boarded with the Bueckert family so that she could take her grade twelve. After graduating from Normal School, she attended evening classes whenever possible at the University of Manitoba and University of Winnipeg.

What a fabulous year it was at Normal School! She enjoyed living in 306 Rupert Hall with her friends Eileen Barkley and Margaret Keir.

Beth Douglas, our music teacher, believed that everyone can and should sing. What stood out about her were her bubbly, joyous personality, her infectious laugh, and her ability to instill into her students the expectation and confidence that we could accomplish anything with love, hard work, and fun.

Mr. Lightly, our six-foot seven-inch (201 cm) tall vice-principal, arrived at the door of the classroom where Miss Norton was eloquently teaching our Class C how to read to children. Tiny Miss Norton answered the knock at the door, dramatically looked straight ahead, and then ever so slowly looked up—waaaaay up—to Mr. Lightly's smiling face. After the laughter had stopped and the two educators had completed their discussion, Miss Norton calmly—without cracking even a little smile—sat down at her desk and continued reading Rudyard Kipling's *The Elephant's Child.*

We shivered with enjoyment as we heard about the crocodile—in the great, grey, green, greasy Limpopo River, all set about with fever trees—pulling on the nose of the elephant child until it changed from a boot–like nose to a useful trunk. The drama and delight helped all of us grow as story-tellers and teachers. Peggy still *loves* to read to children.

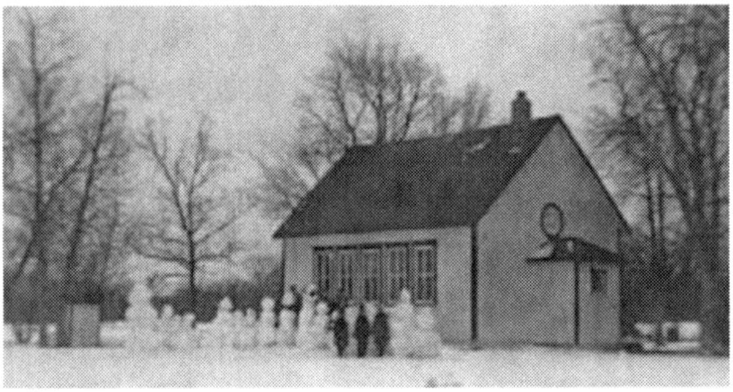

14. Cheval School

Peggy was a permit teacher at Cheval School, in Morden, in 1949–50. She had eleven pupils in grades one to nine, the eldest of whom was eight months younger than her own sixteen years! She returned to that school in 1951–52 following her year at Normal School. Again, she taught grades one to nine.

From 1952 to 1954, she taught grades one to four at Poplar Point. Her class consisted of forty-eight children till Christmas, when the twelve in grade four were moved to the next room because the classroom space heater "cooked' the children sitting near the stove, but left the ones sitting beside the north windows shivering!

From 1955 to 1960, she continued with grade one and grade two—usually thirty to thirty-eight students—at Argyle School, in Winnipeg School Division #1. Since the Immigration Hall was in the school area, most children over age six living there for the three allowable months started off their Canadian education in Peggy's classroom. Everyone had some amazing experiences.

She spent half-time at a Transcona Community Club private kindergarten from 1963 to 1969. Government funding of kindergarten in Manitoba began in September 1969. Until then, many small, often in-home, kindergartens provided some pre-school group experiences for children.

Peggy worked in Transcona-Springfield School Division #12, from 1969 to 1998. She was a kindergarten teacher in 1969–70. Then, until May 1972, she was primary supervisor in the system. For the balance of her time with the school division, she was assistant superintendent.

For all these positions, the only interview that she ever had was for the position at Poplar Point, where she and her dad found the chairman of the board, Gordon Kitchen, pitching hay behind the community hall. Mr. Kitchen asked her one question, "Do you like children?"

She responded, "I *love* children!"

He immediately stated, "You've got the job!"

Peggy was invited to fill all the other positions which she held in her thirty-eight years as an educator. She feels very blessed by the opportunities that she has had in her life.

Vera Derenchuk, superintendent of Division #12, believed in Peggy's abilities and gave her the opportunity for twenty-four years of satisfying work in education. She also helped Peggy through some very difficult personal events in her life.

As part of her responsibilities as assistant superintendent, Peggy frequently spoke to the students "graduating" from grade six. She encouraged them to approach life with curiosity, imagination, as well as love and caring for all whom they encounter in their lives.

She has advised young people wishing to become teachers to enhance their love of children, to be always curious, imaginative, and understanding as they provide the opportunities for learning how to learn for their pupils.

Her personal situation of having an abusive alcoholic husband and three children—who were her priority—made it very difficult to attend university for the length of time needed to earn a degree. As a result, she was the only member of the Manitoba Association of School Superintendents who did not have a degree. Mostly, she relied on common sense!

She divorced her husband in the 1970s. To prepare for a court appearance, she purchased a book, handled all the paper work herself and acted as her own lawyer. The actual proceedings took all of eleven minutes. Although all three children function normally and well, they all have some of the difficulties that are associated with adult children of alcoholics.

As a child, she enjoyed reading *Little Women*, by Louisa May Alcott. As an adult, she liked *Julian's Cell*, by Ralph Milton.

Ralph is Peggy's brother. He changed his name from Ralph Milton Friesen to Ralph Friesen Milton when the manager of the radio station where he was working—about 1953—told him that his name sounded too German and, that if he wanted to continue in his job, he had to change his name. Ralph has expressed regret many times that he did change it. He had a wife, two children, and an excellent work reputation before it became acceptable to be named Friesen in media circles.

Dr. Ralph Milton has worked in broadcasting and media in Asia, Africa, Canada, and the United States. He is the author of eighteen books. On the internet, Ralph publishes the popular e-zine *Rumors*, which uses liberal doses of humour to communicate a lively faith. Co-founder of Wood Lake Publishing, Ralph lives in Kelowna, B.C., with his wife and friend of fifty years, Beverly, a retired United Church minister.

For pastimes, Peggy enjoys singing in her church choir, interacting with their thirteen grandchildren, travelling, reading, camping in their Volkswagen camper, and gardening.

She is involved in several community activities. In the Transcona Memorial United Church, she serves in the choir, on the official board, and as representative to the Winnipeg Presbytery, and as member of the Hymn and

Worship Committee. She is a life member of United Church Women and a member of the Transcona Friends and Neighbors Study Group.

Peggy has enjoyed and learned from pilgrimages provided by the Vancouver School of Theology (VST), http://www.spiritual-pilgrimage.com, led by Dr. Gerald Hobbs and Dr. Lynn McNaughton. On one trip, forty-four pilgrims travelled to Ireland. They learned about the incredibly deep religious faith of the early Irish people as exemplified by their amazing burial sites. The pilgrims also experienced the energy and faith of the modern day Irish people as they work to eliminate harsh and horrible memories and traditions stemming from the extremes of poverty and wealth of their ancestors.

Jim and Peggy followed the advice of Brother Ralph. “Register. You’ll like it. Bev and I are going again.” He tossed a pamphlet on their kitchen table. Therefore, in June and July 2000, they travelled from Lindisfarne to Coventry on their first pilgrimage with Gerald and Lynn of VST. It was an incredible “Study Tour to Britain”. This was the first of four study tours that they have taken in a series entitled “Claiming Our Spiritual Heritage”.

In 2003, they experienced their Spiritual Heritage in Europe from the Rhine valley to Geneva. She and Jim continued their journey by train, visiting Salzsburg, Vienna, and Prague.

Prior to their 2005 VST study tour to Ireland, together with Bev and Ralph and friends Art and Oriole Veldhuis, they rented a van and explored Northern Ireland. In 2007, the study tour to France and England was entitled “A Singing Heart”. It was absolutely marvellous.

Along with several others, they travel from Winnipeg, and have formed a tradition by starting their trip to Cuba. They have pot-luck dinner gatherings both before and after their journeys to share their learning, books, and pictures and to watch appropriate videos and DVDs that relate to their travels. She has detailed pamphlets and summaries of these travels. There is also the web site, which provides much information.

All of the trips described above would not have happened if not for a United Church led study tour to Cuba in January and February 1999. On this two-week journey in which they lived in the middle of Havana in the Luyanno Presbyterian Church, sleeping in pre-Castro student dormitories, they visited schools, day care centres, hospitals, farms, and a government building—with speeches by the Cuban officials. They attended a fabulous concert in the Havana Ballet Concert hall, slept in thatched roof cottages at a Pentecostal Retreat Centre, swam in the turquoise water off the beach at the United Church House near Varedaro, visited church people in their homes, and had many other incredible experiences. Here, Peggy met the most wonderful man—Jim Lawrence.

As they travelled in their ancient Pastors-for-Peace school bus, Jim and Peggy found that they were gradually spending more and more time together. As they talked, they discovered that they were living very similar lives—twenty miles (32 km) apart. They sat together and talked all the way home from Cuba. A few days later, Jim appeared at Peggy's door with a bouquet of pink roses. Both persons knew that they wanted to spend the rest of their lives together. Jim proposed to Peggy—on his knees—at a grandaughter's birthday party.

They were married on June 26, 1999, just five months after they met. The three ministers from their two churches, both choirs, four music leaders, and a completely full church of family and friends sang Beethoven's "Joyful, joyful, we adore you!" as the couple walked down the aisle with all seven of their adult children and their partners and all thirteen of their grandchildren. They enjoyed a marvellous potluck reception in the downstairs hall as everyone brought food or a contribution to Habitat for Humanity instead of the traditional wedding gifts. Their children and grandchildren all like each other and happily gather at the Lawrence house or a local park in summer for various celebratory gatherings. Despite some medical problems, Jim and Peggy feel most blessed with having truly joyful lives.

Peggy would suggest that visitors to Canada should go to Winkler, in southern Manitoba. The residents—mostly Mennonite—have invited and welcomed people from all over the world to come, live, and work in what has become a thriving city.

Dr. Bill Blaikie has been the Member of Parliament of her constituency for twenty-six years. He is an ordained United Church Minister who has always refused to compromise his principles. He has earned the respect of all the members of Parliament. He is now teaching "Religion and Politics" at the University of Winnipeg. Peggy considers him to be a great Canadian.

"To thine own self be true, and it shall follow as the night the day, then thou canst not be false to any [man] one." Everyone in the whole world is equally loved by God and this belief must direct our attitude and life style. This states her philosophy of life. She urges all to love their neighbours as themselves.

Peggy has lived in Transcona, a suburb in the east of Winnipeg, in the same bungalow for over forty-nine years.

21

Shirley (Fulmore) McCracken

What a bad night it was! Try as she might, she cannot forget the embarrassment. She had not been feeling well when she arrived for the annual Christmas concert at Edgeworth School. Usually, the children would perform a Christmas pageant. However, since this year was during World War II, the children performed a patriotic one instead. Each student portrayed someone who would be helping in the war effort. Shirley had the honour of being a nurse. Before she could complete saying her part, disaster befell her. She fainted —for the first time in her life! Her current acting career was suddenly halted. Her parents whisked home to bed and administered her with a bitter dose of quinine.

Shirley was born at Edgeworth, Sask.. Now, she and her husband live on a farm near Ogema, Sask. Her first school was Edgeworth School, where she obtained her grades one to ten, but she studied grades nine and ten by correspondence. Then she took grades eleven and twelve at Caronport High School. After attending Manitoba Provincial Normal School, she studied at Briercrest Bible Institute, in Caronport, Sask., for one year.

Her teaching career took her to Wild Rose School District, Parry, Sask., as a permit teacher; Parkland School District, Virden, grades one to nine; back to

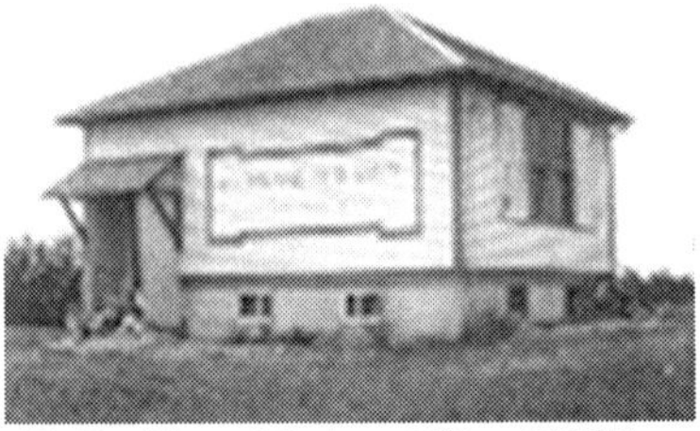

15. Parkland School Div. #2197

Edgeworth School, grades one to eight, but with few students; Margaret School, Margaret, grades five to eight; and Dahinda School, Dahinda, Sask., grades three to five. Her other important profession was that of homemaker.

Ever since she was a child, she has read everything on which she could lay her hands. She is still an avid reader. As a result, no favourite title has ever emerged.

In addition to reading, she enjoys working puzzle books and sewing. There are other things which she would like to do. However, she has a form of anemia, for which there has been no determined cause and which requires the taking of iron intravenously, and also chronic lymphocytic leukemia, which requires no treatment. Thus, she does not have much energy for walking and other physical activities.

In the community, Shirley has taught Sunday school, has been a leader in a 4-H club, and has been a member of Women's Institute. In the 4-H work, she taught such subjects as values, mineralogy (including lapidary), photography, and sewing.

When she was teaching at Dahinda School, a tall grade five boy was heading toward the door of the school one day with a garter snake in his hand. Shirley saw what he had in mind. How she rushed to reach the door first! The school had no basement, but it did have cold air vents in each room. Thoughts of what "fun" there would be if that snake were to slither down one of those. When that lad held the snake straight out from his shoulder, it reached the ground. Shirley stood her ground at the door and would not allow the boy to take his reptile specimen into the school. Reluctantly, he had to take it away.

When the four children were still in elementary school, the family took a trip to Australia. It was an educational experience for the children and parents alike. Colleen, in grade four, came home from school so very disgusted on the first day. She had a man teacher for the first time. She could not understand a word that he said because of the different accent. In addition, she could not even read his writing, which was actually bad. How awful that was for her! Children adjust quickly, and so did this little Canadian girl.

Shirley's husband Jim did carpentry work during the fifteen months that the family spent in Australia. They had gone to that country to look for farmland and would have moved there, except that the prices were too high. Thus, they returned to Saskatchewan.

Another memorable trip was the one to Niger, a West African country, to visit their daughter Colleen, who was doing missionary work there. Although Shirley and Jim thought that they knew what to expect, they were not prepared for what they actually saw and heard. Housing was generally very poor. They stayed at a farm school and had satisfactory housing.

The guard had a grass house with grass fence around it. One day, a little girl playing with matches set fire to the fence. Someone nearby grabbed the fence ahead of the burning part and tore it down to avoid the fire from spreading to the house. Afterwards, the fence was rebuilt.

Tony, another missionary there, took the family to a bush village where one of the nationals invited them in to look at his tomato plants. Something was destroying them. Such an invitation is a privilege, and not usually done. They can grow tomatoes and other vegetables. On market day, women would pass by on the road with huge baskets of tomatoes on their heads. Bicycles would be seen with live chickens tied to the handlebars and headed for market. The mourning of the death of a loved one in some of the villages was so melancholy and piercing to their ears.

The water supply was a problem. Women carried water from dirty pools which may be stagnant. This was used for laundry and for cooking. The people did not always have a nearby stream for a source of water. The school did have a well. For the missionaries, the water had to be filtered, and for babies also boiled. The women could reach a 200-foot (61 m) deep well (not at the school) by walking along a sandy trail. A bull, hooked up with a rope around it, would pull up a big container of water.

The weather was pleasant, with the coolest temperatures being in the high 50s (14°C). They left before the hot season started late in February. At the time, it was the dry season. The land in the region, known as sub-Sahara, was flat and sandy, but there were trees.

Closer to home, the family was filled with awe as they viewed the natural wonders of Grand Canyon in the southwest of the United States.

Shirley and Jim would recommend visitors to come to Saskatchewan to enjoy the view provided by the wide open spaces of the prairies. To some, there is nothing exciting about it. Her family lives in the hills of the rolling prairie and knows what to show a visitor to that area of the province. They have hosted numerous visitors from abroad who were simply engrossed when sitting at the tops of the hills and looking out over the "flats". They could hardly pull themselves away from the panorama.

Her advice to teens in general is to be true to God and you will be true to yourself and to others.

The classroom has changed considerably from when she taught. If the person is really determined to teach and is a mature individual, she would likely tell him/her to go for it. She cannot think of any favourite teacher, only one very "unfavourite" one! She usually liked them.

She tells about their family of Colleen, Joan, Jeff, and Stan. Colleen is married and has two sons (one married). Her husband works for the State of California in waste water management. Colleen did volunteer work in Long Beach. She spent a year in Liberia before getting married and going to Niger, where she did volunteer work in the school. In Monrovia, Liberia, she taught religious training to high school students—with one hundred fifty in a class!

Joan married an immigrant (now Canadian) from Romania. They live in Regina. Joan received 91% on her licentiate in piano from Trinity College in London, the school's highest mark up to that time. She is on the last lesson on her CGA course. She is financial advisor in a government job (property management). Her husband had his Masters in Civil Engineering degree—but no jobs here—and he is working for an office supply company, setting up and repairing equipment.

Jeff did a short term mission in Benin, met a girl from Switzerland who was teaching him French, and they were married in Saskatchewan. Her parents came for the wedding. She is also now a Canadian citizen and Jeff has taken out Swiss citizenship. They have two sons.

Stan married a Canadian-born girl. She has cystic fibrosis, has had a double lung transplant, and is doing very well. Stan is an agricultural technician (farm machinery mechanic). They live in Moose Jaw, Sask.

Dr. Henry Hildebrand, first principal of Briercrest Family of Schools, was an encouragement to her in her faith and life. He related very well with young people, tolerated no nonsense, but did encourage his students.

She especially liked it when a Normalite teacher would say, "Half of you have been permit teaching and know what I mean. The rest of you will soon learn when you get teaching." Oh, the poor "other half"!

In Normal School, she was in a group that met for Bible study with Jerry Hildebrand. One evening was set aside for roller skating. She had never been roller skating and very much wanted to go. Unfortunately, that was when she had received smallpox vaccinations. Twice, they did not take. However, on the third time—when she wanted to go with the group—it took. How disappointed she was when she had to miss the fun!

Miss Ring, our health teacher, insisted that everyone in Manitoba knew what lice were like and had seen them. Someone in a class ahead of hers had never seen lice, and Miss Ring cut that person down. Shirley was very tempted to say that she was from Saskatchewan and she had never seen lice, but refrained from doing so. If she had, it would have been interesting to have heard Miss Ring's response. She noted that her shy classmate from Ontario also did not respond. Maybe, he had seen lice, or, perhaps, he also preferred to keep still as she did.

Shirley is a Christian and firmly believes that following God is the best way to live—and die. She also feels that the family is very important.

Ogema, the community where Shirley lives, was awarded the trophy for the best sustainable development throughout all of Canada in the 2005 National Edition of Communities in Bloom.

Communities from around the world which are doing the most to address issues ranging from pollution to conservation and poor housing were named at the annual finals of the International Awards for Liveable Communities held over in November 2008 in Dongguan, China. Ogema received a silver award in the category for communities having a population under 20,000.

22
Ethel (Galloway) Currie

Who says that the prairies are a vast stretch of flat, boring land with no beauty? The Rocky Mountains have their form of beauty, and the prairies have theirs. Let us enjoy a September trip through part of western Manitoba and eastern Saskatchewan with Ethel.

We shall commence our drive at Brandon, located at the junction of the Trans-Canada Highway and #10 Highway. We travel north to the town of Minnedosa and on to the entrance of Riding Mountain National Park, a rise in elevation created by the glaciers of long ago. Throughout the park, we witness the many-coloured deciduous leaves in contrast to the green fir trees.

We continue for a short distance beyond the park to the city of Dauphin. Here, we follow #5 Highway to the west. In the Bield area just east of Roblin, we pass through rolling hills. To the west of Roblin, we come upon the beautiful Shell and Assiniboine Valleys near the Saskatchewan border.

Throughout this section of our trip, we marvel at the splendour of the leaves in their glorious array of colour. To complement this, we behold the fields as they exhibit beautiful blue flax and yellow canola and mustard. Other crops are in their various stages of development. The rolling prairie accentuates the beauty of this painters' paradise.

Ethel was born in Gilbert Plains. She took grades one to ten in Glen Lyon School in the Municipality of Gilbert Plains.

Being a positive person, she, therefore, prefers not to dwell on unpleasant experiences that she may have had in school as a student. However, she does remember an experience that made her very proud and happy. She was chosen for the academic award and the sportsmanship award in the same year. It was a commendable achievement in receiving one award, more so in receiving the second one.

As she attended country schools where one teacher taught all grades and all subjects, she cannot say that she liked one teacher better than another. Each was different in a number ways. She does not remember disliking any one of them.

Normal School to her was a great holiday. She enjoyed the "hut life" with the companionship of the girls. She remembers Miss Pilling and her art classes. Ethel claims to be no artist, but she enjoyed those classes. She also relished the vitality of Miss Douglas in her music classes.

She did all of her teaching in one-room Manitoba country schools. As a permit teacher, she taught for two years in schools near Roblin. Then, after attending Normal School, she spent three years in the Neepawa area.

From the time when she left home to take her grade eleven until she ended her teaching career, she lived with various families in their homes. They were all very good to her and, of course, had a great influence on her life. She was helped in so many ways that she cannot name one particular person who had a greater influence on her.

Ethel decided to leave teaching when she married. However, she did work part time—for an auctioneer, in a fabric store, for a transport company, and in a dress-making shop. Since she raised three daughters, she spent most of her time in her home with her family.

She was involved in whatever her girls were taking part—majorettes, figure-skating, or baseball. For many years, she belonged to the Legion Auxiliary. More recently, she has belonged to the Manitoba Society of Seniors. Over the years, she has made many quilts and afghans for Project Linus Manitoba and Blanketing Manitoba. She also knits mitts and toques for Christmas Cheer boxes and Izzy dolls for orphans of war-torn countries. She was the principal leader of her local 4-H Club for a number of years. During that period, she taught one of the sewing levels each year.

Ethel has been an avid reader for all her life and has enjoyed most of the books that she has read. Although she does not have any really favourite titles, she does like mysteries.

She always enjoyed such hobbies as sewing, knitting, crocheting, quilting, and reading. In addition, she also does painting on plaster cast—villages, ornaments, and other subjects.

Gibraltar was on the itinerary of a trip to Spain. Knowing very little about the fortress, she took advantage of the situation to learn about it. In doing so, she really enjoyed this experience.

The guide was a war veteran and, therefore, was very knowledgeable. While there, she saw two warships involved in the Gulf War in harbour for repairs. In touring the caves, she saw where the military had once assembled. She peered through the portholes where guns had protruded while protecting the harbour and sea. It was amazing to learn of all the activity that occurred inside that "rock". The idiom "as solid as the Rock of Gibraltar" became fact. Of course, no visit to Gibraltar would be complete without observing the antics of the apes.

She feels that the best advice which she can give to anyone, teenager or adult, is to obey the Golden Rule. If one follows that advice, one will not go far wrong.

As teaching was the only profession in which she really participated, other than being a homemaker, she would advise a young person to research the professions and vocations, and be very sure of one's decision. Teaching today is so very different from the "olden days".

There are two people whom she feels contributed greatly to Canada. One was Tommy Douglas, a former premier of Saskatchewan. His influence in establishing the Medicare System should never be overlooked. As one who had a husband sick over numerous years, there is no way that Ethel could have managed to pay for the care. The second person is Nellie McClung. Her work to have women recognized as persons was monumental and resulted in the enabling of women to make the strides which they have accomplished.

At this time in her life, Ethel lives one day at a time, enjoying it, and trying to obey the Golden Rule.

23
Isla (Gliddon) Lawrie

At Normal School, she lived in one of the huts, having a room to herself. One day, on returning to her room, she noticed something amiss. Why was the door ajar? This was unusual as she always closed her door before leaving the hut. Was someone hiding in her room?

Cautiously, she began to open the door. Splash! The plastic glass of water balancing at the top of the door fell, unloading its cargo on her. One of her friends down the hall had placed this booby-trap into the precarious position to create a little fun. When something appears to be out of order, it probably is.

Isla was born in Chater. She first went to school in Molson.

No one teacher could really be considered a favourite as she moved much because her mother was a teacher, although she remembers one high school principal who helped her personally. The frequent moving may have been traumatic for some children, but not for her since she had her mother, piano, and rocking chair wherever she lived. It was just her way of life and it did not bother her as her mother made home wherever she was.

Normal School was a comfortable place to be, as it felt homey and exhibited no class or economical divisions. It took her a long time to figure out that the french fries which were served in the dining hall were actually parsnips. Who could forget a meal of fish every Friday? She frequently boarded the city bus at the campus stop and travelled downtown, with one change on the way. She had good friends and good fun. She remembers going with Pat Enns, Jake Enns, Abe Friesen, and Abram Friesen to the wooded area across street from the campus to bring back a tree, but she cannot remember the reason for this activity. That area is now lined with houses.

Miss Douglas, our music teacher, had the most influence on Isla. This experience of music classes at Normal School broadened her field. Since then, she has been a church organist for thirty years. She liked Miss Carscallen, our physical education and youngest teacher, very much. Isla fondly remembers both Miss Carscallen and Miss Ring, our health teacher. She remembers Mr. Clarke as a former school inspector.

Isla taught near Portage la Prairie before moving to Delta, B.C. In her first permit year, she earned $75 per month and her board was $25. The next year, when her salary was raised slightly, her board was also increased. She taught the son of the people with whom she boarded. One time, when Isla strapped him, his parents were not happy with her. On another occasion, her landlord transported her to school on a stone boat, on which it was necessary for her to stand.

When the inspector took her to see her one-room school near Ladner, B.C., before hiring her, he apologized for the poor-looking facility. As she walked into the building, she noted that it had indoor flush toilets; and, when she opened the cupboard doors, she noted that they were filled with books, pencils, and other equipment. She had never seen anything like this in Manitoba.

She taught for six years, and then she left to raise her family, during which time all lived on a farm. When she returned to teaching, she substituted for a while; but she felt that this was not the work for her. Then, she became involved with school library as a technician. In this position, she worked in the back room, where she performed such functions as processing and cataloguing incoming books, repairing damaged ones, and tending to overdue notices. This work she enjoyed immensely. She was a school library technician, in Delta, B.C.; in Seaquam Junior High School; and in Delta School Board Resource Centre.

As a child, Isla read many books, but none stand out as being a real favourite. It has been the same as an adult because what might be a favourite one year would be replaced by another the next year. She does like English, Scottish, Irish, and Canadian writers, but she has no particular liking for American writers.

She has taken trips to Europe, New Zealand, Australia, the Maritime Provinces, southern United States, California, Yukon, northern British Columbia, and the Queen Charlotte Islands. She has ridden the Alaska State Ferry and took a cruise on the Columbia River. On most of her trips, she did not see anything truly exciting, although she enjoyed all of them.

It was scorching hot when she was in Europe. She saw people carrying bottles of water with them, but Isla had never wanted to do that—until this time, when she saw the value of doing so.

One trip that she enjoyed occurred when she visited her daughter who lives in the North Coast Region of British Columbia. Her daughter was required to travel to the Queen Charlotte Islands on business. After crossing the strait on a ferry, Isla stayed at a hotel several days while her daughter travelled. However, there was time for Isla to be shown much of the islands, which she found to be beautiful. The weather was windy, but otherwise quite good. Overall, it was a wonderful trip.

Another trip that she enjoyed was a cruise on the Columbia River for which she was invited by a friend. At first, she thought that it was too expensive; but, on further considering it, she decided to go ahead and do it. She joined two friends and a group from Alberta at Abbotsford Airport, in the Lower Mainland Region of British Columbia. From here, they travelled by tour bus to Portland, Ore., where a total of 150 persons boarded a paddle wheeler. The boat wound its way upstream to the Snake River at the Idaho border, and then made its way back to Portland. Along the way, the boat passed through locks beside nine dams.

For pastimes now, she enjoys playing the piano and organ, playing mah jong, walking, swimming, gardening, crocheting, visiting families and friends, volunteering in the community, solving crossword puzzles, and reading.

In the community, she volunteers with Deltassist, St. Stephens United Church, Friends of the Library, and two school libraries.

She recommends northern British Columbia as a place to visit. It is so beautiful in the summer. As for the area having a reputation for flies and mosquitoes, she admits that their presence can be noticed. However, there are times when there are virtually none. She suggests that winter is not an ideal time for a visit here unless one is an avid snow person.

She would counsel young people to follow their dreams. They should expand themselves as much as possible by trying new ventures, travelling to new places, and meeting people.

Teaching is different now from the time when Isla was starting out—and also more difficult. As a result, she would not like to be a teacher now. She much prefers the library as it is a more controlled situation. However, she enjoys doing some volunteering at the elementary level. From her experience, she feels that a young person has to be very enthusiastic to teach at this time.

The person whom she feels has had a positive influence on her was a librarian with whom she worked. She helped Isla in her field and allowed her leeway in how she did her work. This librarian became a good friend. Isla also has close ties with the people of her church. They also have helped her in various ways.

She considers Prime Minister Stephen Harper to be a good Canadian leader and she admires him. She does not agree with everything he does, but he has his own opinions and stands by them. This is a good way to be today, especially since many people in high places tend to vacillate.

Her philosophy is to have a positive attitude and not to look at the negative. She has had ups and downs in life, but she has strong family ties and tries to be positive at all times.

24
Evelyn (Graham) Jones

Harvest had begun and a sale of the farm was in the offing. It was also the beginning of the school year, but not the usual one. A farm girl had to go to General Wolfe School, in Winnipeg, for her grade nine. Under the circumstances, it was necessary for her to go alone to settle in the big city.

As fate would have it, she became lost on her first day. However, she eventually managed to reach the school. At 11:30 a.m., a gruff-spoken teacher told the students to go home and to return at 1:00 p.m. Guess what? After being at two schools in the forenoon, she had no clue how to return to her boarding house. However, during the wait, she met a girl who helped her find the way back. How thankful the lost girl was to receive this kind assistance! This traumatic experience has stayed with her for all of these years.

Evelyn was born on the farm, E half 18-4-12 Rural Municipality of Argyle, between Pilot Mound and Baldur. She first attended school at Zephyr, Section 7-4-12, a country school near Greenway.

When she was twelve years of age, she went on a trip to British Columbia and attended school for three weeks in Vancouver. Her inspector at the time felt that it would be educational for her to have a trip for three months.

Since it was not a holiday, she had all her text books, notes, and assignments with her. Her mother, having been a teacher, also felt that it would be useful for her daughter to experience city school for three weeks. In addition to the classes and assignments, she was able to see many sights of the city. This was an opportunity in which Evelyn took full advantage. How many grade eight students of that time were able to take a trip to learn?

Her favourite teacher was Marjorie Meder, who taught her in grades four, five, and six at Zephyr, a country school. The teacher was very fluent in English and taught her students proper use of the language.

As she was a non-resident student at Normal School, she did not take part in many extra-curricular activities. However, she had a good circle of friends among other non-resident students. She recalls being very nervous in one class when she was required to tell about a grain elevator. Although she was a farm girl who had accompanied her dad with loads of grain to a country elevator, she did not know about how one operated or what it was like inside.

Evelyn taught one year on permit at Centreville, a country school between Holland and Treherne in 1949–50, before attending Normal School. After two years of teaching, she left the profession for a while to raise her family, following which she returned to complete thirty-three years of teaching in total. This included six years in country schools in Manitoba and twenty-seven years in Cypress River at the primary level, teaching grades one and two. Her only other profession was that of domestic engineer!

For someone contemplating entering the teaching profession, her advice would be to enjoy the experience of teaching in the primary area. The children in those grades are eager to learn.

A person in Evelyn's life as a teacher was Mrs. Doris Stone, another primary teacher. Her lifestyle created a positive impression upon her.

Her favourite childhood books were the *Honey Bunch* series, by Helen Louise Thorndyke, and the *Anne of Green Gables* series, by Lucy Maud Montgomery. As an adult, she enjoys reading any biographies.

Evelyn would suggest visitors to come to Manitoba in June to see all the canola fields, the greenery of the trees, and the grasses.

She is involved with the Order of the Eastern Star, Red Hat Ladies, and Seniors' Centre activities. She has been a member of Eastern Star for thirty years, seven of which she served as Worthy Matron, the presiding officer. The Order is a ladies' group of the Masonic Lodge. Originally, a woman would have to be the daughter, widow, wife, sister, or mother of a master Mason; but the Order now allows other relatives and a few others.

For pastimes, she likes Scrabble and card games.

25
Joyce (Griffith) Garner

Being one who liked adventure, this young lady applied for a position in Northern Ontario one April. It was an adventure that she will never forget.

Eagerly, she travelled by train to check out the new school. When she arrived, board members took her to see the school and the teacher accommodation. Where was the school? Oh, it had recently burned, along with the books and educational material. She can have a job without a building or resources for teaching.

Was there a place where she can live? Yes, there was one. On close examination, she saw that it was a closet-size room in a makeshift building. Inside this mansion, she saw a bed and a hotplate with two burners. Not being interested in such a rustic life, she told them that the position was not acceptable and that she would be taking the train back south that evening.

The board was not to be stifled. They turned the clocks back and kept her entertained, hoping that she would miss the train. What an ambitious group they were! After a time, two geologists said, "I guess you are staying as the train leaves in fifteen minutes."

No, she was not staying! She has never run so fast in all her life as she did to catch that train. Not even a cheetah would have caught her. Apparently, she was the third teacher who had come to see what the job entailed and had left post haste. As a footnote, it appears as if the board finally woke to the fact that something was not right. They decided to improve the facilities.

Joyce was born in St. Boniface. Before she attended Normal School, all of her education was obtained in Winnipeg. Since she was a serious student, she did not have much time to socialize. However, when she was sixteen years old, she was asked to act as a chaperone for a doctor and his housekeeper. That was a very interesting experience. When she took time off to look after her sister, she was without a job.

Her favourite teacher was Marcel Bonneau, her grade ten teacher and principal. He brought such a fresh approach to learning, making school fun. He taught his children to think, to use their imagination, to create and to explore. Joyce looked forward to each day as her teacher opened a whole new world to his class in every facet of education.

Miss Pilling, our Art teacher, was the teacher who stands out in her memory from Normal School days. It was she who caused Joyce to realize that you can do anything if you go about it the right way and have a positive attitude. Joyce detested art, feeling that she could not do it. Throughout her school life, this was the class which she dreaded most. However, under Miss Pilling's tutelage, she produced some very good work. This changed her attitude towards the subject and taught her that, with the right attitude and excellent instruction, anyone can achieve good results.

After classes one day as she was returning to her residence, she met a nun who was extremely upset. This student had been separated from her sisters and, therefore, could not travel home on her own. Having concern, Joyce accompanied her to her residence. The

Mother Superior thanked her, fed her, and had her spend the night at the convent. She returned to the school the next morning. Until that time, she did not realize that nuns could not be out alone, but had to travel in pairs.

Since she had to pay her own way at Normal School, she was busy working in the cafeteria at school and going home each weekend to work in a general store in her community. That left her with very little time to socialize. Therefore, her memories are chiefly of studying and working. Her goal was to become a teacher, giving her little time for other activities.

After Normal School, she attended University of Manitoba, University of British Columbia, and finalized her Bachelor of Arts degree at University of Windsor.

The first school in which she taught was a one-room school, with thirty-five students in grades one to ten. We can imagine how busy she was. Her school was located in the community of Vivian. From there, she moved to Morris, where she taught grade seven. Then she taught grade one in Winnipeg.

After her four years of teaching in Manitoba, she accepted a position in Kitimat, B.C., where she stayed for three years. Then she supplied (substituted) for a principal and also taught grade ten in Kemano, in the same province. Her next stop was a grade seven class in Prince George, B.C. From there, she went farther north to Yellowknife, N.W.T., where she taught grade nine.

Joyce became more venturesome by going to Australia, where she taught grades nine to twelve in a boys' school in Sydney, New South Wales. While in that area, she also taught in a primary school at Coogee Beach, popularly known as Sydney's Seaside Village.

She had her first experience with an opportunity class at Riviere Qui Barre, Alta., and at Mission Park, a Catholic Public School in St. Albert, Alta. She moved from there to teach in Amherstburg, Ont. She was next the Special Education teacher for Mountainview School, in Stoney Creek, Ont. Her last position was as a resource teacher in Dundas, Ont. She retired at age sixty-five after having spent forty-five years in teaching. She loved her job and regretted having to retire.

Dave Goldman, the principal of Amherstburg, Ont., Public School, had a positive influence on her life work. He showed her how to teach the individual child, even within a large class. Individual spelling lessons were given to children who could go beyond their grade level. They were to be taught at their level. He taught his staff to be energetic, to use imagination, to create with the children, to be willing to change their methods in order to bring a fresh approach to teaching. The teachers worked hard, but they were learning and enjoying their work. As the children progressed, the staff felt rewarded. She and her colleagues attended many types of seminars in the United States, only a few miles away, to learn new methods and ideas. What an exciting and enjoyable time were those seven years for Joyce!

This is the advice which she would probably give to teenagers. Do your best at whatever you decide to do. Enjoy yourself, but be considerate and respectful of others. Help those less fortunate than you when and if you can. Appreciate what you have. Be positive at all times. Keep an open mind, keep learning, and be active as long as you can. Find something you love to do and it will never seem like work. Enjoy yourself; life is precious and short.

She has advice for those considering the teaching profession. Make sure you know what the job entails. Be prepared to teach each child to his or her individual needs. If any child has a disability, do not write him/her off as unteachable. You must do your best to find out how a child learns and give him/her the best education you can. Too many children slip between the cracks—and that is unacceptable! As an educator, it is your responsibility to make sure you give them your best. If you are not prepared to do this, you are in the wrong profession. Also, as an educator, you must keep learning yourself.

Being an avid reader in her childhood, she read everything that she saw: biographies, mysteries, adventure, history, and others. Thus, there was no book which she can claim to be a favourite. She loved every book that she read. Now, she belongs to a book club and reads many types of literature. However, she does not like romance or pulp fiction. She reads to learn and to enjoy new ideas and vocabulary. If a book makes her think, she enjoys reading it. Since there are so many of them, she finds it difficult to isolate one favourite.

She is married and has two daughters and one granddaughter. She babysat her granddaughter for five years on a once-a-week basis.

At present, she enjoys gardening, bridge, walking, swimming, baking, entertaining, attending theatre, and meeting new and interesting people from all walks of life. She volunteers for VON (now Acclaim Health). In the past, she engaged in friendly visiting; but, currently, she is the receptionist for the Foot Clinic. She is also the docent for the Burlington Art Centre, attending art history lessons once a week and volunteering at arts and craft shows and other major events. In addition, she is the vice-president for the women's Probus Club in Burlington.

Wherever one travels in Canada, there is something interesting to see. The Rocky Mountains and the northern and southern communities have beautiful and varied scenery. On the prairies at harvest time, a quilt of yellow sunflowers and mustard, purple chicory, toasty brown wheat fields, and black furrowed earth spread across the horizon. Add to that the pastures with different coloured cattle, sheep, and horses. Ontario and Quebec have winding roads, quaint villages, colourful ports, and low mountains. The Atlantic regions are exciting as one zips along the hairpin roads and views the ocean with colourful villages huddled along the coastline. The barren north with its many lakes, small trees, rocky terrain, sparkling snow, and northern lights has another majestic beauty. It would be difficult to choose one place as each has its own beauty and fascination.

Of all the places where she has visited, she thinks that Turkey had the most interesting archaeology, history, countryside, customs, and people. Every region had something fascinating and exciting to see.

In 1960, having a wanderlust, she took a year off teaching. Her desire was to see what people in other parts of the world were doing and how they lived. As her friend decided at the last minute not to go, Joyce felt that she could travel by herself. She embarked from Vancouver aboard *Hikawa Maru*, a small Japanese ship making its final voyage to Japan. Most of the passengers were missionaries. As it was a Japanese ship, she learned much about their customs and obtained her first taste of authentic Japanese food.

After the ship had docked in Yokohama, she proceeded to enjoy Tokyo, Kyoto, Osaka, Nikko, Kobe, and several other areas. She stayed in a *ryokan*, a type of traditional Japanese inn dating from the Edo period (1603–1868), which served travellers along Japan's highways. Sleeping on the floor and eating meals sitting cross-legged at a low table became routine. When she had depleted the money which she had reserved for her stay in Japan, it meant no more time at the fancy Kobe Hotel. Thus, she went to the Japanese YWCA, where no one spoke English. Here she waited until the freighter came and then left about three days later than expected. This was a challenge, but it was also good experience.

She happily participated in many different experiences in Japan. It was difficult for a young woman who is rather tall to be travelling alone in Japan. At first, she was nervous as many signs at the time said "Go home, American." Naturally, the Japanese identified her as being American. However, she spent three weeks in this country and appreciated the lower prices at the time. In Kobe, she partook of many meals of Kobe beef which she probably could not afford today.

Having completed her visit here, she boarded a Japanese freighter to Australia. That too was an enjoyable experience. There were only seven passengers and the Japanese crew. Fortunately for her, they were transporting silks and toys to Australia. On the return trip, they carried cattle. She was happy not to have been a passenger on that trip.

She spent the winter months in Australia and left when the southern winter approached. She enjoyed Australia immensely; but, at that time, she felt that it was a bit backward as she was used to the "mod cons" in Canada and Australia was behind the times in that regard. She and another girl hitchhiked along the coast highway. They stopped at Brisbane and then went as far as the Coral Reef. On the return trip south, they took the interior highway. There were not so many cars travelling, making it a wee worrisome as they were still hitchhiking. She had a pleasant time in Melbourne, as well. The weather was ideal; the scenery was beautiful; and the beaches were exquisite.

She left Australia on an Italian passenger ship which stopped at every city around Australia and beyond. Thus, the passengers had time to spend in each city, including

Singapore, Jakarta, and Cochin. They disembarked at Aden and went to explore the pyramids in Egypt. They also had the opportunity to ride a camel. Their ship later passed through the Suez Canal. They disembarked in Naples. It had been a month that the passengers had been aboard the ship.

She took her time travelling up the boot of Italy visiting many of the cities and towns. From there, she travelled to Spain and followed a similar routine. She travelled throughout France and Belgium, took a ferry to Denmark, and finally went to England, where she spent a few weeks. She returned to Quebec and enjoyed time there. Finally, she set out for Winnipeg to conclude her trip. Eventually, she returned to Yellowknife.

The trip on the ship had cost her $395, and she saw countries that now exist in name only as they are so different. She does not recognize them. No longer do kimonoed women fill the streets of Japan. McDonald's and other fast food places crowd every city today. The food in Italy is so refined today. Eating hunks of bread with cheese and wine for breakfast is long gone. She was so fortunate to experience this old world, which was not contaminated with North American foods and customs.

She had written home and asked her mother to keep the letters. It was a good thing she did make that request as she lost her diary in Rome. Relying on her memory today would not be as good.

There are many leaders whom she has greatly admired over the years. Mohandas Gandhi and Mother Teresa are two who were outstanding. But, in Canada, she would say Tommy Douglas was outstanding for giving us a wonderful health system and Stephen Lewis for his integrity and humanitarian contributions.

Joyce's philosophy of life is virtually the advice which she would give to an assembly of teenagers.

Class D

Lumina Chartrand
Ronald Fordon
Thelma Friesen
Emil Gillies
John Halirewich
Betty Hamilton
Ben Hanuschak
Aileen Harbottle
Thelma Harper
Marlene Harriott
Muriel Harris
Wilma Hedley
Henriette Heiget
Olga Hilash
Agnes Hildebrand
Dorynne Hipwell
Odarka Hrycyna
Keith Huss
Lyla Ilchena
Gwen Jackson
Emily James
Vera Jones
Nora Kabernick
Ena Kandall
Dorothy Keffen
Margaret Keir
Mabel Kemaldean
Angeline Kerbrat
Charlotte Kingdon
Katherine Klassen
Mary Klym
Sophie Kohut
Elaine Kolke
Sophie Konowalchuk
Ann Kopetsky
Peter Peters
Gordon Reynolds
Maurice Saranchuk
Dorothy Twilley
John Wherrett

26
Aileen (Harbottle) Huss-Seidel

It was 1950, the year of the Great Flood in Winnipeg. At the time, she was in grade twelve in her fourth year of attendance at Norwood Collegiate. An emergency which affected many people struck! The school was closed in early May because of its proximity to the rising water.

It was necessary for all students to go elsewhere to complete the year. Three methods of transportation supplied the means to reach the temporary school site. First, they took a bus to the railway station in St. Boniface, where they boarded a train that carried them across the raging Red River. Then, they transferred to a streetcar to complete the journey to Danicl MacIntyre Collegiate, where they attended very crowded classes. They would leave home about 7:30 a.m. and would not return until supper time. It was hectic, but it was also an exciting adventure. She did manage to graduate and thus entered Normal School in September of that year.

Before she dwells on her life and career, Aileen would like to pay tribute to the person who truly influenced her professional life. Dean Finlay was the principal of Windsor School in St. Vital (Winnipeg) where she first taught after graduating from Normal School. He was in his early forties and, to her nineteen-year-old eyes, appeared quite mature. He had the amazing gift of enjoying each day and also had a robust sense of humour. He gave his teachers, especially those just starting, a sense of security. One knew that Dean would be ready with a kind word of advice and also encouragement. She feels that these qualities became part of her own way of being, too.

Aileen was born in Binscarth. Her parents, Lawrence and Kay Harbottle, were farmers; and, for the first five years of her life, Aileen lived on a farm.

At the age of three, she attended the nursery class at the Binscarth United Church. She loved her teacher, the lessons, the singing, and being with other children. Upon returning to the farm, she would enlist her dear dog, Scottie, and proceed to teach him the Christian faith. Sometimes, he would want to lie down but his teacher insisted that he "sit up straight and listen!" It would seem that at such an early age, she had already embarked upon a teaching career.

The family moved to Holland in 1937; and, a year later, Aileen commenced her school life. Miss Pitt was her grades one and two teacher. She wore the most beautiful dresses and large brightly coloured brooches. Again, she loved her teacher, the lessons, and being with other children. As an only child, going to school was a great adventure.

In 1941, the family moved again, this time to Winnipeg, and lived in the part of St. Boniface called Norwood Grove. She attended Queen Elizabeth School for six years. Moving to the city and attending a really large school was a shock for this country girl. It took her almost two years to adjust to the changes. From this experience in her own life, she learned to pay close attention to any new students who came into her class and worked to integrate them to their new situation.

In grade six, the teacher, Miss Christie, read *The Old Curiosity Shop*, by Charles Dickens, to her students. She made it sound so interesting and very exciting and influenced Aileen's interest in reading greatly. Her junior high English teacher, Mr. Radcliffe, was very strict and loved teaching. He made English grammar a serious learning experience. It was at that time when the Department of Education chose a new English text called *Vitalized English*. Mr. Radcliffe denounced that text and used an old copy of an English grammar text book. She enjoyed these classes although some of her fellow students rebelled at the study.

Normal School was a definite change in her life, creating a feeling of freedom that she had not previously experienced in school. She made new friends, most of whom consisted of a small group who did not live in residence. They missed the twenty-four-hour association with all those who did. It was during this year that she met Keith. She remembers thinking the first time that she saw him, "What a handsome man!"

After graduating, she taught for three years at Windsor School, where she met Dean Finlay, to whom she has paid tribute above.

She and Keith were married in July 1954 and went to teach at Whitemouth. She had the grades three and four class while he had the grades seven and eight class. During their five years in that community, Aileen was leader of the CGIT (Canadian Girls in Training). Working with those energetic young women brought much joy to her life.

They have three children—Kenneth, Katherine, and Mary. When the children were young, the family had a cottage at Beaver Creek (north of Riverton) on the shore of Lake Winnipeg. In the late 1960s, there was neither hydro power nor telephone at the cottage. The children learned to build fires in the cook stove and to use an outdoor toilet. They also learned to appreciate the natural setting as they explored the shoreline for hours.

Aileen has had a variety of experiences in education. She taught grade six at Ramah Hebrew School on Grant Avenue, in Winnipeg, from 1965 to 1971. Here she learned about the Jewish faith and took part in many of their religious celebrations. Both Katherine and Mary attended nursery and kindergarten at Ramah and learned basic Hebrew. They attended free of charge because it was school policy since their mother was one of the teachers.

In 1971, they and their three children moved to Waterhen, which is about a four-hour drive north of Winnipeg. She taught grade four and Keith taught grade seven.

Waterhen School had been chosen as one of three schools in Manitoba to be part of a pilot project by the Department of Education. The programme was called Confluent Education and focused on the idea of joining the affective and cognitive domain in our teaching methods. Teachers received training at numerous weekend workshops and two-week long summer workshops. Many of the facilitators were from the University of California, Santa Barbara, where there was a master's programme in Confluent Education. It was during this training that Aileen learned to appreciate her intuitive skills and how these helped her to be a successful teacher.

When they returned to Winnipeg in 1973, she taught grade four at Dalhousie School in Fort Garry for two years. This was a giant open air school and, from her view, was much better than teaching in an isolated classroom.

In 1975, a dramatic change occurred in the family as Keith and Aileen were divorced. That year, she was hired by Frontier School Division to be one of several consultants with the Confluent Education programme. During the years from 1975 to 1978, she travelled throughout the province working with teachers in their classrooms and also leading teacher-training workshops. This was an exciting three years because she was fortunate to visit schools as far north as Island Lake and as far south as Woodridge. As with other consultants, she also continued receiving more training to improve skills.

In the fall of 1978, Frontier School Division granted her a sabbatical leave so that she could go to Santa Barbara to attend the University of California. There were about forty students in the Confluent Programme with only three from Canada. Several students were from Germany, some from Norway, and others from various states of the United States. Aileen graduated in June with a Master of Education degree.

Upon returning to Manitoba, she went to Crane River and taught junior high for two years. In 1981, she was hired as principal of Waterhen School. Ten years had passed since she had taught there; and, during those years, she had gained many valuable skills to help her in her new role. She gives great credit to her human relations training and improved teaching skill to her experience with Confluent Education. The staff worked as a team to run the school.

In 1987, she and Keith came together again after being apart for twelve years, and were remarried two years later. During those years, each had lived in California, visited Japan, and spent months in India. It seemed that their life journeys somewhat connected.

After she "retired", she was invited to be principal of Denino School in Fort Resolution, on the south shore of Great Slave Lake in the Northwest Territories. They were there for almost three months until the principal was well and could return to work. They walked to school each morning in the dark and returned in the dark after school. This experience was a challenge to her skills and experience as a principal.

Her last teaching experience was in 1994 in a little two-room school on Matheson Island in Lake Winnipeg, where she taught the little people—nursery to grade four. Using a highway map of Manitoba, they travelled in their imagination to many different places. It was exquisite fun working with these enthusiastic children!

One of the yearly events that she truly enjoyed was facilitating the Orientation Workshop for the PENT (Programme for Educating Native Teachers) students of Brandon University. Each year in early May from 1976 until 2002, she travelled to Brandon and spent the day at the university. It was so exciting to meet the many young people from reserves all over Manitoba and to encourage them on their educational journey.

She and Keith have five grandchildren. Their oldest, Kristin Huss, lives in Edmonton; Kyle and Trent Huss live just down the street; and Robbie and Katie Brown live about twenty minutes away. All four of the local ones are very fond of animals and all four are active in Scouts. It is wonderful to see them growing up!

She leaves the reader a thought to ponder. While attending the University of California, the students were required to read the book *Man's Search for Meaning*, by Viktor Frankl. That book had a profound influence on Aileen. " ... man should not ask what the meaning of his life is, but rather he must recognize that it is he who is asked." What has she done in her life? She hopes that she has had a positive influence on other people and left her tiny spot on this planet Earth a little better than when she came.

27
Wilma (Hedley) Treloar

There were no big, yellow buses in those days—but there was a car van to transport the children during the warm months. Members of her family and other families crowded into three rows—including twelve of all sizes in the back.

"Hey, get off my shins!" How cosy it must have been! As well, two big girls and a small girl squashed into the front seat. It was impossible to crowd in their dinner pails and homework books. These were tied together by belts and placed inside a homemade wooden box on the back of the car. All aboard!

In winter, the car van was replaced by a sleigh van. The trip of six miles (10 km) was covered much more slowly. In the spring when some roads were soft, neither vehicle was viable on occasion. In such a circumstance, they were able to wallow through the mud in a van that had high wooden wheels.

After arriving at their destination, Hamiota Consolidated School, everyone could breathe and stretch normally again and collect their belongings. It must have been more fun travelling to and from school then—for both students and drivers—than nowadays in the modern buses.

Wilma was born at Hamiota and obtained her grades one to twelve in that community. Prior to attending Normal School, Wilma worked in the Royal Bank of Canada, in Hamiota.

In her childhood school days in Hamiota, she was an eager participant in December concerts. The popular school concert was held on the first Friday of December. Proceeds from it were donated to the Children's Aid. She also loved the Christmas concerts at the local Chumah Country Church.

The church building has an interesting history. It was opened in 1903 and closed in 1953. In the following year, it was moved to another site. Today, a cairn, built in memory of the pioneers from Ontario who settled in the area in 1881, marks where it used to stand.

Despite knowing that she could never be a part of the glee club, she still appreciated Miss Douglas' cheery classes. However, it was the speech choir under the capable direction of Mr. Turner which attracted her. This experience was an asset in her teaching days.

When Wilma was a timid grade one pupil, she was very frightened of the school inspector, Mr. Clarke. She does not recall why she was. So years later, guess who she had as a teacher—and appreciated? He was no other than the former inspector at her school. Mr. Clarke was now teaching Classroom Management at Normal School. She now saw him in a much more favourable light.

She is most grateful that God provided her with a wonderful roommate: Ethel (Galloway) Currie. The girls arrived at Normal School from farms in different parts of the province. Ethel was from Gilbert Plains and Wilma was from Hamiota. They have remained good friends over fifty-eight years since and have travelled together.

A highlight of Normal School was the Christmas pageant. It was a delight for her to be a participant.

Following an enjoyable year at Normal School—between teaching years—she attended a summer school at Gimli and a summer school in Winnipeg. The latter included an advanced sewing course at the technical school, in the old Ford Building on Portage Avenue.

Between 1951 and 1953, she taught grades one to six at Cameron School, near Minnedosa. In the school year 1953–54, she taught grades one and two at Brookdale, a village near Neepawa. In the following year, she taught nineteen pupils in grades one to eight at Harrow School, between Rivers and Brandon.

As a child, she enjoyed reading the *Green Gables* books, by Lucy Maud Montgomery. Many years later when a daughter resided in Prince Edward Island, Green Gables was a great tourist attraction. As an adult, a favourite book was *The Robe*, by Lloyd C. Douglas.

For many years, she has loved to sew, knit, embroider, and read. She also spent much time in preserving food, gardening, and picking saskatoon berries. In recent years, she discovered that she can paint scenes with oils. More recently, she has assembled pictorial albums of her various family lines for future generations.

She has taken a daring step, one with no room for error, when she decided to cut her great-grandmother's crazy quilt into sections, and repaired and rebound heirlooms for family members. She was able to locate history books which provided information of this dear lady whom she never met.

Wilma was a Women's Institute member in Rivers for thirty-six years and, later in Alberta, for another ten years. Being a farmer's wife near Rivers, she became involved with the local hospital guild, her local church, and teaching 4-H sewing. She found that being involved with 4-H as a teenager and later as a leader most interesting. She participated in numerous 4-H trips, which were highlights for her.

Because one of her daughters was living in Prince Edward Island, Wilma made trips there. These allowed her to follow the progress of the Confederation Bridge to New Brunswick. A week after the opening of the bridge, she accompanied another daughter and family, travelling by motor home, to the island. They were high enough to see over the bridge walls to enjoy the view of the water.

She highly recommends any tourist—from home or abroad—to enjoy the fabulous autumn colours of the trees in eastern Canada.

Because she grew up in years when there was a scarcity of money for many people, she exhorts young people to spend carefully, to avoid debt as much as possible, and to be able to savour some travelling in our wonderful country.

Wilma believes that good teachers are born teachers. She taught for only four years as she felt that her family—which eventually included five children—required her to be at home. She has never regretted that. Farming was a good and versatile way of life.

It has saddened her that the teaching in schools has been restricted in recent years because of lack of discipline. She has been closely watching families—many of whom are Christian families—who have opted to homeschool their children. She is amazed with these children's capabilities, their respect, their knowledge, and their training. Wilma has attended various large homeschooling conferences. Yes, grandparents are encouraged to attend, also. To walk into a huge arena and observe thousands of young people in navy and white dress code, parents appropriately dressed, and everything well-organized was a sight to behold.

She particularly remembers her only high school principal, Mr. Ruttan. He taught algebra, geometry, physics, and chemistry—all subjects that required methodical and neat paper and blackboard work.

Wilma appreciated the influence of Shirley Fus, who was a pianist for a large Calgary church and who directed a seniors' hand bell choir. For many of them, they had never participated in an instrumental group prior to this time. Wilma loved it when they went to play at nursing homes.

She appreciated the leadership exhibited by Mr. Moorhead as our Normal School principal. He believed in his students, many of us fresh in from the country communities. Sometimes, it was not book learning we obtained at Normal. It was more the opportunity to live with and socialize with one another in preparation for going into new communities and situations. What really impressed her was Mr. Moorhead's faithfulness in returning from his church service in order to say grace at our delicious Sunday noon meals.

She believes that God has put us into this life to serve others as best we can, wherever we are located. This is her philosophy.

28
Henriette (Heiget) Leduc

What does a teacher do when the students refuse to work? Does she rule with "an iron fist", or does she sit back and let events take their course? When she was in grade six in a rural school, she had a teacher who was not strict. The result was that the students were mischievous.

One time, they decided that they would not work on their assignments. Therefore, they lined up at the blackboard and stayed there all afternoon. They were on strike! There was no real issue other than they wanted to see what would happen. Apparently, nothing happened that day, as far as they were concerned.

Henriette was born in St. Claude. She obtained her elementary schooling at Barron School, a rural school located eight miles (13 km) north of St. Claude and twenty miles (32 km) south of Portage la Prairie. Then, she went to St. Claude for grades nine, ten, and eleven, followed by her grade twelve at Notre Dame de Lourdes.

When Henriette was in grade eight, she had health problems. Her teacher, C. Bellec, took her aside after school hours and taught her a method for focusing and one for studying. What she learned from those sessions guided her for the rest of her life. As she struggled through high school, a teacher in grade eleven showed approval for her work. This helped her to gain confidence.

Leonie (Rey) Philippot helped her with her studies. When Henriette arrived at the St. Claude School from a rural school, she was lost and bewildered. Leonie observed this and went to chat with the new student. The two girls became instant friends. They completed high school together and then they went to summer school. They were also together during and after Normal School. Henriette considered her friend delightful and outgoing.

She particularly remembers Mr. Turner, our speech teacher at Normal School. He showed how to make teaching language enjoyable. He did this with his interpretation and intonations of literary poems and novels.

She feels that life at Normal School was lax, but very full. There were organized games outside the school and in class—though some were the usual ones. There was a time when all classes organized culture plays. These ideas showed her how to have students work and perform together, as occurred in her Christmas concerts.

She took her Bachelor of Education degree at the University of Winnipeg during the time when she was teaching adults with learning disabilities.

She was a permit teacher at Emberly School, a rural school near St. Claude, prior to attending Normal School. After that, her first assignment was at St. Jean School, another rural school, near Haywood. From there, she continued her rural teaching for two years at Grange School, near Cypress.

During her teaching in a rural school, the students organized and conducted a Christmas concert with her guidance. This was a memorable event for rural residents. Parents helped in setting up the stage and trustees bought presents and goodies for the students. The evening ended with Santa Claus delivering the presents.

In 1954, Henriette married John Leduc and subsequently raised four children. She substituted in St. Claude and area schools before moving to Brandon, where, again, she was a substitute teacher. These schools included St. Claude town schools; rural Kenneth School; Pinkerton School, in Treherne; and Dandurand School, in Haywood. The ones in Brandon were George Fitton, St. Augustine, and St. Michael's Academy.

Outside the teaching profession, she worked at a hospital in Brandon and then in a store. In Brandon, she was active in Navy cadets, Brownies, and Girl Guides. When the family moved to Winnipeg, she also worked in a store.

In 1984, Henriette and her husband travelled to Europe. Their main destinations were France and England. In France, she noted a ritual at mealtime. There would be a different dish for each food that was served. However, in England, the same plate would be used for all foods. This was more like the custom in Canada. She also noted that the climate and the old traditions were different from those in Canada.

For visitors from another country coming to Canada, she would show them the city of Brandon and its surroundings. The hills and valleys make the scenery awesome, especially in the fall when the harvesting of the fields is in progress and the trees are changing colour. This is a sight which no one can forget.

Her advice to teenagers would be clear. When in school, do your best, and learn all you can as you search for your career. When you have obtained that dream, follow it by working, studying, and being serious.

If you choose a teaching career, make certain that you enjoy children's views and their hang-ups. Listen to them and try to understand how they understand their surroundings and then teach them accordingly.

Pierre Elliot Trudeau made a great contribution to Canada when he was Prime Minister. What he accomplished for education is still practised. He introduced French immersion into the schools. Now, young people have become more tolerant of different cultures. Youth understand that speaking a different language is an asset at work, in travel, and in socializing.

When she was in elementary school, she liked *Call of the Wild*, by Jack London. As an adult, she enjoyed *Snow Falling on Cedars*, a novel by David Guterson. Currently, her hobbies include quilting, puzzles, and sorting out and arranging family albums.

In life, one has to realize one's nationality—Canadian! In Canada, we belong to a multicultural society. We, as a result, should respect others while observing them in their lifestyles. In doing so, we can understand and not judge; therefore, our lives will be more peaceful and happy. With this advice, she states that her philosophy of life is to show interest in others as she realizes that she is not "an island unto herself".

29
Keith Huss-Seidell

> 'Why are we here?' I ask myself. 'What are we to do? What can we be other than ourselves with nothing to teach old pros?' I consider statistics we present merely as a mesh to hang part of our story.
>
> I have little interest in just reeling off anecdotes. I would rather get a sense of character development. Some might parallel my own; some will probably be different. Is there some general amalgam that cut us out to be educators? Early life background emotions and attitudes might present many clues.
>
> I'm willing to help stir up the gist of the old Normal School spirit that has brought us together once more.

Those are Keith's words as he introduces a capsule of his life's story.

He was born in a St. Boniface hospital. In 1930, Keith's parents were homesteading in southeastern Manitoba on the edge of the Canadian Shield and surrounded by heavy evergreen forest.

They had a few acres of barely arable land to grow hay for the draft horses which they used to haul marketable timber by sleigh. The forest, far from civilization and a regular road, was the main source of the family's livelihood. There were neither machines nor sawmills. The cabin and bunk houses for the woodsmen were all hard hewn. The homestead shut down with the winter breakup.

For a little boy, it was a winter wonderland. How fascinated Keith was with the men, mostly single and from many different cultures! They were kind and considerate to him when he wandered into their quarters. He remembers that they curbed some of their usual rough language in his presence.

In summer, the family moved closer to the railway line, which ran along a little river valley and a water pipeline from Shoal Lake, in Ontario, to Winnipeg. This light railway, the Greater Winnipeg Water District Railway, was used in maintaining the pipeline and also served as the only means of transporting goods into the area. It was back to the homestead in winter.

By the age of seven, it was time to go to school, so Keith was sent to Maison Chapelle Preparatory School for Boys, a boarding school located in St. Boniface and run by the "sisters". His mother was Protestant and his father, who had been educated by the Benedictines in Bavaria, was nominally Catholic. Religion was not an issue, but education was.

With no-nonsense teaching, he received a solid first four grades of education. He retains one old faded report card—third in class, A+ in religion, and so-so in deportment. Maybe most important, he loved his teacher. Decades later after the school section had closed, he met her—now Sister Superior—and she said, "Yes, I do remember you as that clever little German boy." He claims that she had an immense effect on him at that age as his classroom teacher.

Keith remembers being interested in history—which was mainly about French Canada founders and missionaries, as might be expected. Why did the lessons end with the Plains of Abraham battle? He could not comprehend that approach to Canadian history.

Life in an institution, by its nature, was sometimes lonely for one so far from home. One year, he stayed there for ten straight months with no visitation—absolutely none. The playground was unsupervised. He and a few aboriginal students usually stayed on the edge of the playground while the majority French kids played their games. Off classroom time was not very inclusive for those who were left out.

During World War II, the men who worked in the woods were less available, making it necessary for his family to move permanently from their winter quarters to a new home along the little Boggy River. Keith's sister was old enough to walk with him to the one-room school two miles away (3 km). The teachers were either permit, "unqualified", or both since teachers were scarce during wartime. Work was easier to find elsewhere under better circumstances.

Meanwhile, his eldest spinster aunt was a teacher in a one-room school sponsored by the Anglican Church on an Indian reserve, 40 miles (64 km) by water from road and civilization. With his parents' consent, his aunt borrowed him for company.

Comforts of life were minimal. He attended class; but his aunt, fearing tuberculosis infection which was rampant, would never let him play with the Indian children. Yet, he observed their life and, by osmosis, sometimes, felt and acted more like them and at some variance from his aunt's Victorian ideals. She was good to him, but he yearned for more. He still has a letter which he wrote, fantasizing meeting a boy companion by a stream where they watched the sunlit coloured pebbles and fish in the water swirls of the stream.

One day, he came across a pen pal column in a weekly newspaper. Being interested, he wrote a letter about having ridden in a genuine birch-bark canoe which was paddled by an old Indian man who also taught him how to make bows and arrows—all true. What was unexpected was a flood of responding letters from various parts of the English-speaking world. Some suggested material visitation with great interest. Poor Keith! He did not know what he should do—it was too much. He cannot remember having answered a single letter.

Back to his home eleven miles (18 km) west of Falcon Lake, there was only a trail to reach the lake. He remembers going there once by horse and seeing only one cabin along the whole lake.

Later, his father helped build a gravel road and then pavement, which is now Highway #1 East, part of the Trans-Canada. He made his living as "road boss" on the 70-mile (113 km) section from Richer to the Ontario boundary.

Keith returned briefly to the local school and then again away from home to the most available high school, which was at Teulon. There was a boarding home for boys and one close by for girls. For four years, he lived with an average of fifteen boys, most from distant places.

From being an only boy at home, it meant that he learned much about socialization with boys from many different backgrounds. No cultural amenities were provided; but they played games, had endless conversations, kept up their interest in girls, and borrowed each other's musical instruments.

Keith belonged to a small band and even played at a few local dances. The boys alternately gave the matrons respect and a hard time. He had earlier read avidly *Tom Brown's School Days*, by Thomas Hughes, which had an impact on him; but this was different in actuality.

For him, school was secondary. He did not apply himself as much as he should have, especially after a competent staff almost totally resigned and the replacements were not themselves very disciplined. The students went from a strict school to one with too much freedom for the times. He feels, though, that the staff did the best that they could. The students even went on strike at the boarding home.

Were things partly influenced because of the war? Probably they were. He had no grievances from home and signed his own attendance and report cards.

He joined the air force cadets and, later, the army reserve. It was certainly a period of adolescent fervour and learning, but no harm came from their adventures. Because of the way in which he studied, he barely graduated from grade twelve.

He met John Ryan there and began a lifelong friendship. Both boys decided to go teaching on permit. They remember one teacher at the school with fondness, John Norquay, the descendant of a Manitoba premier. He looked somewhat like Santa Claus with a moustache, but no beard. He was jolly and very even in disposition through the vicissitudes of the school and the boys' antics.

There has been a long tradition of teaching in Keith's family. His Grandfather McNiven was principal in Rivers when he died. While in Winnipeg, he was a founder of the Manitoba Teachers' Society. Four children, including Keith's mother, became teachers. One of his stepfather's brothers was head of a Normal School in Bavaria, Germany.

Ah, permit teaching! This year was his first big responsibility of work—for $1,000 per year. His destination was a one-room school twelve miles (19 km) west of Lac du Bonnet. His dad drove his truck, taking him and a month's supply of food over mud-rutted roads. They found the place with difficulty—no reception; but near the school was a teacher's log cabin cottage.

Inside the building were a heater, a bunk bed, an enamel wash basin, and a kerosene lamp. Outside, there was a little firewood which he cut. Later, he borrowed from the one and only neighbour a team of horses to haul wood. Within a month, Keith took his meals at the same neighbour's place—a welcome relief.

Supplies in the school were minimal, for example, not enough readers. He had grades one to seven, with a large primary class. The older siblings helped their young teacher to teach the youngest children the three Rs. Not all beginners spoke English on their arrival at school. The inspector arrived about a month later, stayed for an hour or so, and then dismissed the class to go partridge hunting—and never seen again.

On one rare occasion, Keith had to go to Winnipeg. He was dropped off at Lac du Bonnet and then proceeded to walk the twelve miles (19 km) to his school in time for Monday morning. Halfway back, he came to a small village where a three-day Ukrainian wedding was taking place. He met his neighbour there and was invited to partake of the festivities.

He does not recall all of the events, but time passed —and, two days later, he continued his journey. How he marked the register, he does not exactly remember either; but whatever he did or did not do, did not seem to matter. As the old saying goes by those exiled in Siberia about the law, "God is in His heaven and the czar is far away."

John Ryan permit taught similarly cross-country with no connecting roads. The two young men did not meet each other, but Keith still has about a dozen letters, up to fifteen pages long, which they exchanged about their tough circumstances. There was plenty of humour about events, about teaching theories, and about a philosophy of life in general.

John had distinct plans for the future—university, professorship, travel abroad—and he did all those things timely and systematically. Keith, on the other hand, had the philosophy and curiosity for learning, but largely for where it took him at his own pace and inclination, not that which was set by the usual education and work practice.

Normal School was a distinct, delightful, and wonderful learning adventure—with not much of the formal part for him. Meeting so many bright-eyed and bushy-tailed idealist companions as equals on the journey was of more interest. He feels that our enthusiasm affected the teachers more than theirs did the students.

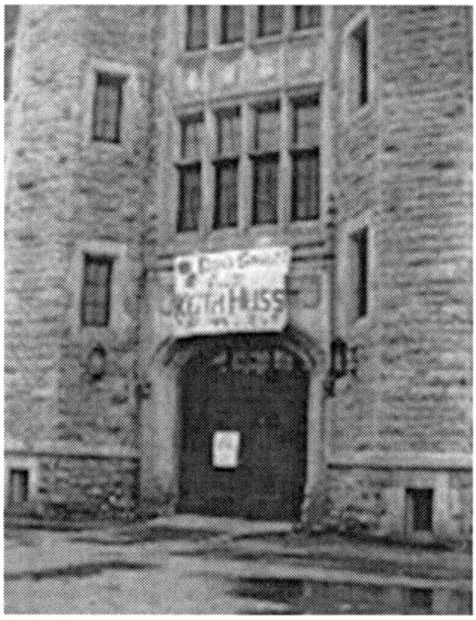

16. Campaign Poster

Keith roomed with John and Harry Rudy, the latter from Balmoral, in the Frontenac dormitory, a wing of the main building. They talked many late nights while they dated girls on other nights. There was a girl-boy ratio of at least 3:1—which was to the boys' advantage.

Usually, Keith had to sleep in someone's class, often that of Mrs. Turner or Miss Ring. In Mr. Herron's class, he read *War and Peace*. None of the teachers seemed to appreciate his needs. He was fortunate and grateful that they did not fail him. He had no problem with passing in the summer schools.

He liked art, physical education, and sometimes Mr. Turner's class for entertainment. The Normal School administrators, Mr. Lightly and Mr. Moorhead, complemented each other, liked their students, and worked in their interests. However, the chef was cranky and some of the students made life miserable for him.

Keith provides a list of his post-secondary education and his teaching assignments—all in Manitoba: permit teaching near Lac du Bonnet in a one-room school in 1949–50; Normal School 1950–51, including two weeks practice teaching at Portage Correctional School for Boys; Hutterite colonies at Waldheim and New Rosedale; grades seven and eight at Whitemouth for five years, during which he helped to write an MTS salary schedule; Norberry Junior High in St. Vital for five years; sabbatical at University of Winnipeg; Glenlawn Senior High in St. Vital for two years; grades seven and eight in Waterhen Community School in Frontier School Division; two summer schools in Confluent Education at Winnipeg and Brandon; principal of Camperville Elementary in Winnipegosis School Division; principal of William S. Patterson Elementary in Lord Selkirk School Division; social studies consultant for the Dept. of Education; liaison officer at University of Winnipeg with Dean Clake for the Dept. of Education; adult education training from Frontier College, in Toronto, Ont.; taught mostly functionally illiterates reading at Stony Mountain.

Normal School was also delightful because he met Aileen Harbottle. They were married a few years later and spent their first five years together teaching at Whitemouth.

They enjoyed their newly built apartment first home. Often, and especially on weekends, they scooted cross-country between A-class roads to eighty acres (32 ha) of forested land and their log cabin along the same river where Keith had grown up.

Overall, teaching at Whitemouth ranks first among his experiences. Whitemouth was a quiet unruffled community with solid citizenry. This was reflected in their children who were eager to learn. They respected their teachers highly and were willing to work diligently without much persuasion.

Aileen had grades three and four and also was the CGIT leader, with most of the girls coming from Keith's class. They had many new adventures with their leader "Twinkle". Nearly every class day in the spring term, Keith raced the boys to the best spots for pickerel fishing.

An elderly lady, Mrs. Godolphin, taught grade one. Her youngsters followed her like a flock of snow birds, even after she left the school to return to her quaint little home. She was just as kind and loving to her colleagues.

Her husband Will was second generation Old English stock, with old world charm and manners. He was an artist who had left his family business when they wanted him to be sensible and settle down. He did study the great painters, many of whose works were to be seen in London. When he had depleted his money, he was too proud to seek help, and thus stayed on for years without contacting his family on either side of the ocean. He had to live in the Bohemian section in the city out of necessity —and maybe by inclination. Eventually, he came back, put away his paint pots—as he said—married, raised a family, and "kept his nose to the grindstone". When he retired, he and his wife moved to Whitemouth.

A decade later, Keith and Aileen met them, and by then he was his old artist self. Keith identified with his wide-ranging mind and with his idealism still aflame. He was a philosopher in a large inclusive sense. Will did not always suffer absurdities of life well. If he were critical, it was always in a reparative manner. He had lived for a time on the other side, a Bohemian lifestyle which, at that time, was looked upon as lower class. He knew that people in "that class" were basically the same as anyone else, but more honest. Keith thought of him, for want of a better word, a spirited guide, because he was more intimate with Keith than his own parents were. Will quickly responded, "Don't call me that, Keith."

As you can see, Will Godolphin meant a great deal to his teacher friend as he did to others. The two men spent many hours together, being closer to each other than to their respective families. He was a rare character who loved poetry and natural things with equal passion.

It took Keith so long to complete his Bachelor of Arts degree that one of his last professors was his friend John Ryan, who taught geography at University of Winnipeg. The further he proceeded toward his degree, the better his grades became. Pursuing his idea of education, he picked, dropped, and even failed courses—anything to continue free-wheeling open-ended means of acquiring learning "from inside out".

He wanted to major in psychology, but behaviourism was in vogue; and he finally balked at taking the required statistical rat-course. He was more interested in such psychologists as Carl Jung and his approach to what humans were and why they behave as they do. That was a "no-no" in the psychology department.

Therefore, he switched his major to geography and took as many full and half courses as he could. He came near to the gold medal award even though he had not reached for it. He was more flattered when two of his professors commented that he was the best-read student across whom they had ever come.

Keith had read thousands of books by this time—non-fiction mostly and course unrelated. Earlier, in addition to Carl Jung, he had studied the works of Aldous Huxley and Bernard Shaw. Coincidentally, all three were born on July 26, as was Keith. He still reads voraciously in general and has specifically studied metaphysics and mysticism. Far Eastern life and religion have been of periodic interest connected with travels which he made.

From being principal of a brand-new school in Comperville, he signed as principal of William S. Patterson Elementary School, in Clandeboye, within Lord Selkirk School Division. It was the only open-air area school in the district and the superintendent wanted new blood to make it work.

Keith had trained in Confluent Education—an affective model of education that emphasized both head and heart. The superintendent cherry-picked a group of teachers that was compatible with this style of teaching and close cooperation. Everything worked out well. The school became very community-oriented with the help of volunteers both in and out of the school.

One year, they doubled the school budget for extra office, science, and sports equipment through various projects. One of Keith's concerns was that the staff was being raided for "higher" positions—for example, administration—all men, it so happened; but before he left, he persuaded a well-qualified woman on staff to compete for the position. She did apply and received it.

He then took a position as social studies consultant with the Department of Education. When he arrived, one of the well-known school superintendents, who had visited the school while Keith was on staff, asked him, "Why would you want to do that? That's the kind of school I'd like to switch to."

It so happened that the inspectorate was being phased out at the time. However, the inspector was right in a way which Keith did not expect. He found the new position somewhat lifeless with no bustle of students around and without the reality of working "where the rubber hits the road". Working days and nights in revising curricula was no compensation for the kind of satisfaction of live teaching.

His last teaching of any significance and challenge was instructing adults at Stony Mountain under contract with an organization called Frontier College in Toronto. Here, it was rewarding to help men become literate, which greatly enhanced their opportunities in locating jobs and being participating citizens. By this time, he was becoming burned out.

Over a year before pension time—age fifty-five—he decided to travel extensively. He changed his name from Huss to Seidel (his mother's married name before divorce) to "psych up" his new identification. He explored several countries in the Far East, but mainly India. Next, he lived for six months on a commune in the Sierras of California.

Then, he returned to Canada, a brief expatriate. In Winnipeg, he joined a company of friends, five in all, and purchased a vacation property in Vernon, in the Okanagan Valley of British Columbia. For five years, he was the manager on site—a wonderful experience.

Then, he and Aileen met and, two years later, remarried. They had been twelve years apart. That ended the gypsy and communal life experiment. Majority family roots lay in Winnipeg and Aileen had kept their original home.

He and Aileen have always had lake or country property; but in 2008, they sold their old mission and cottage manse at Carrick. They had converted the church into a studio workshop, for clay sculpturing and other activities. On their two acres (0.8 ha), they created a rock garden, artesian-fed ponds, and a facsimile oriental garden. They still retain an old family acreage in common. For vacation, they often go to the west coast; but Winnipeg is their base.

30 Emily James

She loved his history classes. Her teacher would stroll into the classroom, perch on the corner of his desk, and demonstrate that history is not only something of the past, but something that can be exciting and relevant to the present. He did not need to rely on a textbook. He knew history!

This man was Mr. Meldrum, her principal at McCreary High School. He had a very positive influence in this student's becoming a teacher. She was a very shy girl, but his encouragement and his belief in her helped her to take that giant step into the unknown world. He was a role model for a girl who decided to make teaching her profession.

Emily was born in McCreary. She took her first eight grades in a country school at Norgate, and her high schooling at McCreary.

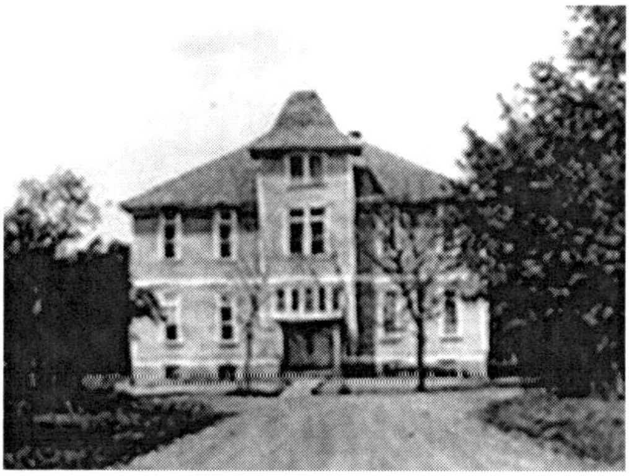

17. McCreary School

She grew up on a farm which was fairly isolated. Thus, her memories of Normal School are about all the girls—so many. She made good friends. The sessions with them in her room were something very new to her. She really enjoyed every minute of it. She has kept in contact with a few of the friends from those days. Meeting them at the reunion at Gimli in 2006 was a wonderful experience.

She remembers Mr. Chidley, our practical mathematics teacher at Normal School. She was always amazed with the manner in which he could work so deftly with mathematics.

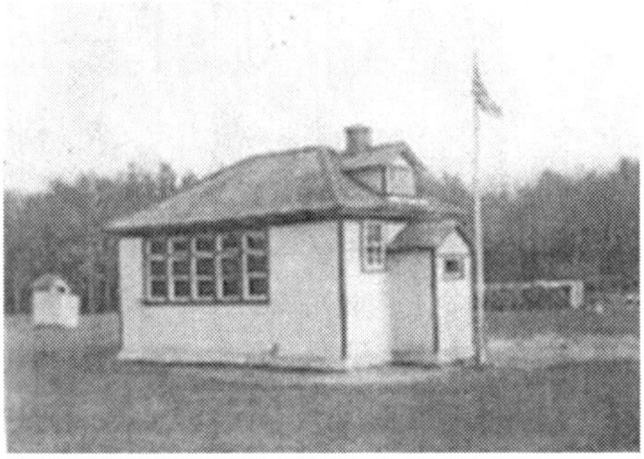

18. Turtle Plains

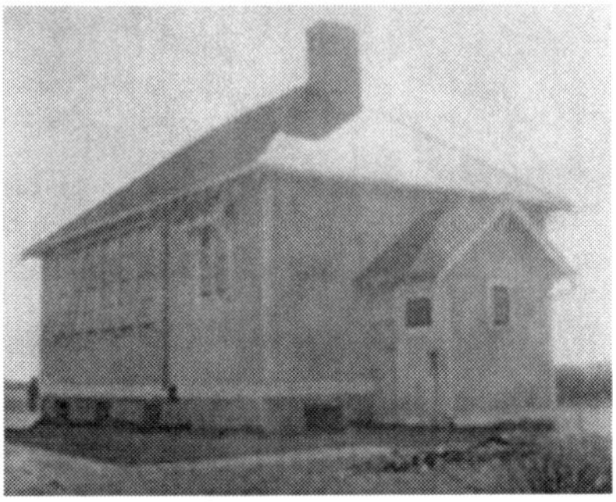

19. Osprey School

After she graduated, she taught in country schools at Turtle Plains, Osprey, Victoria, Bower, and Meadows—all in Manitoba. Emily taught for fifteen years. She has three children—one girl and two boys.

Emily has numerous hobbies. She knits toques for the homeless and crochets blankets for the Linus Project. Painting and making cards provide her with enjoyment. She is an oil painter of landscapes and still life, but she feels that she is very amateur.

Although she has not joined many clubs, she has helped with Awana at church. Awana helps churches and parents worldwide to raise children and youth to know, love, and serve Christ. Based in the Chicago area, Awana is the only organization with fully integrated evangelism and discipleship programmes for ages two to eighteen that actively involve parents, church leaders, and mentors.

She is also a member of Overcome Outreach. This is a twelve-step programme for people with problems, using the twelve steps of Alcoholics Anonymous. The main sources of information are the Serenity Bible and the Life Recovery Bible. These Bible translations are the same as other versions, but the explanations are for people in recovery. People who are not believers would probably have a problem accepting the general method of recovery, but the programme is open to anyone whether the problem is over-eating, anger, gambling, or anything in between.

Emily has always been a great reader, so it is difficult to pick a favourite book from her childhood. She enjoyed *Black Beauty*, by Anna Sewell, and *Tom Sawyer*, by Mark Twain, among others. Today, she enjoys reading Christian books and has many favourite authors. One book that really stands out is *Dana's Valley*, by Janette Oke and Laurel Oke Logan.

In 1984, she and her husband flew to England because her aunt had passed away without a will and they were her closest next-of-kin. They travelled from Land's End, in Cornwall, to Newcastle, in Durham, meeting Emily's remaining relatives. They were known only by the correspondence that kept families connected. She has not seen them since then. Some have since passed away, but she still keeps in contact with the rest.

They did not go sight-seeing—only "people" seeing. They did not realize how very close they were to Stonehenge and Hadrian's Wall. Therefore, they missed them—and survived.

She would suggest that tourists visit Canada's Prairies, especially Manitoba. In summer, there are numerous lakes throughout the province where people can fish or use a boat. In winter, there are skiing, ice fishing, skidooing, and many other winter sports. The scenery is beautiful and varied. It is a wonderful place to live or to visit.

Emily would give teenagers the same advice which she gave her own children. Get involved with youth groups and be active in sports. If you cannot for some reason play the game, there will be something you can do. Stay away from drugs and alcohol and have nothing to do with gangs. Become active in your church. Help those who cannot help themselves.

For those contemplating the teaching profession, she would admonish that they not go into the profession for the money. If their main focus not be on the children, they should consider another field.

She feels that Pierre Elliot Trudeau made a strong negative impact on Canada. She did not like his underhandedness and his smugness in the way he governed. He appeared as though he did not care about Western Canada and, thus, changed Canada forever.

Her health failed her in 1973 and, thus, she was unable to teach after that. She looked after her mother for eighteen years until she died in 1997, four months short of being one hundred years old.

Basically though, Emily's life has been good. She is no longer the shy girl that she was in Normal School. Thanks to Al-Anon and other twelve-step programmes, she is now a different person.

Her philosophy in life is to please God. In everything that she does, she puts Him first. She brought up her children to believe in Him, and has done the same for her grandchildren and her great-grandchildren. She is teaching them to love the Lord. Her prayer is that they will follow the teachings and not stray.

31
Vera (Jones) Skayman

Living in small quarters can be interesting provided one does not have claustrophobia. When one moves alone to a new town, this situation may occur, especially if the school board does not have much to offer or there is a scarcity of available accommodation elsewhere.

One such situation arose when a young teacher moved to the town of Hamiota to assume her new position. There was a bed available so that she had a place to sleep at night. There was a hot plate to use when cooking. That did limit what she could prepare and having a guest for a meal. Very little else in the line of furnishings could cram into that one-room apartment.

After she had spent some time residing in this set-up, a Good Samaritan came to her rescue. Another young lady living in the community felt that she could share her apartment with this unfortunate resident. How thankful the young teacher was in being made this offer! It did not take long for her to accept the opportunity for change. It was an experience that she could never forget.

Vera was born in Glenboro, one of eight children in her parents' family. Saturday was grocery shopping day for the family. So off to town they went—covering the eight miles (13 km) with horse and cutter, if it were winter. If they were fortunate, they were able to see a movie at the local theatre. Her dad always bought some candy for the children—no matter how tough the living situation was.

She commenced her education in a nearby rural school named Mimer, which included grades one to eight. In summer, she walked five miles (8 km) a day with some of her brothers and sisters and other neighbours along the way. In winter, her dad drove them to school with horse and sleigh—and many blankets. Sometimes, the temperature was forty degrees below zero and the horses were up to their bellies in snow. Every year, there was a new permit teacher. And there was a very scary principal —Mr. Lockhart.

An unpleasant memory was the outbreak of head lice, which spread throughout the school. The head of each infected child was treated with coal oil; and then, the lice were combed out. What an unpleasant task that was! There was another disagreeable situation as some new immigrants in the area loved garlic. It was so strong that it would almost knock a person over.

She remembers in elementary school playing fox and goose during the winter. This was a tag game played on two concentric circles drawn out in the snow. In the centre was a safe haven. From this spot, radial spokes extended to the outer circle. Tagging could take place on the circles and the spokes, but not in the centre haven.

A memory of life at Normal School was the experience of sleeping in a bunk bed in Radisson Hall. She reserved the top bunk and she did not sleep walk. As long as she had a ladder, she had no problem. Her co-partner was Florence Chambers from Belmont, near Glenboro.

Our Normal School teacher whom Vera particularly remembers is Mr. Clarke, who taught classroom management. She describes him as being stern, but with a good sense of humour.

Prior to attending Normal School, she was a permit teacher in the rural Stratherne School where she had grades one to eight. The school was located near Wawanesa. Immediately following her year at Normal School, Vera taught grades two and three in Hamiota School for two years. Then, she changed her profession to that of a farm wife, living not far from Hamiota.

As a child, she enjoyed reading *Call of the Wild*, by Jack London. As an adult she liked *The Proud and the Free*, by Janet Dailey.

Today, she keeps active by participating in curling, bowling, and golfing. Although she likes to golf and to bowl, curling has been the love of her life. She did win some trophies during her lifetime, but the highlight of her life was going to Gimli in 1994 with three other "fun-loving gals".

They were playing for the Provincial Golden Gals title, a category that is for ladies over sixty years of age. Her skip's name was *Little* and that of the opposition in the final game was *Small*. Guess what! Vera's rink won—and the headlines read, "Little too much for Small." The picture of the winners was placed on the wall at the Keystone Centre in Brandon.

Seven out of eight of her family members were curlers. She has a photo of the four Jones sisters and the three Jones brothers plus a neighbour who participated in a male versus female challenge match. The girls won—and love to brag about their accomplishment.

Vera and her sister flew to Newfoundland and were bussed around to see the sights of the province. They enjoyed seeing a different scenery and different ways of living. She remembers the thousands of pine trees along the narrow road leading out of St. John's. They were pretty; but, after a time, the visitors would have liked a change.

While in St. John's, they visited the Citadel, from which they marvelled at the view out over the large expanse of water. They went out on a boat and did some deep-sea fishing, but no bites. They also saw many fishing boats and lobster traps. Everyone had to try their "Screech"—a strange kind of terrible drink. They found that the people are very jolly and laid back. However, the ladies felt that they would not enjoy the climate of Newfoundland.

When they had completed their visit, they travelled all the way to Winnipeg by bus. Surprisingly, they did not find the bus ride home too uncomfortable as the passengers were allowed to explore Nova Scotia, New Brunswick, Prince Edward Island, and Quebec. It was a long, enjoyable trip home.

Vera recommends that a traveller in Canada should visit the International Peace Garden, near Boissevain, at the U.S.-Canada border, in July or August. Enjoy the extensive variety of wild flowers, trees, and shrubs abundant in this garden. The flowers are at their peak during this time.

Her advice to teenagers is to practise respect and to do unto others as they would have others do unto them. They should work hard and live life to the fullest. For anyone considering the teaching profession, she says to go for it.

The teacher whom Vera particularly remembers is Erla Nattress, who taught all subjects and was friendly, approachable, and willing to spend extra time.

She is very appreciative of help given to her and her family by Al and Paulette Shewfelt since she moved to Brandon in 1987. Much of her time has been spent helping her two handicapped children who live together. Her son Glen met Al at his first job. They have been good friends for the past twenty years. They go to hockey games and have coffee out together. The Shewfelts take the whole family for car rides and short trips. These two deserve a medal. They have been a great help to Vera.

In her community, she volunteers with the United Commercial Travellers (UTC), a service organization or club which raises money for their community and gives grants to those in need. They support Cor Enterprises, which is a workplace for the mentally challenged. She helps to sell daffodils in a local mall and collects donations at Christmas for Helping Hands, an organization which supports the Soup Kitchen and other projects. Anyone who has a worthy project can apply to UCT for funds. Bingo is one of the organization's largest projects.

She likes former British Prime Minister Churchill for his toughness. Although he was not Canadian, his leadership during World War II had an effect on Canada and the rest of the world.

Her philosophy of life is to do unto others as you would have others do unto you. She recommends that everyone should work hard, play hard, practise respect, love well, laugh much, and live life to its fullest.

32
Ena (Kandall) Sparrow

She was working at the United Grill in Brandon for two summers when she was in grades ten and eleven. The grill was located on 10th Street, just south of Rosser Avenue. She rented a room from an elderly woman who lived on 11th Street.

One night as she was walking home after her shift, she noticed that a young man was following her. She was terrified! Therefore, she ran home as speedily as she could. The house was dark! On entering it, she found her landlady sitting in the living room without any lights on.

Ena tried to be calm as though nothing unusual had happened when her landlady spoke to her, but she was so afraid of that young man. She hurried directly to her room upstairs. When she felt that she could do so, she cautiously peered into the cold darkness outside. Was he still looking for her? Yes, there he was! He was looking at the next house. Maybe, he had thought that she was in it.

The next day, she told her employer of her frightening experience. That was not going to happen again! From that time, he walked her home at night.

She met her colleague from the grill, Wilma Shadlock, thirty-five years later. Now, they have picked up their friendship again. Still, she has chilling memories of that unnerving experience.

Ena was one of five children—also including her brothers Kenneth, John, Sandy, and Arthur—born to John and Albertina Kandall, who had emigrated from Finland to Canada.

When they came to Rosendale, her father worked on the Canadian National Railways (CNR). Three years later, in 1935, he transferred from the Rosendale station to a foreman's position at Exira, a short distance north of Austin. He travelled to his work by jigger. There were frequent freight and passenger trains passing over the line, which was close to Ena's home. Because of the proximity of the house, hoboes often stopped to ask her mother for food.

The three-bedroom house was painted by the railway crew members. There was no electricity or telephone at the house. The family used a wood or coal stove for warmth, a kettle for tea or coffee, and a side boiler for the stove to provide hot water. They used a barrel of ice and snow for the water, using a big kettle to heat it on the stove. Coal-oil lamps provided light for the house. With their battery radio, they could listen to western music, drama, and Hockey Night in Canada. A well near the house provided the water for every use. The house had a summer kitchen; but in the winter, the living room became the kitchen. Of course, they had outdoor plumbing with an outhouse.

One night, one of her brothers set a fire causing severe damage to the house and a nearby shed. With the help of neighbours, the fire was eventually extinguished with water. However, it was necessary for the family to sleep on blankets on the grass that night.

The children would visit a bachelor farmer, Mr. Gatley, who lived across the tracks from their house. They felt that his house had an unpleasant odour from his cats that would sit on the oven door for warmth. When the children would upset outhouses on Hallowe'en night, they avoided this farm as Mr. Gatley had threatened them with a shotgun. They did enjoy hunting prairie chickens with him. She and three other young girls liked to play hide-and-seek with him.

Her family purchased bottled milk from the nearby Anderson farm. It was Ena's job to walk across the field and through a wooded area at night for the milk. One evening, the farmer's handicapped son waited for her behind the barn and tried to catch her. She discarded the bottle and set off for home at her top speed. Thereafter, she followed the road instead of taking a shortcut.

Ena obtained her grades one to eight at Springbrook School District and grades nine to twelve at Austin School District, both districts in Manitoba.

The children walked for one mile (1.6 km) along the railroad or walked or rode their bicycles one-half mile (800 m) along the road when they went to school. Once when they were walking on the rails, they saw a train coming. Quickly, they moved as closely to the steep ditch as they could. The train slowed down as it needed to stop at the coal dock and the water tower.

When the train had come to a halt, the crew in the caboose invited the children in. What a thrill that was! How many young people have such an opportunity to see inside a real caboose? They showed the children what was there and offered them sweets and fruits for their lunch. All were eagerly accepted.

When she was ten years old, she had an accident at the school. At noon, the students would play at an old farm site which had a creek. They would sometimes paddle in the water. One afternoon when the bell rang and they were running to the school, Ena caught her leg in barbed wire. This resulted in a deep three-inch (8 cm) cut on her leg. When she arrived at the school, her brother John rushed her home and covered her wound with a bandage. She did not visit the doctor for stitches.

Her brother Sandy went to school early to start the fire. In winter, it was so cold and there were piles of snow everywhere. Sometimes, the children would have a ride to school by neighbourhood horses and wagon or their dad would give them a ride on the jigger for part of the way.

Her name is *Ina*, a Finnish name, which is pronounced "EE-na". One of her teachers would pronounce her name using a long "I" instead of a long "E". As a result, she decided to spell her name Ena so that people would pronounce it properly. How many of us have had a similar problem with the ways that teachers have mispronounced our names?

Her Dad had a small barn with a cow, some pigs, chickens, and a pony. The children used to gather hay for the livestock along the road and railroad. One day, Ena and two of her brothers were playing hide-and-seek around the haystack. They climbed to the top, but Ena tumbled off and cracked a rib when she landed on the ground. Her family took her to the doctor, who taped her ribs. She does not remember how long that she was bound by the tape, but she does remember how ripping it off hurt.

Since her Dad worked on the CNR, she had a pass on the railroad. She took accordion lessons in Winnipeg, using the free passage to go to and from the city. From the train station, she would take a taxi to the studio, which was beside Eaton's store on Portage Avenue. After the lessons, she would walk back to the station on Main Street to catch her train.

When she was in grade nine, she had to walk or bicycle for two and one-half miles (4 km) to Austin High School. If she wanted to go out in the evening, it was necessary to walk back to Austin and then walk home again afterwards. She and her friends would go to a movie, a dance, or outdoor ice-skating. Ena was invited to a costume dance in Austin one night. She dressed as Daisy Mae Scragg, of Dogpatch. She wore a green blouse with black dots and a skirt and she was bare-footed. Her partner, who dressed as L'il Abner Yokum, was so shy that he participated in only one dance.

One summer night as she was bicycling home, a transport truck stopped and the driver offered her a ride. Ena did not want to go with the men in the truck. Therefore, she told them that her house was nearby, when actually it was not. She biked into the farmyard at hand and stayed until the truck had left. In the meantime, the farmer's dog barked at her. She was so frightened! When she felt that it was safe, she pedalled her bicycle as hard as she could until she was safely at home.

At Normal School, she worked in the kitchen to earn a little money. She participated in such sports as softball, volleyball, and hockey and won awards. She was a member of the choir and took part in stage plays. She felt that our principal, Mr. Moorhead, and his staff of teachers were very good.

After graduating from Normal School, she was hired by the Turriff School, in the Forrest School District. In Forrest, she rented a room from Mrs. White, for two years. In the third year, she and a high school student rented a small house. To further her education as a teacher, she attended summer school in Gimli. There were such sporting activities as volleyball, baseball, and swimming in a wonderful setting beside Lake Winnipeg. She did have classes, but it was an enjoyable time, also.

She joined the Forrest Church choir and can remember the school Christmas concerts which were held at the church. During her time at Forrest, she met Edward Sparrow at the choir. They married in 1954 and settled on the farm.

Ena had no experience as a farmer when she and Edward married, but she learned to drive the truck and tractor. She fed the cattle, chickens, pigs, and horses and milked the cows. It was a valuable experience, except when a horse kicked her. She experienced a very sore stomach for a while.

She and Edward had four children: Robert, Joanna, Sandra, and Cathy. Between raising their family, housekeeping, gardening, and farming, they kept very busy. She helped with the Forrest 4-H club as their children were members. She also helped with the Sunday school classes at church. The children took piano lessons and gymnastic lessons.

After being married for twenty-eight years, she was divorced. She moved to Brandon where she worked at the Eaton's store in the jewelry department and then in the clothing department. She continued working there until the store closed eleven years later.

In her home, she works in pottery, enjoying the making of such items as vases, bowls, plates, and other art work with the clay. She also does pencil drawing and painting. She has a small vegetable garden, but mainly a flower garden, with the latter having been in the Community for Blooms display.

She enjoys visiting family and friends in Manitoba, Saskatchewan, Ontario, Alberta, and British Columbia. She has been able to visit Ireland, Scotland, England, and some parts of the United States. Since her daughter Cathy lives in Ireland, she has had the opportunity of visiting that country a few times. Ireland is a wonderful place! Since she has travelled within Canada, she recommends this country as a beautiful place to visit and a lovely place to live!

Her philosophy is to be happy and enjoy one's life.

33 Peter Peters

What is one person's enjoyment may be another person's misery. Occasionally, some young boys are guilty of that type of amusement. Being ticklish may provide a motive for instigators.

He was fifteen years old and in grade nine, taking his grade by correspondence at the school. Word went out that he was very ticklish. One day, three boys, ages from thirteen to fifteen years, decided to have fun—at the other boy's expense. They crept up behind him, grabbed him, and threw him to the ground. While holding him to the ground, they sought out his ticklish spots and set to work. The more he squirmed, the more they worked on him. They did not stop after one minute, but carried on for at least ten minutes! It was so much fun for the aggressors.

The victim claims that this was his worst ten minutes in school to that date. Having survived the ordeal and being released, he rushed to his desk, packed his books and supplies, and made a bee-line for home—never to return to that school. He completed his grades nine and ten by correspondence at home. This very dramatic experience became a laughing matter at school. To this day, he shudders at the memory of it.

Peter was born on a farm seven miles (11 km) northeast of the town of Killarney. He began his education in a rural school in Victoria Lake School District, which was southwest of Killarney and two miles (3 km) north of the U.S. Border.

It may have been the most notorious school in the province. In nine years, the school had ten different teachers—mostly permit teachers. Mr. Clarke was the school inspector for most of those years. He knew the school well and visited it more often than he may have visited other schools. Sometimes, he would come when the RCMP were there.

Because of a job commitment, Peter enrolled a few days late at the Normal School for the 1950–51 school year. The teacher for the first class for Class D that Monday morning was Mr. Clarke—the same Mr. Clarke who had been inspector. When the new student entered the classroom somewhat timid, he sat down at the only vacant desk in the room. It was located at the back of the room on the far side from the door.

When the teacher came in, he noticed a newcomer in the corner of the classroom—and he walked halfway down the aisle, looked at him, pointed his finger at him; and, in his usual Mr. Clarke style, spoke only two words. He clearly said, "Victoria Lake", turned and went to stand at his desk. There was no smile attached. If Peter had been a gopher, he would have very quickly "dug a hole" and crawled into it.

Ben Hanuschak and Peter were on a kitchen duty team at Normal School. Their job was to peel potatoes—not a bowl of potatoes as one would at home—but a 100-pound (45 kg) sack. He had never seen a mechanical potato peeler. Although it saved considerable manual labour, it also wasted much of the potato content. The potatoes would roll around on the peeling disc until all the skin was removed. The result was that the peeled product was round like a ball or oval like an egg. That was how the chef, Mr. Cartwright, wanted them to be.

Following one year of teaching in a country school in the hamlet of Lena, south of Killarney, he and his wife Helen farmed for the next twenty-five years. Then, he was a shareholder and manager of Boundary Fertilizer Limited—a chemical and fertilizer retail outlet six miles (10 km) south of Killarney—for thirteen years. After that, he owned and operated a 4,500-square-foot (418 m^2) gift and general store in Killarney for another thirteen years. During the above fifty-one years, Peter spent twenty-five years in a pastoral ministry in a fairly large church in Boissevain.

When he was a chemical fertilizer dealer, from 1979 to 1992, in one twelve-month period he won volume sales and good service awards from different companies. These awards included all-expense-paid trips to Germany, Quebec City, Las Vegas, and New Orleans. Previously, he and Helen had enjoyed a fourteen-day cruise on the *Nordic Prince* from Miami, Fla., to the coast of South America and back. This included stops of one day at each of eight different Caribbean islands.

Their trip to New Orleans and surrounding area was a very fascinating, educational, and exciting trip. The history of the area, the mansions, the food, and the many amenities made it a very memorable experience.

In the prime of their lives, they travelled considerably, mostly on the North American continent.

Peter recommends visiting Manitoba during October and enjoying three of the many, most beautiful areas of this part of creation, for example Whiteshell Provincial Park, the Turtle Mountain provincial parks and the adjacent Peace Garden, and a drive north through Flin Flon, eastward to the Paint Lake area near Thompson, north to Lynn Lake, and finally back south to Winnipeg.

Options for children's books were, to his knowledge, very limited when he was a child. He learned to speak English when he started school—and he learned to read soon thereafter. Even "The Reader" was very interesting and very exciting. He learned to know two children, Jerry and Jane, whom he had not known before.

In recent years, he has read about one book per week. He finds biographies and autobiographies very interesting. One particularly fascinating book is *Blood Covenant*, by Michael Franzese. This is the story of Mafia boss Michael Franzese, who actually left the Mafia and lived a very inspirational and productive life.

Over the years, he has worked in more than one dozen volunteer organizations. The most recent has been Big Brothers. Approximately five hundred children in Winnipeg have a big brother or a big sister. Peter has been with his "little brother" since 2004. In 2008, he was honoured by being chosen as Winnipeg Big Brother of the Year. He was very surprised to receive this award, and he does not feel that he deserved the honour. Both big brother and little brother appeared on the Hero of the Week programme of a Manitoba television station.

Peter enumerates six points for teenagers to consider in regard to their future. Be goal oriented. Be focused. Reach for the top, but do not step on others to gain it. Share your talents and resources with others. Do not envy those who are three or four rungs ahead of you, and be compassionate toward those who are unable to climb. Keep a daily journal and make it into good reading for the future!

He offers four points for those interested in entering retail sales. Be honest! Cause your customers to do your advertising, as this is much cheaper and much more effective. Do not keep two sets of books, since it is not too difficult to deal with Revenue Canada if an "honest" mistake has been made; however, by observation, he has learned that the “smell” of fictitious numbers really draws their attention. Be good to your employees because, if you are, they will respond by being good for your business.

He had numerous good teachers prior to attending Normal School. Mr. Victor Tesson taught his two favourite subjects, namely, mathematics and chemistry. This man was kind, friendly, and easy-going; and he taught his subject material so well that learning was a joy. In fact, he was the only teacher who had ever invited his entire class to his wedding. Then when the class celebrated its 50th anniversary, he came from British Columbia to join his former students in Manitoba!

Peter attended Mennonite Collegiate Institute at Gretna, a private Christian high school, for his grades eleven and twelve. It was three hours by car from his home. In those days, going home for Christmas and Easter was customary.

Mr. Schaefer, one of his teachers, was a father figure to him during those years when he missed his parental home. This man was also an ordained minister, Christian educator, and brilliant historian. He had a heart for each of his students, being interested in the emotional, the intellectual, the social, and the spiritual well-being of each of his students.

Mr. Schaefer impacted his life in numerous ways, and this impact was a long-term impact! Four years after Peter’s graduation, Mr. Schaefer officiated at the wedding of Peter and Helen. This couple was blessed to share love and life for over forty-two years.

When Peter and Helen operated the gift store in Killarney, they tried to stock as many as possible of the unique items that were normally not found in the usual gift stores. They did carry a large inventory of Ty products, i.e., beanie babies and beanie buddies. In fact, they had the second largest inventory of these products in Manitoba. Beanie babies caught the attention of both children and adults. Beanies were collected, traded, and hoarded. They had sales of beanie babies in nine of Canada's provinces and eleven states of the United States.

One Monday at 11 a.m., a Lincoln with a Biloxi, Miss., licence plate drove up and parked at the store front. The four passengers were in their eighties. The two grandmas were collectors. They were in search of the most sought after Canada "maple" bear. They entered the store and inquired if there were any "maples". Happily, Peter responded, "We sell them, but we are out of them presently, but we'll have some in a week or two."

The retail price of the "maple" was $9.95, but since the store was always short, they did accept $100 bills from those who wanted some. However, to make it more "legal", Peter and Helen had the policy that in order to buy a Maple for $9.95, the customer had to buy sixteen much less popular beanies for $9.95 also. These customers made the purchase, which came to a total of $717.95. On paying, they were so surprised at the low value of the Canadian dollar. Therefore, they spent a few more hundred dollars.

There was a more interesting part of this story. The grandmas had begged their husbands to come to Canada to purchase maples. The husbands agreed on the condition that they would enter Canada at Emerson, south of Winnipeg, and head west until they located the desired collectibles. As it happened, Killarney was their first stop in Canada. Since their mission had been accomplished, they had to return home. The grandmas had hoped to find the "maples" somewhere near Vancouver! Two weeks later, the "maples" arrived at their condominiums in Biloxi.

Lee Clark was the Member of Parliament for Peter's constituency, Brandon-Souris, in the early 1980s. It was during the years of usurious interest rates of up to 22% and more. Many farms and business people were hit very hard. It appeared that banks enjoyed "eating for lunch" those who had considerable lines of credit at the bank to keep their business or farm afloat. There were many failures and foreclosures in those years in rural Manitoba and Saskatchewan. Mr. Clark was unusually helpful to any who looked to him as a mediator between themselves and the bank. He served a large constituency with sacrificial care.

Peter has revived a childhood hobby of interlocking puzzles—one thousand pieces or over. In October 2008, he completed the most difficult puzzle that he has ever seen.

He sums up his philosophy of life into three main points. The 40 or 63 or 82 years we live are not the end of the day. Each of us was created for a purpose which would extend beyond the last breath. While we are here, we may enjoy life to the fullest.

We need to care for others to the best of our abilities and resources. We need to be accountable caretakers of the earth on which and from which we live. We must leave our community and the world a better place than it was when we came. One's joy and happiness to a great extent is proportional to the joy and happiness we bring to others. If we throw our "bread" upon the water, it will come back to us.

34

Dorothy (Twilley) Shewfelt

Imagine having fifty-seven children on the roll—but fewer desks! From the standpoint of seating, it was good that everyone did not attend on the same day. However, the children lost valuable time for learning. Some children go to school by walking, some by bicycle, and some by horse; but these children paddled canoes—when there was no ice and snow—to reach their destination. Their school was across the lake from some of the homes.

She taught at a school at Nelson House Indian Reserve, on Footprint Lake, about 70 miles (113 km) northwest of where the city of Thompson would later be developed. It was under the auspices of the Anglican Church of Canada. The only student not from the Nelson House Reserve was the son of the local Hudson's Bay store manager. Dorothy lived in a small room in the same building as where she taught.

The teacher found this school to be her most interesting one. She could accept children in grades as high as she could go; however, very few were past grade four. She had a few students as old as sixteen.

The children seemed to have little to eat as they brought no food with them. It was either the church or the federal government that sponsored a cookie-a-day programme. Actually, the cookies were hard biscuits. There was one per child. They were so hard that the children would slam them on their desks to break them. One wonders how nourishing they really were. In February, the supply ran out. Dorothy wrote to the authorities asking for more. The response was that there were no more. It was so frustrating for her.

She loved working at that school. She also loved the children. The authorities instructed her not to use the native language in the school, a policy which now is in question. She told her students about the restriction. However, she added that, on the weekends when not in school, she was on her own. She invited the children to speak to her in their language whenever they saw her, as she wanted to learn the language. She left that school with a vocabulary of twenty-eight words, but she has forgotten them through lack of use.

Dorothy was born in Swan River. She began her education in a rural school in Roaring River School District and obtained her high schooling at Swan River Collegiate, in Swan River.

She was boarding in town to attend high school when World War II ended. It was not a happy time for her. Her favourite cousin had been killed three days prior to peace having been declared. While everyone else celebrated in the streets, she walked six miles (10 km) to be with her family at the farm.

She particularly remembers Mr. Lightly, our vice-principal and social studies teacher at Normal School. He was a wonderful man who took a personal interest in each student with a new batch of greenhorns each year.

She found that Normal School, for many, was a place of such fun and gentle first venture into the world. The students formed a special fellowship that has remained strong over the years.

After attending Normal School, she obtained a diploma in fine arts at University of Manitoba. As a permit teacher, she taught one year in McVey School District, near Swan River, and at Nelson House First Nations for seven months. After Normal School, she taught in Neepawa, Pilot Mound, Winnipegosis—all in Manitoba—and in Keewatin, Ont.

Her first school had no indoor plumbing, no drinking water, and no telephone. A pot-bellied stove that used wood provided heat. There was no problem in regard to frozen ink bottles since most of the children were still using pencils, not pens. Very few books existed for a library. There was a barn for the horses used by children who had to come from a distance. One evening shortly after school was out, a bear was shot on the playground. That provided a little excitement and concern.

After being married, Dorothy helped her husband with farming and in a TV sales/service shop. One day, a lady from Swan Lake First Nations drove twenty miles (32 km) to their shop. Her young son had taken a kitten while his mother and dad were purchasing a television in the store earlier. She required him to return the kitten and to apologize for having stolen it. Dorothy told them that they could keep the kitten. The mother refused because there was a new baby in their home. She also wanted the boy to learn from the incident. Dorothy had noticed that the kitten was missing. She was duly impressed with this act.

She did some substitute teaching and art teaching—oil painting, clay sculpture, and cake decorating. She also wrote free lance articles for rural newspapers in such Manitoba towns as Carman and Manitou. Friends in Saskatchewan informed her that the stories had also been picked up by a few local newspapers in their province. These were mainly human interest stories. She also won a writing contest and her essay was aired on

CBC radio. Following this, she was asked for more humourous articles for radio.

As a child, she particularly liked the Lucy Maud Montgomery books; but she would read any books that she could obtain. As an adult, she likes the science fiction stories by Isaac Asimov and books by Amy Tan. She usually has two or three books being read at one time—fiction, non-fiction, and something humourous for when she cannot sleep at night.

She used to like to travel, camp, and cross-country ski; but she has slowed down to dancing, golfing, floor curling, and paper tole.

In her community, she has served on the United Church board, in Sunday school, and with United Church Women. She has also served with the Parent Teachers Association, with 4-H, community clubs, and Meals on Wheels, in a Personal Care facility, and in the Red Hat Society.

On a trip to Australia, she learned that the Aussies do not like the Brits because they felt a lack of support during a certain World War II battle. She saw such differences as the species of animals in Australia, but there was nothing significant that she felt was outstanding.

She was more impressed with the number of sheep which she saw in New Zealand. In fact, there are more sheep than people in that country. When she set out from home, she had been more interested in Australia than in New Zealand. However, after visiting both countries, she was more impressed with New Zealand.

She would suggest a visitor to Canada tour the Swan River Valley, in Manitoba, as it is beautiful, bountiful, modern, and developing. In addition, it is not as influenced by the United States as southern areas of the province are.

For one Remembrance Day, she suggested that each teenager go out and shake the hand of a war veteran to say, "Thank you, and we are glad you survived to be part of our future." The veterans must have felt most appreciative when approached by those young people.

Anyone who is entering the teaching profession should begin by being strict with only a couple of rules. Ease up later when it is appropriate. The teacher will learn what rules need to be added and should work them out together with the students.

Miss Ruth Esplen was her grades two to five teacher in a rural school. She taught Dorothy all that she needed to know about how to handle thirty-five to forty students in grades one to eight in one classroom.

Dr. J. Boxall taught her how to use self-hypnosis. This knowledge helped her through childbirth, panic attacks, depression, and insomnia.

She feels that Tommy Douglas was a great Canadian leader. Where would our healthcare system be without his work in bringing it about?

Her philosophy is to judge only thyself—and not too harshly.

Class E

Grace Gorrie
Walter Hucaluk
Eddie Janzen
Hardy Kehler
Alex Klimchuk
Stanley Kokorudz
Nick Kosinsky
Verna Krayeski
Viola Kroeker
Ann Kubas
Evelyn Kuchta
Denise LaFleche
Evelyn Lambert
Lucille Lanthier
Gladys Lawrence
Bill Lebedeff
Dorothy Lee
Sylvia Lee
Florence Legal
Yvonne Legal
Isabel Lepesko
Margaret Lindsay
Agathe Loeppky
Gertrude Loewen
Helen Loewen
Helen Rose Loewen
Juliet Lovoie
Donna Lusignan
Yvonne McArthur
Jean McClelland
Irene McFee
Gwen McIntosh
Joan McLaren
Lois McLeod
Nesta McLeod
Noreen McLeod
Mary Myrowich
Viola Rankin
Greta Sarchuk
Sister Eva Marie
Sister Joseph

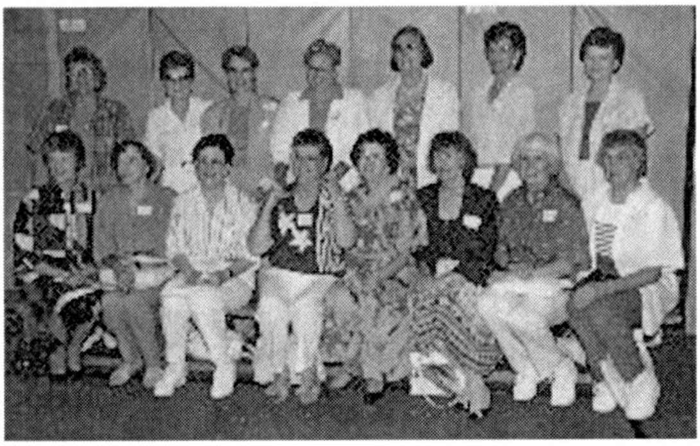

20. Class E

35
Sylvia (Lee) Haverstick

One warm, pre-examination June day, a young man caught a bat and brought it to school to show his classmates. Any live animal—especially one with wings—in any room has the capacity for creating excitement. The creature flew around the classroom and then clung to a clock near a girl's desk.

That morning was mathematics review—students were required to write difficult problems on the blackboard and then these would be solved and discussed. It was ironic that the girl who was tops in mathematics would have so many problems to be written on the blackboard. Possibly, her knowledge of bats was limited to the things people say they do.

Sylvia was born in Swift Current, Sask. The first school which she attended was in Swift Current; but she acquired most of her schooling in Crandall. She earned a Bachelor of Arts degree and a Bachelor of Education degree from the University of Manitoba.

A favourite teacher was Florence Gendreau, who taught French and several other subjects at Crandall High School. She expected much from her students, but was always pleasant and smiling.

At Normal School, Sylvia particularly remembers Mr. Clarke, our classroom management teacher. Although, at first, he struck fear into many young students, she did eventually enjoy his dry sense of humour.

She shared a room in Thompson Hall with three other girls. This particular room had the only window that could allow late-comers to enter the dormitory safely without being reported. This led to some interesting scenarios.

Sylvia was a classroom teacher for one year in Beulah, followed by three years at Sanford. Then, she married in 1955. The rest of her teaching career was spent in Winnipeg School Division #1, where she took library courses and became a teacher-librarian.

Marcel Pelletier, a fellow teacher, had a positive influence on Sylvia's work. As a young teacher in a large city school, his approach to teaching and his attitude were inspirations to her.

When she was a child, she enjoyed reading *Charlotte's Web*, by E. B. White, and when an adult, she enjoyed reading *Trinity*, by Leon Uris. Today, Sylvia enjoys reading, playing bridge, going to hockey games (time with her grandchildren), and attending movies.

Organizations in which she is involved include Wildewood Golf Club, Fort Garry United Church, and Delta Kappa Gamma Society.

An amusing incident occurred at a Christmas concert. A skit called for a pet cat. This created no problem as many students volunteered to bring their pets to the concert. However, the noise and the excitement of the concert backstage were too much for the feline, and the docile cat became a wild tiger! After its performance of being pulled from a box, it made an early exit and bolted home as rapidly as it could scamper.

Sylvia's trip to Australia was memorable. The highlight was the visit to the homes of the Aboriginal people in the desert area. Although very few now live there, she wonders how they have managed to exist in such a hostile environment. The lack of water is so crucial and, although their need for and use of water is different from our perception, the Canadians could not imagine being able to extract sufficient from the plants, shrubs, and trees in an area that was so dry and hot.

Food, too, was difficult to procure; but the whole group seemed to agree that the roasted kangaroo tail was a bit more palatable than facing the huge grub that the guide dug out of a shrub and ate to prove that it was a good source of protein.

She suggests visiting Manitoba, especially the prairie part of the province, in September and October. Although it may not be as colourful as some other parts of Canada, the prairie is unique because of the harvesting scenes; the gathering and migration of huge flocks of geese, ducks, and other birds; and the beauty of the prairie sunsets. The warm, hazy days of autumn are to be enjoyed before the onslaught of cold winter that follows.

Her advice to teenagers in relation to their lives in general is to respect their parents, to listen to them, and to pursue their education as far as possible.

Her advice to someone wanting to enter the teaching profession is to be a student always as one is constantly learning. Each child is different and should be recognized as such. A teacher should be aware that there will be new methods, new materials, and new staffs. Patience and a love of children and for reading and learning go far in making one a successful teacher.

She feels that Lester B. Pearson was a leader who made an important contribution to Canada through the part that he played on the world scene as Minister for External Affairs and as Prime Minister.

Her philosophy of life is the golden rule: “Do unto others as you would have them do unto you.”

36

Jean (McClelland) Tully

She was not an early riser; but during the practice teaching period, it was necessary for her to rise earlier than usual in order to eat breakfast before going to the school where she was working. One morning, as she was drowsily proceeding across the campus in her usual mood of desiring to be back in her comfortable bunk, she heard a greeting, "Hello!"

Coming partially back to reality, she looked around at eye-level; but she saw no one. Thus, she continued her trek toward the dining-hall. "Hello!" her greeter repeated. However, this time, she realized that the voice came from a lower plane than eye-level. Then she saw the source of the greeting. On the ground by the path, trying to attract her attention was a crow.

How foolish she felt! In her mind, she had a clear choice: either to return to bed and finish the dream and eliminate the crow, or to acknowledge that the stupid bird could really talk. Now, she was wide awake for breakfast.

Jean was born, and lived her first nine years, at Rosebank. She started school at Rosebank; then moved to Erinview, in the Interlake Region; and then to Mulvey School, in Winnipeg. For high school, she spent a couple of months at Gordon Bell High School and then completed matriculation at Stonewall Collegiate Institute.

She earned her Business College education from Angus School of Commerce, in Winnipeg; her teaching diploma from Normal School; and her Bachelor of Arts degree and a post-graduate Bachelor of Education from Brandon University. She has various other diplomas and certificates in personal development.

She left school after grade eleven and taught for a year on permit, then went to Business College, after which she returned to take her grade twelve. She had such a good time that year. She was old enough and had enough teaching experience to know exactly what she wanted from the year (not necessarily high grades).

She participated in all of the extra-curricular activities that were available—which were not many in Stonewall High School, but numerous unscheduled ones. She helped organize activities, took up causes, and drove the principal "crazy"—but she had fun.

Her all-time favourite teacher from high school was Miss Gillis. She was her senior English teacher in grade eleven and grade twelve. She was interested in and respectful of each of her students. In a time when unauthorized opinions were not solicited, she encouraged wide-ranging discussions about any part of the course. Personally, she was warm and caring; but she expected everyone's best efforts. The only punishment was her disappointment when her students' best did not occur.

Our Normal School teacher whom she remembers best is Mr. Lightly, vice-principal and social studies teacher. He was so funny and sharp and the kindest person. His interest in each of us was real because he always remembered who we were, even years afterwards.

Jean telephoned him the second year after leaving Normal School. After she identified herself, he replied instantly, "Oh, the Rabbit Point Flash." (Rabbit Point was her first school after Normal). She had not been in touch with him in the interim, except for a class or two he taught at Gimli Summer School. He set the bar quite high as an example to us of how to respect and relate to our students.

She remembers life in the dormitory: the camaraderie, the jokes, and the fun. One time, Sister Joseph solemnly confiscated Hardy Kehler's lucky rabbit's foot, tucked it in her habit, and blandly agreed when Jean told Hardy that she had not taken it, but that she knew that Sister Joseph had. Hardy would not believe that story! Three days later, she showed him the foot. Jean will never forget the look on his face at that moment. Sister Joseph also used to snowball Normalites in the yard and then look angelic when they turned around and could not figure out who had thrown the snow.

She particularly remembers the singing in the class of Beth Douglas, the dancing after school with Hart Devenny, the drama productions, sneaking in after curfew, hiding others during bed check, getting to know the non-resident students by waiting on tables for lunch in the small dining room, cruising the second basement and finding a working phone. This was where she and Gwen Jackson made all of their telephone calls to set up dates for the Aggie spring dance between our students and the Aggies. How difficult it was to have access to a telephone in the office!

Other memories include studying in Assiniboine Park during the summer and walking through the park to catch the bus or streetcar on Portage Avenue, and riding up on the service elevator with one of the workmen to see the view from the tower of the main building of the Normal School. It was a particularly carefree year for Jean and one in which she made lasting friendships.

She taught on permit in two one-room schools: Park View (near Eriksdale) and Phipps (near Stonewall), both of

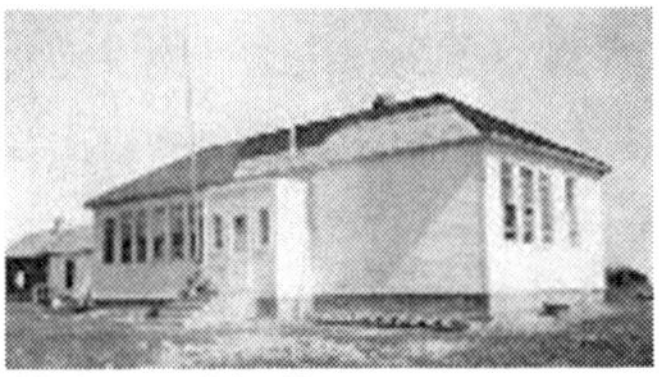
21. Loon Straits

which are long gone. After Normal School, she taught for one year at Rabbit Point, a one-room school on the east side of Lake Winnipeg, and at the High School at Loon Straits, as principal, also on the east side. She then taught at Snow Lake and became principal there by default near the Easter break.

After a seven-year break to marry and to raise three children, she taught for one year at Oakville and substituted for a maternity leave during the following year. Following that, she taught at the high school at Reston, then studied for—and received!—her Bachelor of Arts and Bachelor of Education degrees. This Bachelor of Education was basically pre-Masters, and is no longer given. She completed this in two years at Brandon University plus some summer schools.

Later, she moved to Neelin High School, in Brandon. Her husband, Ken, acquired his teaching certificate in counselling, following which they moved to Minnedosa, where Jean taught senior English and was a coordinator for the high school teachers in the division.

On leaving Minnedosa, she was hired by the Manitoba Department of Education and seconded to Frontier School Division. For five years she was one of six staff of the Confluent Education Programme. She travelled to many schools, conducting demonstration lessons and workshops with parents, trustees, educators, and students.

Jean then travelled for her own consulting company, leading workshops in school and band governance, in personal growth, and short educational programmes, including many pre-employment courses.

She has worked in Adult Education continually since, spending more years in teaching adults than she did in teaching youth. The rewards of teaching are many and so gratifying. Her company received many contracts to work with people, young and old, who had never graduated from school.

In the good old days of fishing at Alert Bay, B.C., many of the boys withdrew from school at about thirteen years of age to earn more money in three months than their teachers did in a year. These folks needed to be retrained, and overcoming their resistance to school again was a true test of humanistic education training. The gratitude for the opportunity to learn, after the initial resistance, was quite overwhelming.

The preparation which she had to do all this was her five years in Confluent Education. What an eye-opener for Jean that was! She thought that she was a good teacher—and she was—but she was so much more effective after all that she learned in those years and since. After that experience, she has worked both alone and with Ken in numerous Aboriginal communities, doing education or business training. These had wonderful highlights.

One of the highlights, among the many in her life, was a high school reunion in Minnedosa. It was twenty years for the grade twelve class that she and her husband had taught—and what a time there was with hugs and appreciation for one another! Her pension is satisfactory, but that experience is the real reward.

Another memory that she treasures is when she and Ken attended the wedding of her husband's grand-niece. Five of her former students—now adults and with professions of their own—were also in attendance. It was a memorable reunion. Two or three of them became teachers. One wore high heels on her first day of teaching because Jean had always worn high heels.

She also remembers driving across Lake Winnipeg in the winter in a rickety old car, with a wood heater in the back seat and the window open to let the smoke out. The wind was blowing, not a full blizzard, but there was not much visibility. They knew that there were two cracks open in the ice, but did not know where they were since ice cracks move erratically. Neither her mother nor her children have ever been aware of the complete story of that trip.

She has ridden with bombardiers and dog teams, flown in ski-equipped planes, and sailed in fishing tugs or small skiffs—or whatever was going. She has run across rubber ice that bowed like an elastic band under her feet. It was an adventure every day on Lake Winnipeg, and wherever in the North that she travelled.

She has had many experiences in her life besides teaching. She and Ken raised three boys and are good friends with them now. Both taught their sons in high school. They have run businesses; built their own house; and travelled and worked in the North, which they loved.

She attended university when she was thirty-eight years old, in part because of her fond memories, not of what she learned academically, but of interacting with other people in a learning situation in Normal School. She believes that the experience of going to teach on a permit and then having our experience legitimized at Normal contributed to her adaptability and enjoyment of change and taking chances, which has led to a fulfilling life.

Anne of Green Gables, by Lucy Maud Montgomery, was a childhood favourite book. Now, as an adult, she relishes reading any book written by Rudy Wiebe, and good crime novels.

She enjoys reading, singing, and directing choirs. Recently, she has begun to find pleasure in cooking as she has discovered many interesting new foods with which to work. She has liked to walk, but a problem with one leg prevents her from doing that now.

She has never joined service clubs. However, she did join professional associations throughout her career and served on them in various capacities. The first one was the negotiating committee of the Manitoba Teachers' Society, in Brandon. Her first experience was a challenge. The teachers could not convince the Board that they had only one submission. They told the teachers that no one negotiates that way; the first position is always out of line.

She has sung in choirs for many years and has led most of them. She has always been a member of the United Church of Canada and is presently past chair of the Church Council for Brechin Church, in Nanaimo, B.C.

Other interests include organizing fun activities and volunteering to distribute food for the local food bank, which has a satellite distribution site in her church. She writes biographies of church members that are published each month in their newsletter.

She and Ken volunteer with CESO-SACO, the Canadian Executive Service Organization. They have participated in many assignments with aboriginal folks.

A different assignment was in Azerbaijan, a small country on the west side of the Caspian Sea, just at the top of Iran and beside Armenia. Her assignment was to help open a business academy. As with most of these things, that is not exactly what she did. However, they were in the country for a month and made many friends and acquired a thorough grounding in Azeri culture and history.

Every weekend their interpreter took them on a field trip to see something of their culture. For instance, they saw a Zoroastrian Fire Temple as it used to be during the days of the Silk Road. Their counterpart made sure that they saw the whole background on Zoroastrianism, even though the citizens are mainly Muslim. However, having been under USSR for ninety years, they are quite secular.

Different also was lamb as a staple meat. Jean is still in touch with their interpreter.

Vancouver Island at any time of the year is the area of Canada to visit. There are so many different aspects, including climates and environments. However, if time be short, she suggests visiting Tofino or Ucluelet on the west coast of the island. In summer, one can swim and surf. In winter, it is storm-watching. It is wise to reserve ahead, particularly if interested in storm-watching as this is a very popular activity. There is caving, whale-watching, skiing, hiking the West Coast Trail and many other trails, kayaking, golfing, and sailing. These are all-year-round vacation spots, but they do not have the crowds of many other hot spots.

Jean often addresses teens, or chats with young people. Her advice is to take every opportunity you are offered to experience something, for example, a job or a trip, as long as it is legal, even if you think you may not be able to do it. Someone offered it to you, thinking you would be up to it and may know you better than you know yourself and your capabilities. In general, go against the flow. If a thing seems not to fit you, do not do it. When you are interacting with people, try to fit into their shoes and then judge if what you are going to do or say will help or hurt. If you ask for advice, listen and weigh it. If you did not ask for it, it is likely better to ignore it.

If you be a people person and wish to teach, Jean would encourage you to explore the job for a day or two by asking to sit in with a teacher whom you admire. Do not go into the profession solely for the time off and money because the time off dwindles away very quickly, and the money does not ever make up for the angst, anguish and frustration you will experience if it not be your passion.

During her training in personal development as preparation for her work in Confluent Education, many people were instrumental in making a big change in the way she thought and reacted. However, the one perhaps most influential was Dr. Tony Stickel, a professor in the Social Work Department of University of Calgary. He spent many weekends with his students, teaching them and experiencing with them Gestalt Therapy.

Jean learned that each of us is complete within ourselves. All we need is to allow our natural understanding of our mind and body to respond to whatever is confronting us. Thus, she needs to wait for others to call upon their own resources before she undertakes to solve their problems for them. Answering other's questions or quarrels without presenting options is counter-productive, even for the littlest child.

Since Jean has a degree in political science, she could analyze each leader's political achievements. Despite the qualities of such leaders as Tommy Douglas, Lester Pearson, and others, she would choose Pierre Trudeau as a great Canadian leader, not for the usual reasons, but that he made it all right to lighten up a bit, have fun in ways our Puritan outlook had not allowed. She thinks that he gave us a psychological freedom that may be as far-reaching and life-giving as the Charter.

Jean subscribes fully to the following statement created by another person: "Life is not a journey to the grave, with the intention of arriving safely in a pretty and well-preserved body, but rather to skid in broadside, thoroughly used up, totally worn out, and loudly proclaiming—wow—what a ride!"

She has within her all that she needs to accomplish the above or anything else that she chooses. All that she needs to do is to learn to access it. If she looks after her own needs, without limiting others the access to having their needs satisfied, there is no reason for regrets or conflict. On top of that, the glass is half-full.

37

Irene (McFee) Coleman

The teacher and her students were preparing for the annual Christmas concert in her first school. The practising went well until she became aware that two of the oldest boys were not singing. Everyone was supposed to sing. The boys were determined otherwise. How could this young lady—fresh out of grade eleven—persuade them to participate?

She instructed them to stay after school and then sing to her. After she had dismissed all the other students, she told them to sit and think about the situation. At 4:30 p.m., she would hear them. They sat and thought. The time had come for their rendition. They stood their ground in defiance. Their teacher did likewise. Who would win?

The time limit was extended to five o'clock. As the time ticked away, it started to become dark in the classroom as there was no switch to turn on lights. It became darker. The teacher waited to see how the boys would react. Darkness became too much for them. The two boys strolled up to the teacher's desk. She was still there. They sang for her. Now, all three could walk the two miles (3 km) home—together.

The boys had met their match. There was no more trouble from them.

Irene was born in Winnipeg, the third child of eight born to Carl and Pearl McFee. Her mother was a school teacher and her dad was a farmer in Grosse Isle. He also drove the school van, drawn by horses, for all of her school years. Her schooling took place at Grosse Isle, except for grade twelve, which she received at Stonewall Collegiate.

She has a vivid memory as a little girl of the day when King George VI and Queen Elizabeth visited Winnipeg in 1939. The students of her school went to Winnipeg by train to see them. What a very memorable occasion it was for her!

She remembers another school experience which was not pleasant. She did love to skate and to play hockey. Then one day, she unexpectedly passed out on the skating rink. What a frightening experience that was! Fearing another such incident, she curtailed her playing hockey to an occasional time until she joined Normal School girls' team under the coaching of Gladwyn Scott.

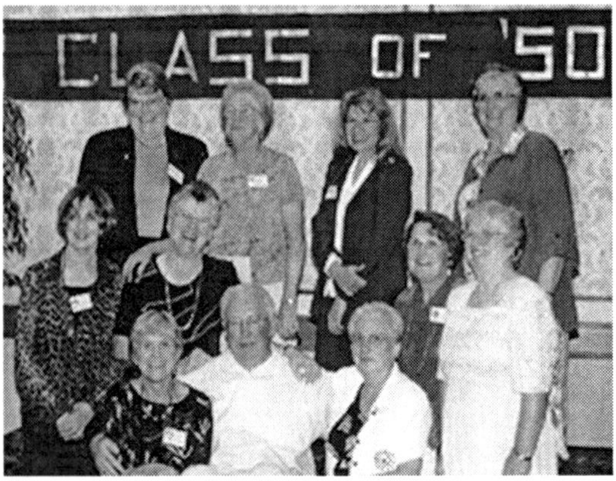

22. Ladies' Hockey Team

Following completion of grade eleven, her plan was to go into the nursing profession, but she did not yet meet the minimum age of eighteen. Since permits were issued to grade eleven graduates at that time, she decided to try to earn some money so that she could enter nurses' training.

In her permit year, she taught at North High Bluff School, near Portage la Prairie. There were twenty-five students in grades one to eight. She boarded with a family that included eight children—and she had one of them in each grade. Since she came from a large family herself, she was used to a big family. It was a learning experience in that first year. She always claims, "I learned more than my students."

In the following year, she returned to high school to take her grade twelve since she had not made as much money as she had hoped.

Then in 1950–51, Irene attended Provincial Normal School. She resided in La Verendrye Hut. She enjoyed the friendships formed in residence and was pleased that many students were placed in schools not far from her school. These students have continued many years of friendships.

Although she lived only twenty miles (32 km) from her home town of Grosse Isle, she lived in residence in order to save money. Thus, she did not go home every weekend. Consequently, she was asked to fill Mrs. Savage's position in the dining hall on weekends.

Through this position, she became acquainted with many students. Her duties were to sign in working students, check tables, and generally help with meals. It meant that she worked only on weekends instead of every day—for even more money. She felt blessed to have acquired this job. Normal School was an interesting experience; but having taught for that one year, she found much material was irrelevant to country schools.

Barclay School, in the Darlingford area, was her first assignment after Normal School. She had eight grades and, eventually, a grade nine by correspondence. She remained here for three enjoyable years, really appreciating the community and their acceptance of her.

Christmas concerts were the highlight of the school year. Teachers were often judged by their concert performances. These did bring the community together.

Many of the people were willing to offer services of sewing costumes, playing piano, and even playing Santa Claus.

When she terminated her contract at Barclay School, the neighbouring school board of Darlingford approached her to fill a vacancy in grades six, seven, and eight. As she had plans to marry the following year, she accepted the challenge. Junior high students are another "age group". She did enjoy the challenges which she faced. She found it interesting that students in this age group are either with you or against you, but preferably with you.

Her next teaching position was a rural school, Grassmers, near Stonewall. This was to fill a position following the resignation of their teacher in October. Irene was asked to teach here until the board could hire someone else. As it turned out, she remained until the end of June. She managed to juggle her little daughter during this tenure.

She spent the next several years raising her own family of five—four girls, including one set of twins, and one son. This also was a great challenge in providing educational experiences for them in sports, music, the arts, and the 4-H programme. All of her children were exposed to the exceptional programme. They gained very valuable social skills and went on trips—rewarding experiences that they would not have had otherwise.

The saying "once a teacher, always a teacher" was true for Irene because education was her top priority. Learning to do a job well and taking pride in accomplishments were instilled into her children and her students. Then, her husband of nineteen years passed away. Her greatest desire was for all her children to graduate from grade twelve. Her goal was achieved!

Following the death of her husband, she and her children moved to Morden. There, she held the position of librarian at the Morden Collegiate for seven and one-half years. Her family became involved in many community activities. When they had finished such activities as choirs, 4-H, operettas, Irene was ready to drop from organizations herself. Nevertheless, she still does volunteer for a few of them. Now she spends time in entertaining seniors.

It is difficult for her to name a favourite book as a child because she enjoyed reading so much at that time. Then she read those books to her own children. There was always library time for them. She did like Nellie McClung's series of books. Now that Irene is living in Manitou, the home of this author, the books bring new meaning to her.

The most memorable trip that she has taken was to the east coast of Canada in 2000. She and her family travelled in a fifth-wheel vehicle with her sister and her brother-in-law. Since they left on May 29, they we were a little early for campgrounds and they also missed the icebergs. She learned so much about this unique area of Canada—so much history and many places to see and many things to do. They were away from home for one month, and it was an enjoyable trip all the way. She would suggest anyone should see this area in mid June.

In recent years, she fulfilled a dream of learning to play the violin. She and a friend of her age took about one and one-half years of lessons. However, they soon realized that what they were learning was not the type of playing which they wanted. Since both had learned to play by ear, they began to work with fiddle music. They have since been playing in three music groups—mostly at senior centres, local hospitals, and other social events.

She mentioned that some of her friends of the past would remember her by her first married name, McElroy.

Class F

Margaret Allen
Henry Dick
Waldimar Enns
Mervyn Farough
Jerry Hildebrand
Audrey Jack
Lois Leigh
Eileen MacDougall
Rose McColl
Betty McMahon
Eva Mair
Helen Maksimchuk
Stella Mandzuik
Jean Mayberry
Edward Maza
Wilma Miller
Ruth Mooney
Margaret Moore
Emily Moroz
Alice Morrison
Bernice Morrow
Jack Morton
Eva Muir
Eleanor Murray
Jackie Naven
Isabelle Neeley
Jim Norrie
Lena Nykolaishen
Doreen Olafson
Cecilia Olson
Delphie Olson
Doreen Olson
Hank Otchanash
Ai Otsu
Emilie Paswisty
Verna Perry
Helga Peters
Rose Phillips
Dave Semenko
Julius Skuben
Sister Brigette
Sister Mary Emile

38
Henry Dick

It was his very first car! A brand new Volkswagen Beetle. How proud of it he was! So passionate was he with it that he became absorbed in repairing it and others as a hobby. Then he turned his attention to the collecting of insects. Beetles, to be exact! In 1971, he constructed a camper from tin and wood. This he placed onto a 1971 six-passenger Volkswagen truck. He still had the passion. The follow-up was a trip to Disneyland in southern California. All five of his family lived in it throughout the journey.

While in that state, he met a retired policeman from New York. Yes, he was driving a Volkswagen camper. This fellow traveller asked if Henry were armed.

"No," replied Henry.

"I retained my Colt that I neglected to turn in to the force when I left," the former policeman announced.

"Have you had to use it?" inquired Henry.

"No, but I'm not going to give a dope-head my life for just a small trinket for which he might want to kill me," he replied.

In 1927, Henry's parents migrated to Canada from the Ukraine. His mother travelled westward via the Atlantic while his father travelled eastward via Siberia, the White Army, asylum in China, and then to Canada via the Pacific. They were eventually reunited in Saskatchewan. His father's name was registered as Dyck. Somehow, Henry's name was registered as Dick, and it was never corrected. Even though his given name is Henry, his parents called him Hein in the interest of efficiency at calling their brood of nine—at one syllable each.

Just imagine! His first day of school happened at Rapid Advance, a one-room school located nine miles (14 km) north of Young, Sask. He entered academia at age seven from a very isolated, dust-blown, three-room house on the desolate prairie—and speaking only German. One would think that 1938 would be a great challenge for him, especially with the imminent threat of World War II. But not so! A grade nine correspondence student came to sit with him to translate for the young newcomer.

Being born at Young and being fed locally milled whole wheat bread and attending Rapid Advance School spelled "advantage: Henry". This was instant progress—so he thought. By lunch time on his first day, one should have witnessed his communication skills in his second language. Little did he know what he was learning!

When he and his friend were outside eating sandwiches from their syrup pails, he spotted a man climbing out of a basement that he was digging for a teacherage. Little Henry noticed a split in the seat of the man's pants and drew it to his attention by saying, "Mister, you have a hole in your a--."

The man looked at the little fellow, and, with a twinkle in his eye, said, "So do you!"

Henry checked his pants as well as he could and, finding no hole, proceeded to be shocked at such an outrageous lie. He had not recognized the vulgarity.

His grade three experience was the one that settled his career choice. The teacher had such an engaging approach that he decided that very year "that a teacher he would be."

Henry graduated from high school in 1950, together with Hardy Kehler, Peter Peters, and Peter Klassen. Their paths crossed at Normal School the next year. P. J. Schaefer, principal at their alma mater, stands out as being very instrumental in his life for his influence in shaping and directing Henry. His passionate dealing with both English and German literature really had soul. Shortly after ordaining his student as a lay minister in their church in 1969, he died and Henry had the honour of being one of the speakers at his funeral.

In Normal School, it was again the principal who stands out in his memory. Mr. Moorhead deserves recognition for his patience and understanding. Although his name was Duncan Bruce, Henry wondered if the name Enza had some association with him. When he walked into the boys' dormitory during an episode of horse-play, he could have lectured them or even expelled them for failing to be the disciplined characters that would be expected of mature leaders in education. He was recognized in a poem in which a student humorously described his entrance into their building as "Influenza".

It was 1955. Alberta was fifty years old when Henry was teaching in one-room Willow Lake School, eighteen miles (29 km) south of Medicine Hat, Alta. Craig, an orphan boy in grade three and short for his age, rode to school on a full-sized horse—bareback. He would use the steps of the school to mount his steed, and then head home at a gallop. As the teacher stood at the window and watched, he saw a bit of heaven between his seat and the horse at every bounce. What a rider that little boy was!

In the 1950s, several Janz brothers, graduates of Prairie Bible Institute, in Three Hills, Alta., created Janz Team Ministries, a faith mission for evangelism in

Germany in the German language. In the course of time, they added Black Forest Academy, a grade one to twelve school, using the Saskatchewan curriculum. Nestled in the village of Kandern between Freiburg and Loerach in Germany's enchanting Black Forest, the setting provided the group with a wonderful year of working with 124 high school students from eighteen different countries where their parents were serving.

While Henry was involved in the school, Mary took her daily two-mile (3 km) walk through fairy tale woods and past storybook villages to a big old World War II military building, now a dormitory for students, where she helped to prepare food.

The school building, a three-storey clothing factory, was converted into classrooms to serve the academy. The old wooden warehouse nearby served as a gymnasium and chapel space.

When a German guide took the group on a walking tour through the village, Mary and Henry understood everything that the leader said. The translator relating items to their fellow staff in English did not translate everything that the guide said. In response to the question from a tourist asking about the group of the English foreigners trailing behind, we heard the guide say, “Oh, they come from Black Forest Academy claiming they are a Christian ministry, but I think they are a cult.”

Their rented house was close to a church whose bells in the tower frequently chimed. It had no built-in clothes closets, and electricity ran on 220 volts. On the narrow old streets, the German drivers made no allowances for Henry’s driving errors or for his ignorance but were very quick to lecture him liberally. The stories about “the wall” impacted Henry and Mary to the extent that they decided not to go to see it. Instead, they enjoyed many ancient ruins easily accessible along the many hiking trails.

Haying on the steep hillsides was done with a three-foot (91 cm) wide sickle power mower. Long-handled wooden rakes were used to bunch the hay to be loaded by fork and muscle power onto farm wagons drawn by horses or small tractors.

Whenever they espied a maple leaf flag in a German car during that year, it managed to make them emotionally homesick. Imagine that! They must be Canadian, eh?

As a child, Henry read *Singing Wheels*, a story set in Scotland. Even as a senior citizen, he can still feel the loneliness of those moors as the scenes linger in his heart. Now, he does not remember an outstanding book as much as he does such authors as Dr. Clarence Jordan and Chuck Swindoll, whom he likes very much.

Besides earning the degrees of Bachelor of Science and Bachelor of Education and teaching from 1951 to 1996 in Manitoba, Alberta, and in Germany, he also worked as an electrician's helper. His longest teaching tenure was in a church school, Mennonite Collegiate Institute, in Gretna, for twenty-three years.

His electrical work in Calgary, Alta., lasted only two years. It came to a shocking end when he experienced a near electrocution.

Since 1986, when the first grandchild was born, Henry has switched his hobby from beetles to that of keeping a record of daily events. When each of the nine grandchildren reaches sixteen years of age, he presents a book of that child's biography transcribed from his diary. What a wonderful way this is of capturing his illusive memories!

To their grandchildren and to other youth, he would say, "Lead a life of prayer, of exercise, and of working with integrity."

To those who aspire to teach, he would say, “Give it your all and don't be lazy because nothing resembles death more nearly than inactivity. Should you get tired, as you sometimes will, take a sabbatical if you must; but don't you quit.” Such a life has resulted in the following equation for him, “Enjoyment equals involvement.”

He never met Mackenzie King, yet he considers that former prime minister as one who made an important contribution to Canada, one that affected Henry personally. Mr. King held the front door of our country open for Henry’s mother to enter and the back door for his dad. Now, here the son of these two immigrants is—a first generation Canadian!

Preparing his submission for this chapter has been a wonderful exercise in flashback. There are many knowns as well as many unknowns in this intricate web of life.

Henry and Mary have been married for fifty-two years and live in a seniors’ home in Calgary, Alta. He works as a caretaker and she carries on her job as a food demonstrator person at Safeway and Costco stores in Calgary.

39
Jerry Hildebrand

She was a persuasive grade school girl. She was a jealous rival whenever there was a competition that included Jerry. This time, it was an egg-colouring contest with all of the children vying for top honours. Who would win?

At Jerry's house was stored some chocolate-coloured barn paint. It was ideal for the task. After using some to paint his hard-boiled egg, he asked his sister to prepare some icing for it. After he had administered that, he borrowed his mother's cake decorating set to trim the egg. He neatly trimmed a horizontal ribbon of icing around it, and then he squeezed a beautiful flower on top. It actually looked like a commercial Easter egg—good enough to eat. His masterpiece was ready for the competition!

All of the decorated eggs were placed on the chalkboard ledge in the classroom to be judged by all of the children. At recess, just before the judging was to be done, the rival girl set out to persuade her classmates to vote for her egg so that she would be voted winner. She did this by stating negative remarks about the entries—all but hers. Would the children be intimidated by her?

Normally, the voting was by show of hands. Thus, the antagonist could see who voted for or against her entry. However, there was a flaw in her plan. Mr. Giesbrecht, their very perceptive teacher, saw what was developing. Therefore, he called for a secret ballot. He handed each student a piece of paper on which to write the number of the egg deemed to be the best. After the votes were counted and the winner was announced, the girl was devastated. Her egg was not the winner! Her chief rival, Jerry, received first prize. Mr. Giesbrecht had taught the whole class a valuable lesson of life.

Jerry was born in Winkler, in the Friedensruh district of the Winkler trading area. He started school in the Blumstein School, about five miles (8 km) southwest of Winkler. His post-secondary education includes a Bachelor of Theology degree from the Mennonite Brethren Bible College, in Winnipeg; a Bachelor of Arts degree from the University of Manitoba; a Master of Arts degree from the Wheaton Graduate School, in Wheaton, Illinois; and a Doctor of Missiology degree from Trinity Evangelical Divinity School, in Deerfield, Illinois.

His first language is Low German. However, he is fluent in English, High German, and Portuguese. He had two professions—teacher and minister/pastor—working in these professions in Canada and Brazil.

He and his wife Marjorie were in missionary service in southern Brazil for almost sixteen years. During that time, they were involved in evangelism, church planting, and mission administration. Jerry was the field treasurer for several years and later was the field leader. While in the latter position, he travelled to such countries in the Caribbean area as Haiti, Dominican Republic, and Trinidad and Tobago. In Haiti, he was touched by the extreme poverty and by the fear that is generated in people by the Voodoo religion.

The two most memorable experiences of his life's work are connected. It was a memorable day when he was ordained to the ministry on Sunday, June 26, 1955. On June 26, 2005 (also a Sunday) he and Marjorie, under the blessing of God, celebrated fifty years in the ministry. They are to be commended for their commitment.

One of the greatest accomplishments that he has made in his life's work was that of being the first Executive Director of Missions for his denomination, the Evangelical Mennonite Mission Conference of Canada, after he and Marjorie returned from the mission field in 1976. In the following nine years at that post, he had the privilege of bringing structure to that office.

On the negative side, he feels that he allowed his work to take him away too much from his family. Two men have since succeeded him as directors. Thus, he feels that someone else could easily replace him, but no one else could be a husband and a father to his family.

At Normal School, he lived in Strathcona Hall, where Jack Morton was the hut captain. He recalls a couple of experiences from the 1950–51 school year.

Candidates were nominated for the various offices of student council in each of the two terms. In the second term, Jerry was one nominee for the office of treasurer and Leon Stocki from Class II was the other. One assembly was arranged to have each nominee for office give a "campaign speech." Leon was an entertaining speaker. He facetiously wanted to impress the audience with his political campaign experience. He stated he had had experience in "running" since he was eight years of age. That was when the neighbour's bull took after him! Despite his speaking ability, he was not elected treasurer. Therefore, Jerry became treasurer for the term.

Another memorable Normal School experience came as a result of having been chosen valedictorian. Mr. Harold Turner, the speech instructor, was placed in charge of grooming Jerry for that occasion. That was as much a grueling experience as it was a grooming experience!

He had to write out his entire valedictory. When he presented it to his instructor, Mr. Turner tore the paper to shreds and sent his student back to rewrite it. That happened not once, but several times. Towards the end, Jerry was ready to throw in the towel.

When the teacher was finally satisfied, he asked Jerry to memorize it. Next, he took his student to the Knox United Church where the graduation exercises were to be held. There, he had him make a practice run with the speech. Mr. Turner went up into the balcony and sat down in the seat farthest away from Jerry. If he could not hear every syllable of every word distinctly, he stopped him and made him do it over again. What a humbling experience it was! However, as Jerry now looks back on his training, he wishes that he had had that kind of teacher in his homiletics class in seminary!

After the graduation ceremony, the Turners, both instructors at Normal School, came to congratulate him. Miss Norton, the English literature instructor, said to him, "I have never heard Robert Frost quoted better." Jerry had quoted a few lines from Frost's *Mending Wall* in his valedictory.

One person who has had a very positive effect on Jerry is Dr. Carl Braun (Class J in Normal School). The two met late in their grade eleven year in high school. Carl was assigned a seat right beside him. The new student was as shy as they come! The first thing that virtually struck awe in Jerry was Carl's exquisite handwriting.

Eventually, the two students did become acquainted and soon were close friends. Carl later excelled as a teacher and received an honorary Doctor of Laws degree (LL.D.) from the University of Manitoba, in Winnipeg. He has challenged Jerry to excellence many times. Carl was

Jerry's mentor when he worked at his doctoral dissertation and helped to take off some of the sharp edges in his presentation.

Apart from the incidents already mentioned, he adds that he had pleasant memories of all the instructors he had, albeit some with a chuckle.

It was reported that he delivered a very inspiring message for the Sunday service in the former Normal School auditorium at the 45th anniversary of our year. At the 50th anniversary, in Brandon, he was asked to repeat the valedictory address to the Normalites and their spouses who were present.

His philosophy of life is quite simple. Trust in the Lord with all your heart and lean not on to your own understanding. In all your ways acknowledge Him and He will make your paths straight. (Proverbs 3:4-5)

For a hobby, Jerry enjoys woodworking. He is a handyman and loves to putter around. He does take an unusual exception to doors that do not function properly. They tend to irk him. As a result, he readily offers his services to correct the situation.

40

Lois (Leigh) Moore

Information for this chapter was submitted by Lois's children, who, in addition to their own memories about their mother, provided what Lois had written for her grandchildren. Lois passed away in January 2009.

The farm girl had never seen the big city of Winnipeg, had never ridden on a streetcar, had never been on a Greyhound bus, and had never really been away from home on her own. Here, she was riding by herself from Medora, in southwestern Manitoba, to that big city to fulfill her ambition of becoming a teacher. That experience would have been very traumatic for some girls—and boys—just out of high school, but this girl found it exciting.

Lois was born in Medora. She was homeschooled and took some correspondence courses. Like the others whose stories appear here, she obtained her teaching certificate from Normal School in 1951. Later, she attended summer classes at Gimli.

She taught in Waterloo for two years, boarding with Jack and Ruth Meggison. Her next school was at Pennisula, which was near Melita, for one year, boarding with Harry and Mary Champion. Her third school was Northfield School, near Wawanesa, for two years, boarding with Bill and Mazie Shearer. Outside of teaching, she did home care later in life for fifteen years until 2000.

When she was a child, she enjoyed reading *Betty Zane*, by Zane Gray. In her adult years, she would read any books written by Nellie McClung.

Her hobbies consisted of sewing, cooking, and genealogy. In her community, she participated in Seniors Independent Services, Genealogy Society, 4-H, and square dancing

The remainder of this chapter was written by Lois for some of her grandchildren for a project on which they were working at school. She entitled it "Memories of My Year in Normal School".

> Labour Day weekend 1950 was a busy, scary, exciting time for me. I was achieving my dream of going to the only Normal School, or Teacher's College, in Manitoba. By the end of June 1951, I hoped to achieve my lifelong dream of being a teacher. My mother had attended Normal School in Blue Earth, Minnesota, where she had grown up. Neighbours my mother's age at Napinka, Manitoba, and Medora talked about attending Normal School at Manitou, Manitoba; and that is what I would have to do to receive a teaching certificate. The strange word *Normal School* goes way back to after 1066 when the Normans from France had overrun England.
>
> Anyway, here was this country bumpkin of a person who had never been to Winnipeg, never ridden on a streetcar, never been on a Greyhound bus, never really been away on her own before riding by herself from Medora to Winnipeg. Exciting!!
>
> Anne, an older friend, who had completed a business course at Success Business College and was working in the city, met me at the bus. She got a taxi, my luggage was loaded, and we drove the six or seven miles to the site of the school. Now, the Canadian Mennonite University, or the CMU, occupies the area. During WW II, a group of airmen

called Wireless No.3 trained here. The bus that ran there was still called the Wireless No. 3 bus. The H huts and the huge gym that were built during the war were still there. Years before the war, a marvellous, huge four-storey building had been built here as a residential school for the deaf. Now, the teachers in training were using all of the buildings for residences (300 of the 360 students lived on the campus), classes, recreation, and all else that was needed to make a happy community. To the east, the south, and the west was undisturbed poplar and oak bush and to the north a golf course for half a mile and then the Assiniboine Park and Portage Avenue. Many a time we would walk across the Park to catch a bus or streetcar or to return home from an outing downtown. The bush around the campus made it seem as if I were still in the country.

Well, Anne established me at the Manitoba Provincial Normal School, or the MPNS. Then she returned to her home. I was on my own. The lone person that was registering the dozen or two holiday registrants had placed me in a single room at the north end of the east upright of an H hut. The two uprights had rooms down both sides with a hall in the middle so there were four rows of rooms in each hut. There were only four single rooms and they were at the north end of each upright. The crosspiece that joined the uprights together housed the laundry, the showers, and the sinks—no bathtubs. Residences in the main building had tubs. There were running water, showers, and washing machines—very new items for many of us. I soon learned to enjoy showering. And, oh! there were electric lights. The Medora farm did not have electricity until the fall of 1951.

A girl from Regina (Marjorie Woods) registered that night and was given the single room across the hall from me. We agreed to support each other as if we were sharing a room. Thus began a friendship that lasted a lifetime—she passed away a few years ago. The following weeks I got acquainted with, worked with, played with, and lived with so many groups that were different from the Anglo-Saxon / Flemish culture that I knew. There were the Ukrainians, the Mennonites, the French, the born and bred city students, the war veterans, the way Northern Canada students, ten nuns wearing their habits (they were non-resident students), a Japanese fellow, and a Chinese girl who had been uprooted with her family from British Columbia to Alberta during the war. A fascinating mixture of people! Over a hundred of us were together for our fifty-fifth reunion. The friendships have carried on over the years.

Then there were classes. The subjects were: Social Studies (how to teach), English 1 (how to teach), Physical Education, Art, Classroom Management, Childhood Development, Library, Maths A, Maths B (remedial), Health Education, English III (remedial), Music, Science, English II (the spoken word, improvement of individuals speaking, speech choirs) and Basic Techniques. I learned the most from English II. I became a clearer speaker, learned how words should be formed and developed confidence. Basic Tech did little to prepare me for the classroom. Recently, a fellow classmate of mine watched her grandchild train for a teacher at Brandon University. Her opinion is that now the students do not learn any more in two years than we learned in one.

Some of the things I took part in were the debating group, the speech choirs, learned to skate on the campus open air skating rink and to swim at Sherbrook Pool, and made money serving meals in the dining hall. There were streetcar and bus rides downtown and always somebody to visit with. It was a great year. I am thankful for it.

41

Rose (McColl) McIver

Whenever young teachers think about teaching, there is an initial tendency to lump all children together, thinking of them as malleable clay which they, as their mentors, will be able to mould into accomplished little scholars, being justifiably proud, at the end of the year, in handing out report cards—passports, actually—for sending these students triumphantly on their way into the next grade.

However, as teachers shortly discover, their students are anything but a homogeneous little group; indeed, no two of them seem to be made of the same kind of clay at all. In short, these children before us are very much like everyone else in the world, each arriving in his own shape and colour and size, and each with his own peculiar quirks and quarks and funny, distinctive personalities.

In her early teaching career, Rose had two of these "distinctive" young personalities in one of her classrooms —two little boys who sometimes just about drove her "wacky". She had to learn as quickly as possible how to deal with these miscreants in order to keep discipline in her class, with a semblance of learning taking place.

Those were the days when students, after they were assigned their work in class, were expected to settle down quietly, and do it, with no talking, or "fidgeting around".

However, one of them (whom she will call Barry) had his own funny, little peculiarities, coupled with a tremendous sense of humour, which Rose usually enjoyed—but not when everyone was supposed to be working on lessons.

As might be expected, his desk was stationed right at the very front of the teacher's desk, where she could keep her baleful eye on him. However, as she moved about the room helping individual children, she would quite often become spatially removed from any effective influence on Master Barry. He had an active mind and acute hearing; and, if anything in the classroom caught his attention as being funny, as happened many times in a day, she would immediately hear from the front of the classroom, "Too-shay, Mon-soor Poo-sy Cat!", and there would be Barry, laughing delightedly, while taking a wide swipe in the air with his pencil, mimicking the sword fight between the Cat and the Mouse, as depicted in the television cartoons. That was sufficient to set off the entire class!

Today, with a much more lenient attitude toward the disciplining of children, this would be thought of as nothing, but in those days it was somewhat unnerving for a young teacher, especially with a watchful, sober, no-nonsense principal stalking the halls. It was, indeed, a somewhat harrowing experience for this teacher. Nevertheless, Barry, despite his sometimes madcap antics, remains to this day firmly entrenched in her memory as one of the most delightful students whom she ever taught, likeable in every way—and she still remembers him fondly. She wishes him well today. "Too-shay, Mon-soor Bar-ree!"

Such was the teaching world into which Rose, a little country girl from Gladstone, was apparently destined to step, with nary a shade of foreboding of all the Barrys and other delightful little mischief-makers whom she would encounter within a few short years!

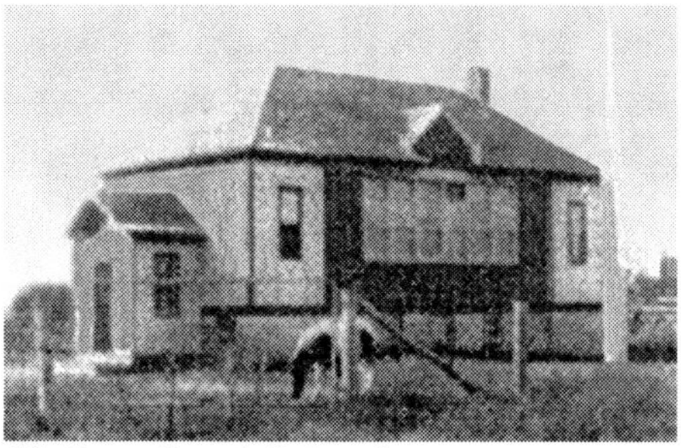
23. Bear Creek School

As a March child, Rose was born in the frosty month of February, entering the world a month early—the first, and one of the few times in her life that she has managed to be early—in her parents' farm home, near Gladstone. When she was six years old, she began attending Bear Creek School #762, which was eight or nine miles (13–14 km) away from the town.

Even though the name of the school might suggest a very rustic and unsettled area, this part of Manitoba had been settled and farmed for quite a number of decades by the time that she was born. Situated in the parkland area of the province, the land had long been cleared of trees and bush, and the farming carried on there was a mixture of growing cereal grains and raising cattle.

The school was a one-room building which had been built about twenty years prior to her enrolling. Thus, it was still called "the new school", as opposed to the original "old school", constructed of logs, now humbly serving as a chicken shelter on a neighbouring farm.

The "new" school was regarded by everyone in the district with much pride. It had a large classroom, with elegant blackboards along two sides and a long row of large windows along the east side to let in plenty of light for the scholars. In the basement was a furnace which never did work well, and therefore, heat for the classroom was supplied by a large tin heater at the back of the classroom. A tin guard surrounded it, over which could be draped an assortment of wet mitts, socks, toques, and any other article of apparel which needed drying.

The classroom had a small room at one end, optimistically designated as a "library", while at the other end were two cloak rooms. In between was a stairway, leading down to the door opening onto the "front" yard.

This was quite an important part of the school yard, because, right in front of the school—the very epicentre of their educational universe—was the flag pole, majestically displaying, in all kinds of weather, a large Union Jack, indicating to all and sundry that this was an official school, organized by the Province of Manitoba, in the Dominion of Canada, and under the aegis of the British Empire, and that young Canadian scholars were there at work, being educated by their government on behalf of King George VI.

At a distance further on from the school was a large and handsomely-constructed barn which had been built to shelter the ponies and horses used as transportation by many students; while at a discreet distance away from the barn were the "outhouses"—one for the girls and one for the boys.

Certainly a practical necessity, these little buildings also provided a pleasant destination and diversion for students sometimes wishing to escape the odious tasks of memorizing the "times table" or the learning of the capital cities in South America. An arm waving in the air, with the request, "Please, may I leave the room?" was the magical formula, similar to "Open, Sesame!" which provided ten or fifteen minutes of heavenly respite for most students at one time or another.

Not all children went to high school in those days, as grade eight was regarded as a practical education for most farm families. However, Rose was one who did. After taking grades nine and ten by correspondence lessons from the provincial Department of Education, she took grades eleven and twelve in Gladstone High School. Her father was adamant that she should acquire a "good" education leading to a profession, just in case she ended up "marrying a drunk" and having to support herself and a little family! Happily, that scenario did not occur for her; nevertheless, she has always been thankful that she had parents who had their daughter's future in mind well ahead of time.

She applied to enter Normal School to prepare herself for a teaching career. Money was in very short supply in her family; thus, it was a blessing for her when her bachelor Uncle Curly gave her a gift of one hundred dollars to provide for augmenting her meagre wardrobe for her "Normal School Education".

Thus provisioned, off she went to Tuxedo to obtain her training for a career that, while it had its ups and downs, provided nevertheless, quite a marked degree of satisfaction and independence for her throughout the years. It also enabled her to meet and socialize with many wonderful children, their parents, and many people in other professions and vocations in various parts of the province of Manitoba.

Normal School was interesting in a number of respects. Since she had no brothers or sisters, the opportunity to socialize with other young people of her own age was a golden experience. She is quite certain that she was a complete exasperation to many young women in residence who had to put up with her juvenile antics during that year.

However, on one hand, she learned to grow up a bit during her time there, while at the same time, other residents learned a bit of long-suffering, and most learned to get along with each other with a fair amount of grace. Many good friendships were made which, in retrospect, is probably the most beneficial outcome of any experience.

One of the customs which was extremely beneficial to some students at Normal School was the opportunity to work for one semester in the dining-room or in the kitchen. This provided students with a little badly-needed extra cash and, of course, that was always welcome to anyone. She became acquainted with Ben Hanuschak, Duane Duff, and Walter Hucaluk, amongst others, as they worked in the kitchen, keeping all the cooking utensils and pans clean. Rose was one of the students who worked in the dining room, setting and clearing tables for the evening meal.

Here is where she encountered the notorious duo, Harry Rudy and Johnny Ryan. These two delightfully zany fellows regularly sat at her table, having been assigned there for supper by the dining-room steward. These guys, full of fun, and entertaining though they were, sometimes exasperated the life out of Rose.

One of the regular suppers each week was spaghetti and meat balls. Nearly everyone agreed that the meat balls and tomato sauce would not win any blue ribbons at the Cordon Bleu School in Paris—or anywhere else, for that matter—but the students generally ate them anyway to stave off hunger.

However, that did not include Rudy and Ryan, who utterly refused to eat those meat balls, and instead, hid them under the upside-down cups! At the end of supper, Rose would clean off the table. When everything looked clean and tidy to her, she would sign out. The next morning, there would be a tow-row because the cups, now to be used for breakfast coffee by someone else, were full of ancient meat balls. She was then in trouble with the dining room steward! From that experience, she learned that what looks right is not necessarily as it appears to be, and that it was much better to check those innocent-looking cups before she left for the night.

Among the Normal School staff, the member whom she enjoyed and from whose instruction she benefited the most was Miss Douglas. Her vivacity and enthusiasm for music was an inspiration to Rose, later giving her the confidence to do choir work, including musical festivals, with her classes in subsequent years of teaching. She considered Beth Douglas to be excellent because, among her other attributes, she was truly an encourager and was a good example for all of her students.

Rose taught for a total of ten years, the first few in rural Manitoba, and later, in city schools in Dauphin and Winnipeg. After she married, she taught in Moose Jaw, Sask., for five years. Here, she worked with various primary grades and was a travelling music teacher for junior high grades for a time. During her teaching years, she attended university classes at United College in Winnipeg and at the University of Regina.

However, somewhere along the way, two little boys came along, and she decided to stay at home and "be a mother"—a decision which she never regretted. As her little boys were growing up, Rose involved herself in the community in various ways, which resulted in a number of interesting experiences from time to time.

In the early part of the 1980s, numerous refugees from Vietnamese and Cambodian Communism found haven in Canada, and many Christian churches either sponsored them or helped them to learn about their new home. At various times, she would teach English to mothers and children, or be a taxi driver for people with medical appointments. Once, she was commissioned to scout around in Regina for the best buys in used coffee shop equipment for a fledgling doughnut shop.

For a period of time she was a "teacher" for a student attending a welding class at the Provincial Technical School. Rose was not a welder by any stretch of the imagination; but in the evenings, her new Laotian friend would bring his textbook over to her home, and she would explain, in the best way that she could, with diagrams and simple words, just what all those puzzling terms and words meant as they went through his lesson for that day. As the weeks went by, she became quite an expert in welding, and began to think that, if she had her life to relive, she just might be a welder instead of a teacher!

Without doubt, Rose's most memorable experience came when her good friend Nguyet asked her to go to Court with her to be a translator for her younger brother. Apparently, her brother, under the somewhat nefarious influence of an older acquaintance, had gone to Regina with him one night to experience the exquisite and titillating pleasures of several "Ladies of the Evening". They had not counted on the young woman in question taking certain safety precautions such as providing a friend in the trade with the license number of the vehicle used. The vehicle was traced and the young man was charged and had to appear in Court. His English was quite limited, as was that of his sister, with the result that Rose was prevailed upon to be the translator in court.

The entire case was quite messy, with several extraneous complications being involved, and Rose was extremely embarrassed to have any part in the ultimate proceedings. In retrospect, she must admit that nervous as she was long ago when she "walked down the aisle" on her wedding day, she was not nearly so unnerved then as having to walk down the aisle on this particular day toward the prisoner's box with that young fellow in tow, the jaded eyes of the judge watching the whole procession, tapping his fingers on the charge sheet before him, and idly wondering to himself, no doubt, "Now, just how did *she* get mixed up in this?"

Happily, all survived the unsavoury experience of that morning; but the truly positive part of it all was that she still has the devoted friendship of Nguyet to this day —Rose loves her dearly—and she also has the friendship of that rascally young brother, hopefully somewhat wiser, who still visits Rose and her husband occasionally when he is in Moose Jaw.

Probably the most interesting part of her life has been her involvement with politics. In the early 1990s, she became a believer in the need for political change in Canada as envisioned by Preston Manning, and a call to bring government closer to the people in order to ensure more responsible governance.

So, buying a membership in the Reform Party, she volunteered her services as a worker at the local constituency level, doing any and all jobs which would help to promote the party's goals for a new Canada. Her forte became door-knocking and door-talking—something from which most people tend to shy away, but something which she enjoyed immensely. Her attendance at various national conventions and meetings resulted in trips across Canada, where she met many interesting people.

She confesses, though, that her greatest heart-break in life came just recently when she did *not* receive her expected appointment to the Senate of Canada, being prevented by age limitations and considered too old to qualify for the position. Imagine—just as she confidently believed that finally she had "earned her way to the top"! O, the ironies of life! O, the agonies of hopes forever dashed! O, quelle sorrow!

Even though her Senate hopes are a thing of the past, she still works with the political party of her choice, while involving herself with a few other pursuits as well.

Her garden has always been a source of pleasure and she does much reading. In her pre-teen years, a favourite book was *Salvage All*—the story of a young man who, with his orphaned kid brother, salvaged an old, abandoned tug-boat, and the two of them made their living being sea-scavengers. It stirred her childhood imagination, and, even yet, she has longings to be a houseboat dweller and an explorer of the deeps. She always has a desire to explore the water-fronts of whatever city the family is visiting—much to the horror of her very prosaic husband and sons.

More recently, one of the truly interesting books which she has read is *Wanderings: Chaim Potek's History of the Jews*. It details their history from the time of Abram, in Ur of the Chaldees, up to the present time, and is written from the perspective of a modern Jew. Well-written and comprehensive, it is a fascinating book and one which Rose recommends highly.

Something else which she recommends to anyone seeking both beauty and adventure is a canoe trip along the Churchill River system in northern Saskatchewan. Any time in the summer is rewarding, but the early autumn colours enhance the beauty of the rushing river, the breath-taking rapids, and the grandeur of the forest—both deciduous and coniferous—as a living backdrop in this astoundingly beautiful part of the province, hidden to all but the most adventurous souls. However, if you do decide on this unforgettable trip, do not forget to take along a generous supply of either Deet or bear-grease, which ever is handier!

Hers has been an interesting and rewarding life, mainly because of the profession which she chose. She would add that one of the most important pieces of advice which she can offer to anyone, either at the beginning of one's life and career or at the end of it—or, anywhere in between—is the commendation found in the Book of Micah, Chapter 6, verse 8: "What does the Lord require of thee? To act justly, to love mercy, And to walk humbly with your God." This is wise advice to all of us, so that at the end, we may hear those welcome words from our Lord: "Well done, thou good and faithful servant."

42
Wilma (Miller) Furniss

Some people like to place footprints or initials into fresh, drying cement. Wilma and a few friends at Normal School were no different. There was a fresh coat of cement in the washroom of the dormitory.

Now, they were called before our vice-principal, Mr. Lightly, to explain themselves. This administrator did not need the skills of Perry Mason or Sherlock Holmes to solve the mystery. The initials of the girls were clearly portrayed. What kind of punishment would he mete out? His use of kindness as a form of psychology made the girls think and be ashamed of themselves. Here were future teachers who would be setting examples for young children and probably would be having, at some time, to deal with such activity. The girls learned more from his approach than if he had taken severe measures.

Wilma was born in Elm Creek, and obtained her education prior to Normal School in that town.

When she was in high school, a group of students travelled to Winnipeg to attend a presentation of "Hamlet". On their journey home, virtual blizzard conditions with blowing snow arose. The road became impassible. They were stranded in a community twelve miles (19 km) from Elm Creek. How would they be able to complete their trip home? They were able to keep warm in a local restaurant.

Eventually, their knight in shining armour came to their rescue! He was a person with a Bombardier snow machine, which was relatively rare in the 1940s. He was able to transport the students safely home.

Her favourite teacher was Max Parker, her school principal for eleven of her twelve years at school. He taught history and French. He was always fair, had good discipline without ever raising his voice, and played outside with his students at recess. Beth Douglas, our music teacher at Normal School, had such sparkling eyes. She explained that the reason why we have holes in our heads is to make the tones come out right.

Prior to her year of Normal School, she taught in Bertram School District, near Swan Lake. After her year of teacher training, she taught in Midland School District, near Manitou. One day when she opened a cupboard while working at the old Midland School before moving into the new one, she experienced a surprise. There was a nest of baby mice. Quickly, she scooped it all up, took it outside, and hit the young rodents with a baseball bat! Years later, when Midland had a school reunion, she was presented a commemorative. Her former students had not forgotten that day in the life of their teacher, giving her a mouse trap and a rubber mouse. Happy mousing, Wilma!

In her first school, there were a water pail, dipper, and wash basin, which were used by everyone. Since water had to be carried, it was not wasted. There were few materials for teacher and children. They had to purchase some items or make do with what was available. There was a small library with a few books. The children walked during warmer weather, while horses were used for transportation in the winter. Parents would bring their children to school and return for them at the end of the day.

The home where she boarded had a telephone which was on a rural party line. When a call came in, it was likely that most people on the line would be listening in on the conversation.

Wilma met her future husband in this district. Since then, she has been a farmer's wife and has remained in the area. She had grown up on a farm; thus, it was not a big transition from being a teacher to being a farm wife. As a young girl, she did not do much farm work as her mother preferred to do it herself. Her biggest transition was learning to drive the farm vehicles since she had not driven anything before her marriage. Suddenly, she was on her own and had to learn for herself.

She enjoyed reading *Heidi*, by Johanna Spyri, as a child. Life on a mountain fascinated her. In adult life, she found *I Am Hutterite*, by Mary Ann Kirkby, particularly interesting.

One year, she and her husband Vic took a trip to the Maritime Provinces in late September and early October. She had studied the history of these provinces in school and now actually saw what she had learned. The fall colours were spectacular!

She would suggest people visit the Pembina Valley, south of Manitou, either in the spring with the many shades of green or in the autumn with the colourful leaves. Either time, it is beautiful there.

Her advice to teenagers would be to enjoy these carefree years. Be careful who you choose as friends. Listen to the advice of your parents and friends, even though you might not agree with it at the time.

To persons considering entering the teaching profession, she says to go for it! Always be firm, but considerate and kind. Be aware of the pupil's home life because this would have a bearing on behaviour.

She has great respect for an older friend who helped her greatly when she was first married and then all though the rest of her life. She taught Wilma how and when to do things in the garden and gave her advice on the raising of her babies. She showed her how to have a positive attitude toward whatever occurred in her life.

A great Canadian leader was Bert Hall, of Manitou. He was awarded the Lieutenant-Governor's "Make a Difference Community Award" for the Central Region of Manitoba. He was active in initiating community projects and was on the funding board of many national boards, including Poultry Marketing and Keystone Agricultural Producers. He was always a humble volunteer!

For hobbies, she enjoys reading, knitting, sewing, gardening, and square dancing. She has been Health Centre friendly visitor and has been a member of the Anglican Church Women, the Agricultural Society, Parent-Teachers Association, and Red Hat Society.

The Red Hat organization is a disorganized association for women over fifty. Although there is a Queen Mother, there are no offices. The members do not raise money. It is not necessary to take food every time. It is a time for fun for women over fifty years of age. When they attend a gathering, they wear purple outfits with red hats. In her group, in the month of one's birthday, the person wears a red outfit with a purple hat.

When she lived on the farm, she was correspondent for the Manitou *Western Canadian.* She would telephone neighbours in her area and collect any news which they had. Then she would collate all the news and send it to the newspaper.

Her philosophy of life is to keep a positive attitude. Live each day as if it were your last. Do the things you enjoy doing and try to enjoy the other things you have to do in your life's journey.

Wilma feels that all of us should write our own autobiography, including little stories and happenings through the years, for our families to enjoy.

43
Bernice (Morrow) Lewis

In her first year of teaching grade one—in a city school—she had a difficult student. One day, just as she was about to dismiss the class for noon hour, he swung into motion. He grabbed a box of red counters and threw them as high into the air as he could. As they descended, they scattered hither and thither—all over the room. That made Bernice angry! It was such an inopportune time for something like this to happen.

Why was she blessed with a child who could be so disobedient? He could be even worse when the class would go on a field trip. She would not take him unless his parents were willing to go, too. She did not want to be constantly trying to corral this independent-minded child. She did realize, though, that a major cause for his unpleasant behaviour arose from his coming from a broken home.

Bernice was born in Darlingford. Before Normal School, she attended Darlingford Consolidated School, a four-room school having grades one to eleven. She obtained a Bachelor of Arts degree from University of Winnipeg.

A bad experience in her school life was that boys used to like to pick up garter snakes from the school grounds and throw them on the girls. Only once did a snake thrown by a boy land on her back. Oh, what a dreadful sensation she felt! At the time, she was very afraid of snakes. She did not want anything to do with them. The boys were aware of this. Thus, it was more fun for them at her expense.

Like numerous other former Normalites, Bernice enjoyed Miss Norton because of her wonderful story telling.

At Normal School, she stayed in La Verendrye Hut. The comradeship of all there in her wing was outstanding. She enjoyed hanging out in the canteen after study hours in the evening. The year at Normal School was the most memorable of her life.

Her first school was Debonair School, a one-room school located near Roland. There were seventeen students from grades one to nine. The library was very small. The students carried drinking water into the school from a well in the schoolyard. An oil furnace provided heat for the school. A highlight of the year was the Christmas concert. Thus, much of December was set aside to practise plays, recitations, and songs. She taught here for two years. The rest of her career was spent in St. James, a part of Winnipeg, in the primary grades.

In 1985, she was on a tour of Europe and Israel. In Israel, she walked where Jesus walked and had a ride on a large boat on the Sea of Galilee. She does not recall seeing any fishing being carried on. When her group ate after leaving the boat, they were told that the fish served at the meal were from that sea. In Capernaum, a conversation between Jesus and Peter was emphasized. Jesus asked: "Who do you say that I am?" Peter replied: "You are the Messiah." She noted that the town has been modernized.

In Jerusalem, she saw that there is an old city and a new city. The Wailing Wall filled her with awe. People could place their prayers into the cracks in the wall. When in the area, it was necessary for her to have her arms covered. She had no contact with the Muslims, even though she did visit Gaza Strip. At the time that she was there, talk about Muslims was much less. However, she and the other tourists were warned to stay on the prescribed paths as there were land mines in the area.

She also visited Bethlehem. She enjoyed swimming in the Dead Sea. Everyone covered themselves with mud first as it was so hot to walk to the water. She was very fascinated by her visit to Israel. It all made the stories of the Bible come alive.

Bernice recommends Whiteshell Provincial Park, in eastern Manitoba, with its many lakes and beautiful forests, as a Canadian place to visit.

Her advice to teenagers is for them to keep themselves pure so when they enter into marriage, they will have no regrets.

Teaching is very rewarding. It is important to come to the classroom prepared. Each child's life is important and you, as the teacher, are responsible to help to mould each in the truth.

Martha Deason was her grades seven and eight teacher. She taught all subjects in those grades and made each subject come alive. She was fair in every way.

Bernice's daughter Darlene has had an impressive effect on her. She has been at hand, ready to help through the tough times and the good times. She is a principal in nearby Winnipeg and phones every night to relate her day's events and also to see how her mother's day passed.

She admires Steven Fletcher, the Member of Parliament for her constituency, Charleswood-St. James-Assiniboia. Although he is a quadriplegic, he is such a good spokesman in parliament and is also a good listener.

He is the first permanently disabled Canadian to be elected to the House of Commons. Steven has served his community, his university student body, his political party, and Parliament with distinction. Bernice was at a seniors' centre in Headingly, not far from Winnipeg, where he gave an address at a luncheon. A book about him has already been written. Following the 2008 general election, Prime Minister Harper selected him to be Minister of State for Democratic Reform.

One of her favourite books is *Light a Penny Candle*, by Maeve Binchy. For pastimes, she enjoys reading and working crossword puzzles and cryptoquotes.

In her community, she is a member of a Bible study group. She is also a member of the Alpha-Delta-Kappa Sorority in St. James, a part of Winnipeg. This organization originates in Kansas City, Missouri. Most of its forty local members are retired teachers who live in St. James. Very few younger teachers are involved as they feel that they are too busy. The sorority meets monthly and participates in altruistic activities.

A unique experience took place when she spent time in London, Ont., awaiting her husband's heart transplant. There, she witnessed those who were grasping for a few more years of life and also those who did not make it. She was able to talk with some of the patients in the wing where transplant patients were located.

They stayed in a guest wing of a nearby nunnery, Mount St. Joseph, within walking distance from University Hospital. They were treated royally. Many lasting friendships were cultivated at that time. It was a time to show compassion and a time to rejoice. It was such an unforgettable experience.

Her philosophy of life is to do her best always and to be a help to her fellow man.

44
Jack Morton

"Report to the principal's office!" That is what he and three classmates heard. What had they done? On arrival, their principal told them to sit down. That was unusual. They were still wondering what was happening.

Then the explanation was given. A call had come in from a neighbouring high school. They were lacking one rink for their bonspiel. The principal informed the boys that they had been marked in for attendance and that if they should disappear, their absence would not be noticed.

No further invitation was needed. They participated in the bonspiel. Alas! They did not win a prize. However, afterwards, they were caught in "the mother of all blizzards", and came home via the Greyhound bus—after much shoveling on the Arden Ridge.

Jack was born in Dauphin. His education prior to attending Normal School was obtained in Minnedosa. Later, he obtained credits towards a Police Science degree.

In his early high school years, he had an English teacher who really enjoyed her profession. She made her classes a learning environment in which it was fun to be a part. She encouraged participation and interaction.

He has always enjoyed both the written and spoken word, and felt that both Miss Norton and Miss Smith, at

Normal School, helped to increase his enjoyment and ability in these subjects.

When he reflects on his year at Normal School, he recalls that he was an immature eighteen-year-old; but he really enjoyed the experience and relationships that he had. The only outstanding event that jumps to his memory was the fun that the students had with their tableaux in the theatrical productions, *Patterns of Living.*

From 1951 to 1954, he taught in a junior high school classroom in Grandview. His next experience in teaching took place when he was in the RCMP. From 1962 to 1965, he was an instructor in recruit training at RCMP Training Depot, Regina, Sask. From 1970 to 1972, he was researcher, developer, and presenter in the Senior Managers and Executive Development Programmes at Canadian Police College, Ottawa, Ont. From 1974 to 1975, he was police services programme developer and presenter in the Senior Managers Programme at Mount Royal Community College, Calgary, Alta.

As an RCMP officer in the field, he served in three provinces. From 1955 to 1962, he served as a general duty investigator and municipal traffic patrolman in St. John's, Gander, and Corner Brook, N.L. From 1966 to 1970, he was a plain-clothes investigator and detachment commander in Edmonton and Two Hills, Alta. From 1972 to 1973, he was a municipal detachment commander and international airport security commander in Drumheller and Calgary, Alta. From 1975 to 1990, he was police liaison officer, VIP security officer, organized crime officer, human resources manager, operations officer, and detachment commander in Victoria, Vernon, Kamloops, and North Vancouver, B.C.

In the mid 1950s, Jack was stationed at a busy airport in Newfoundland. Work was exciting, and he really enjoyed being responsible for a rural portion of the detachment area. Gander Bay was on the open coast, on the northeast, and included a string of small outports (fishing villages) which constituted the population. There were three ways to reach there in an emergency: by float or ski plane (not practicable for much of the year), by a Gander River canoe, or by a passenger boat from the seaport of Lewisport.

Shortly after Christmas Day, the RCMP was instructed to go to one of these outports, as a result of a sudden death, and to transport the body for a post mortem examination at the Twillingate hospital, where there was a pathologist. Jack was assigned the task.

Early on December 27, he walked down to the boat awaiting him in Lewisport. It was a clear, cold, and calm morning, three weather conditions which are almost never found at the same time on the east coast. He had sailed with the vessel before; but today, the captain was not his garrulous self. He seemed preoccupied, and kept going to the glass (barometer) and expressing serious concerns as it was very low. At sea, this indicates a severe storm is brewing.

They were well into their four-hour voyage; and after a hearty breakfast of fish and brews and steaming tea, he relaxed somewhat. With no seas running, they arrived at their destination early and found that the developing shore ice prevented them from using the government pier. The outporters had made a makeshift walkway using ladders. The casket was on a sled, which the crew pulled onto their boat, using a tossed line.

As this was being accomplished, Jack noticed that the ice was starting to move. On looking out onto the bay, he observed that the ominous sea was rising. They departed for a three-hour trip to the hospital.

The captain hugged the ice on the east coast of the bay, and steamed very slowly. He explained that he did not want to create any spray as the salt water would create ice, especially on any exposed metal portions of his vessel, particularly the metal hand line around the boat. The sea in the open water was now very rough. They had reached the point of no return as they could not go back because there was no shelter. The captain advised Jack that they were going to cross the bay as it was not possible to reach their destination, and that he would land him at an outport. There, a horse and cart would take him and his travelling companion to the hospital across the bay—if they arrived safely.

As they turned to the west, the waves were beam on to the boat. It was necessary for the captain to steam into the wave troughs, and then cut back the engines when the boat crested the waves. By then, the wind was whipping off the wave tops, and Jack soon realized that ice was forming on the boat and it was not as buoyant as before. The lower cabin door swung open. When he looked down, he saw that the crew members were on their knees, rosaries in hand. This was not a good sign!

Jack asked what he might do. He was given a hookless gaff (used for killing fish) and was told, after he was tied to a line, that when the boat was in the wave trough, he could step out of the bridge and beat on the iced hand lines, now as thick as one's thigh. The captain told him that the rope would tether him to the boat if he were washed overboard and that they would not have to search for a body.

At that point, Jack really began to reconsider his selection of a vocation and location. After a few trips onto the deck, he began to develop a rhythm, and the ice began to chip off into the scuppers. He was in a sweat, from either fear or exertion; but his labours were paying off as the boat responded much better to wave and helm. He does not know how long the trip was; but the waves finally diminished in size, and he realized that they were on the lee side of Twillingate Island—and safety.

The pony and cart were waiting as promised. It was now night. The doctor and staff were not waiting; and the following day the facilities were again not available. The examination and report were finally completed. The storm passed, and on January 2, his boat returned to deliver the body for burial, and Jack back to his home port. His date for the annual New Year's ball at the Airport Club had not waited.

If you enter a graveyard in an east coast fishing village, there is often a separate location for those lost at sea, usually with an inscription over the gateway, "For those who go down to the sea in small boats." He now understands the significance of that sentence; but this patrol really reinforced the old Scottish saying: "The best laid plans of man and mice, needs often go astray."

As a police officer, one of his tasks was the VIP security officer for British Columbia, except for the Vancouver area. He escorted prime ministers, heads of state, and—fairly often—members of the Royal Family. When he met Prince Charles, they had a one-on-one session in which the prince presented his expectations, and the officer presented his responsibilities.

His Royal Highness said, "Are you familiar with the naval tenet of 'sailing to the sound of distant guns'?"

Jack replied, "As dismounted cavalrymen, we say 'gallop to the sound of distant guns'. However, for your visits, we will simply change the preposition *to* to *from*." They had a great relationship then and all following visits.

We in Canada are very blessed with so many locations for all occasions. For a visitor in springtime, Jack would suggest a circle trip of western Nova Scotia, including apple blossom time in the Annapolis Valley. In the fall after a few snowfalls on the peaks of the Rockies, a trip south from Calgary to Waterton Lakes National Park along Highway 22 is a treat for the eyes. To see what the west was really like before the European arrival, the southernmost roads in Saskatchewan will be an eye-opener.

He has often addressed youths in schools, scouting groups, cadets, and social settings. He usually talked law enforcement and their reactions to their interactions with enforcement officers. This would lead into discussions of changes needed, and he would try to introduce the concept of affecting changes by working within the systems with which they were associated. If you cannot create the climate of change, then you must abide by those rules that society has democratically chosen, through their elected members.

Jack was very active in recruiting young persons with whom he was in contact in selecting a career in law enforcement. Now, after being on the sidelines for almost twenty years, and having a daughter following in his career, he might be more hesitant in suggesting such a course of action. There have been so many changes in the police service and its relationship with other partners in the criminal justice system that there is little to recognize from his era. Change does not always equate with improvement.

Jack has to go back to his early days as a police officer in a small detachment—his first experience in a small work unit. The officer in charge, E. A. Rose, introduced him to the concept of self learning, with the knowledge that he was there to guide should it be needed. He emphasized the need for group involvement to solve difficult situations and the need for cohesion in a multi-person work unit.

He met Father David Murray, when the latter was the director of the famous Catholic boys' school, Notre Dame

College, in Wilcox, Sask., and who later directed the Canadian national hockey team out of Calgary. He was a dynamic individual, who was prepared to joust against the establishment or status quo if he felt that it was important to do so; but that it should not be done unless he was prepared to offer a viable alternative.

As a child he liked *Trail of the Ragged Fox*, by Pitt Fitzgerald, which was also a favourite for classroom reading during his teaching years. Later, he read fairly extensively such genres as history, biographies, and action novels. He particularly liked Dewey Lambdin's sea stories and Bernard Cornwall's adventure stories.

For pastimes, he plays tennis—outdoors whenever possible—and spends much time with his grandchildren at the ski hill, swimming pools, soccer pitches, and skating rinks. He is a volunteer driver for the Cancer Society and has acted as Safety and Security Chair for the British Columbia Winter Games in North Vancouver. He has been a member of Kinsmen, Rotary, Royal Canadian Legion, and RCMP Veterans, and has been involved in minor sports in all the locations where he has lived.

One should embark on a course of action, and then attempt to reach reasonable goals set in that journey. If the goals are not attainable, do not become frustrated; but appreciate that which you have accomplished in reaching the level achieved.

45
Sarah "Eva" Muir

In the early 1960s, five ladies, four of whom were sisters, drove a car with a roll-down camper to Alberta for a vacation and camped near Banff at Two Jack Lake.

One morning at about 5:00, Eva arose and wandered to the washroom. As she rounded the south corner, she abruptly stopped in her tracks. Lo, a bear was ambling past the building on the other side! How frightened this camper was! Would this unwelcome guest attack her? It was a rapid wash that she gave herself before quietly sneaking back to the safety of the camper. As soon as she had entered, she excitedly whispered to the others, "Do you want to see a bear? Look out the window."

All watched as the bear poked on the exterior of a nearby tent—and finally left. Later, the ladies told the folks from the tent about the bear. One of the inhabitants responded thus, "Why didn't you yell and tell us? We wanted a picture of a bear." Eva was shocked with this comment, but finally replied, "What would have happened if you had poked your head out the tent door? You might have received more than what you bargained for." The lesson here is that you do not yell out when you see or hear something in the wild because the result is unpredictable.

Sarah, known in Normal School as Eva, was born in Winnipeg, but spent most of her years as she was growing up in or near Oxbow, Sask. She started to school at Marconi, Sask., a country school south of Oxbow. Following that, she attended at Poplar, Sask., another rural school. The largest group of students was thirty-two in grades one to ten—with one teacher. Her last school was Boscurvis, Sask., where she was in grades eight and nine. She studied her grade ten by correspondence, following which she took grade eleven in Oxbow and grade twelve in Caronport, Sask. During July and August of 1949, she attended a short course at Tuxedo and then taught at Wicks School, near Pierson.

While attending school at Poplar, she and other children were playing paper chase and run sheep run one day and strayed too far from the school. In the process, they explored an old house. One of the persons sent to find them rode on horseback, ringing the bell for afternoon classes. As a result of the incident, many stayed in for a few recesses afterwards.

At Normal School, our art teacher, Miss Pilling, convinced Eva that she could do some drawing, "as everyone can do some type of drawing." Her scrapbook over the years has been used by her niece, who claimed she had not taken a course on art or art appreciation in her four years at university. The ideas which Miss Pilling provided carried over to the next generation of teachers.

The first year after Normal School, she taught at Crescent School, Sinclair. For the following year, she returned to Wicks School, near Pierson, where she had spent her permit year. After one year there, she returned home to teach at Boscurvis, where two of the three grade one pupils were her twin sisters. Then she spent two years at Souris Flats School, near Glen Ewen, Sask., before continuing on to Polar School, also near Glen Ewen. By then, country schools were in their last days; and, therefore, in 1957–58, she began teaching mathematics and science in two grade seven classes while Miss Cousins taught social studies and English, with each responsible for other subjects, in Brooks, Alta.

In the following year, she took a leave from teaching so that she could spend time in caring for her grandmother. In September of 1960, she returned to Manitoba to teach special education at Pierson and then in nearby Melita for one year.

Over the years, her principals have influenced the way in which she approached special education. At Pierson and Melita, Norman Brown helped her and the inspectors see that many of the students would be staying in their own communities. Eva's task was to help them improve their reading and mathematics skills. As the students became older, the school was able to place them into work situations.

One girl became a proficient seamstress after she had participated in a 4-H club. Later, she was able to work in a few stores, and then the Melita Hospital. From there, she obtained a position in the Brandon Mental Hospital, which she held until her death in a car accident.

One day when Eva was teaching at Pierson, five inspectors came to her room to see how she worked. Norman said afterwards that they were favourably impressed by what was taking place. The students came to her on a part-time basis. During an exam, Eva would read the question and write what the student said. The student then copied that and the home room teacher marked the paper from what the student wrote. Eva attempted to keep these special education students with their peer groups, not in a group by themselves. One young man has performed well over the years and became a good influence within the community.

From 1969 to 1971, she and Jean Woodward embarked on a new adventure in opening a school in

Orange Walk Town, Belize. In the first year, there was an enrolment of fifty-five students. For the second year in a school of grades one to eight and seventy pupils, they had the assistance of a Spanish teacher, who took over the beginners. Long after these two Canadians had returned to teach at Deloraine, they heard that the school in Orange Walk had over 400 pupils. During her two years at Deloraine, Eva took classes in special education at Brandon University, and earned a certificate in that field.

Between the autumns of 1973 and 1976, she stayed at home helping to care for her mother and her sister Lillian. Her mother passed away in 1975, and Lillian, who suffered from multiple sclerosis, was moved to a nursing home in the following year, where she passed away in 1988. Eva and her sister Grace, who also was at home, moved into Glen Ewen. In 1976, Eva organized a special education classroom at Carnduff, Sask., where she worked until retiring in 1988. Grace passed away in 2004.

When Eva was teaching in Pierson, she spent five years with a 4-H club, teaching sewing to the girls. Then in Carnduff, she helped to care for two elderly ladies, each moving to the nursing wing at Sunset Haven in later years.

One of the sets of books which Eva enjoyed when she was young was the *Sugar Creek Gang* series, by Paul Hutchison. The books were about a group of boys in a country school and all their adventures along the Sugar Creek. There is a place in Indiana that has posters showing that the books were written about this area.

Since retiring, she has enjoyed the *Winslow* series, written by Gilbert Morris. The first Winslows came to North America on the *Mayflower*. The family tree at the front of each book advances as the stories progress. Thus, the reader learns more about pioneer days, cotton mill owners, living with the Indians, ranchers, farmers, a circus performer, a sheriff, a wagon train foreman, pilots, missionaries, and doctors. Book 34 reached into the 1930s and 1940s.

Over the years, she has helped make quilts, has done embroidery work, and has grown gardens. Now, she is keeping those in suites and hostel rooms interested in games during the evening hours, and also reports news from her nursing home to two local newspapers.

The trip and stay in Belize gave Eva the realization that we in North America complain and waste much of what we have. We fail to comprehend how blessed we are, and that we can be doing more to help others in need.

She would counsel teenagers to follow their dreams. They should refrain from giving in to peer pressure. They need to realize that each person is important and has value. Since a teacher has a great influence on others, it is necessary to give pupils an understanding that each has abilities which one should find and use, and know that everyone has a purpose.

Dorothy Hughes, nee Jones, her grades seven and eight teacher, instilled in Eva a desire to learn and to do her best. She frequently sees her former teacher, who is in a nursing facility. Her teacher does not remember much; but, when she sees Eva, she always points and says, "She was one of my pupils."

Canada is a large country with a variety of scenery, some of which is in her own area of southeast Saskatchewan. The Estevan coal fields have created a changing landscape. Years ago, it was the digging of underground mines; but now it is huge cranes that pile the earth on each side of a coal seam. It has become a hilly country; whereas, it had been flat. Immense trucks and tractors have created roads on these hills to aid the companies in removing coal. Big caterpillars are now levelling the hills, after which the land is sown to grass. Some of the valleys are filling with water.

Another point of interest in the area is the Alameda Dam, built across a ravine to keep the Souris River from flooding. This is becoming a southeast Saskatchewan attraction. The lake behind the dam has been filled with fish. Every year, a fish derby is held here. Along the northeast side, campgrounds are being established to complement a golf course, which has been in operation since 2005. Also, the Saskatchewan Power Company built Shad Power Station. Here, Prime Minister Stephen Harper's government has helped finance a more environmental way of operating the big generators.

Former Prime Minister John Diefenbaker, from Saskatchewan, one of a number of people who have achieved much for Canada, helped to bring more projects to western Canada. Diefenbaker Lake was named in his honour. Farmers along the lake have been able to irrigate to grow better crops.

Former Premier Ernest Manning, of Alberta, took over *Canadian National Bible Hour*, a radio broadcast that has benefited people across Canada. The programme, now operated by Global Outreach Mission, has been on the air since the 1930s. Premier Manning was born south of Carnduff. One of the broadcasts was aired from a local reunion for the town of Carnduff.

Not everyone believes in the concept about life after death. However, Eva affirms that when her mother was dying, she received a glimpse of something wonderful and was able to let those at her bedside know through a beautiful smile that lit up her face. Even the matron remarked, "I wonder what she saw." This is not an isolated incident as there are many such experiences on record.

Life is a wonderful gift which all should appreciate. Eva is a firm believer in the Bible and lives by the teachings of it. This belief and her ensuing practice of it have been beacons in her life and have given her peace.

46
Isabelle (Neeley) Dowling

As she was preparing her submission to this book, boxes of memories surrounded her as she was about to leave her apartment to take up residence in a retirement home two miles (3 km) away. She has packed all of her treasures and now hopes to add a few more as her life moves into its final stages.

When she looks back over time, good fortune has followed her wherever she went; and, in a life full of adventure, it was hers for the taking. She finds, regardless of the years that have passed, so many memories flood back into her mind on a regular basis, leaving her speechless. She shares a few of these memories here.

Isabelle was born in Dunsmuir, Calif., but left there at the age of one year, and has lived in the Seattle, Wash., area all her life. She started to school in Seattle and attended several schools in the area. Her favourite teacher was Rachel Sealls in a Snoqualmie, Wash., school. She was an exceptional teacher and a very good person, who would help her students, even outside her field.

Her second favourite teacher was her own mother. Her mother was given a scholarship in which she would be sent wherever she wanted to go for one year. She applied for three schools, with Machray School, an inner city school in Winnipeg, accepting her. Thus, Winnipeg came into the life of Isabelle. While her mother taught, she attended Normal School in Tuxedo.

Isabelle was one of the non-residents at Normal School. She drove to school each day, until the snow began to become heavy, after which she travelled by city transit. She really enjoyed attending school there, having much fun; but the system seemed to be quite scary. Nevertheless, attendance at Normal School left a strong impression on her.

She thought very highly of Mr. Lightly because he would talk to her. Since she had problems because the school was so different for her, he tended to help guide her through the year. He was such a fine, outgoing man. A number of years later when Mr. and Mrs. Lightly were visiting in Seattle, they stopped to have a visit with her. She speaks well, also, of our principal, Mr. Moorhead.

Isabelle could not teach in Manitoba because she did not possess Canadian citizenship. Therefore, following graduation at Normal School, she and her mother drove the long way home, touring twenty-eight states and seeing such places as Niagara Falls, the Great Lakes, New York, Washington D.C., and Mt. Rushmore.

After returning home, she enrolled at Central Washington University, in Ellensburg, Wash., to continue her studies in education. In the summer following her first year there, she worked in Seattle to earn money for her second year. She enjoyed her work so much that she surmised that she would probably like this job better than teaching. That ended her potential career in education before she could receive a state teacher's licence. She went to work for a credit union, where she stayed for seventeen years. She loved working in an office and helping people.

In 1958, she married John Dowling, who was born in Ireland and had emigrated to America two years earlier. This alone led to a profound change in her life. When he died in 2006, her loss was overwhelming.

They raised three children: Kathleen, Tim, and Terry. When the boys, who were twins, entered school, Isabelle returned to the work force. She spent her last ten years employed by the U.S. Postal Credit Union. She retired in 1994 after thirty-three years of work, and John retired in 1984 after thirty-one years with the same company.

Throughout the years, the family travelled to Ireland, Scotland, England, and Wales. They visited with John's family and enjoyed the country, customs, and especially, the people. They also made seventeen trips to Hawaii, and two more trips to Ireland. She has always liked to travel, first with her mother and then with her husband—all over the United States, Europe, and the border area of Mexico. She felt sorry for the poor people whom she saw in Mexico, especially the children.

She also has travelled across seven Canadian provinces. Two convent sisters showed her and her mother some of the Great Lakes area of Canada. She and her family liked to take vacations in southern British Columbia. In Canada, she preferred the eastern part of British Columbia and recommends this area to visitors. In 2008, Kathy and Isabelle travelled to Alaska on the cruise ship *Norwegian Pearl*.

For many years up to the present, she and Sister Lumina Chartrand have corresponded to the agony of the postal service on both sides of the border. Some letters have numbered fifteen to twenty pages. Isabelle and her daughter Kathy attended one Normalite reunion and spent a day on the farm of Audrey (Jack) Grier. She met Delphie (Olson) Norberg and Doreen (Olson) Lindquist at the home of their relatives. Mr. and Mrs. Turner, two of our teachers at Normal School, were in Seattle shortly after the birth of her twin boys.

Although she worked in PTA when the children were in school, she was not involved much in community activities as her work took up much of her life. When her husband was living, they did many things together. Today, she enjoys time with her family; and she appreciates the many things that her children do to help her.

Her favourite book when she was a child was *A Girl of the Limberlost*, by Gene Stratton-Porter. As an adult, she has been an avid reader, but no one book stands out as a favourite.

She cautions young persons against wasting their time when in college. She urges them to invest time into what they want to do for their future. They should obtain their education, and then go into the world and make their lives worthwhile.

Her mother was the person who had the most influence on her life. Although many persons have been good to her and have helped her in various ways, no one else really stands out in this regard.

Her philosophy of life is to work hard, to enjoy what she does, and to be able to laugh at things. She has had a tough, but good, life.

To all her former classmates, she wishes for them a good life and good health. For her, this is such a special way to cross the miles and the nearly sixty years gone by.

47

Delphie (Olson) Norberg

Do ghosts frighten you? Mackenzie Hall was on the third floor in the main building at Normal School. The girls were happy there until the authorities decided to move Cecile Droux, Genevieve Grudeski, Charlotte Kingdon, Elsie Murray—the house captain—Delphie Olson, Doreen Olson, and Flora Sampson up to the attic —temporarily, of course. Why was this done? Repairs and painting were needed. Can you imagine such a thing? Their new temporary home, one floor higher—was a monstrous room.

None of these lucky girls had experienced big dorm life previously. On night one, they had just settled down in their allotted spots when there was a ghostly noise. Then, they saw it! A big white blob was sailing around the room! Oh, the screeches of terror that filled that cavernous room! There was a disappearing act as bedcovers enveloped the heads of girls.

Suspicions abounded that Shevaun Smith, roommate of Flora and Cecile, had a connection with the Mackenzie Ghost. She always worked in the canteen. In the yearbook it says, "When Shevy gets going, everyone hides." Thus, she was the likely candidate for "ghostie". The girls also knew that it could have been any other "friendlies" from the other end of Mackenzie Hall.

Delphie was delivered by a local nurse at Sprague, a community in the southeastern corner of Manitoba. For her grades one to eight, she attended the Golden Branch School. From there, she went to Sprague High School for grades nine to eleven. Then, it was necessary for her to transfer to Winnipeg for grade twelve, which she obtained at Daniel McIntyre Collegiate. Since she was a non-resident, it was necessary for her to wait for two weeks until the Winnipeg residents could register before she was allowed to go. At that time, she had to pay tuition. There was no education for all in 1949–50!

She has fond memories of her school days. Because her family lived in a rural area, it was necessary for her to walk two miles (3 km) to elementary school and two and one-half miles (4 km) to high school. There were no buses in those days. She cannot forget the wonderful time that she and her classmates enjoyed at the wiener roasts and singsongs when she was in grades nine, ten, and eleven.

What fun it was for the girls to play soccer and hockey as they competed with the boys who lacked the numbers to play by themselves! Who could forget the old metal lunch pails, which were their companions? Gone are those wonderful days as times have changed—and not necessarily for a better quality of life.

Rose Williams, principal and high school teacher at Sprague, was one of her favourite teachers. She taught grades nine to eleven—all subjects—and was most encouraging for all her students to continue to grade twelve and to do their best to continue with further education. Delphie looks back on Rose's workload and wonders how she could always be so positive. She also played piano and established a choir, which performed at local functions.

Miss Ring was a very memorable and positive Normal School teacher. Delphie served on the health committee and made a number of trips to the CNIB to work. She enjoyed the staff versus students affairs and has good photos of events. In 2008, she attended a quilting show in the Canadian Mennonite University arts and library building, where our Normal School was once located. It now has a large gallery space for art shows. The university has expanded on both sides of Grant Avenue.

Delphie worked in the kitchen serving and cleaning tables all year. Many funny experiences occurred. She still has her yearbook and enjoys looking back at former times and viewing the one compiled for our 50th anniversary.

She obtained her Permanent Teachers' Certificate and taught in Manitoba, except for three years of teaching in Ontario.

For one year, she taught grade one to grade eight at the Golden Branch School, at Sprague, the school where she began her own education. From there, she went to Middlebro School to teach grades one to four, the same school where her sister Doreen was teaching grades 5-8. She taught here from 1952 to 1954.

After that, she taught at David Livingstone School, in Winnipeg, from 1954–56. This school, located behind the old market gardens on Main Street, had an interesting history. During Prohibition days, bootleggers watched teachers go to and from school daily. She liked the staff very much. It was a new education for her!

In 1965, the family moved to Thunder Bay, Ont., where Gunnar, her husband, had transferred. Delphie was able to do much substitute teaching. At Edgewater, Ont., she obtained a half-day principal's relief position teaching in a grade six class. In 1966–67, she taught a grade one class at Redwood, Ont., in a new housing development. She was kept very busy with forty children —and no aides! After returning to Manitoba, she substituted at all grade levels and often at the high school level, giving her varied experiences.

On two different occasions in the 1980s, she was census commissioner for a federal census. This was a new experience of hiring, teaching, and completing. There were 18–21 workers helping her each time. A massive project was completed in 1993. It was a 100-year, 600-page book, with over 1,000 photographs, of the Rural Municipality of Rosser. For the volunteers, it was a success, and, indeed, a learning experience for Delphie.

She has always loved books and art. Her favourites as a child were the works of Jack London and the short stories of Rudyard Kipling. As an adult, she still loves to read. Now, her preference is for historical works by such authors as John Jakes. She has an eight-volume series by him and plans to reread the books.

For hobbies, she enjoys sewing, knitting, crocheting, quilting, hardanger (a Swedish needlecraft—very detailed), gardening, and painting with water colours and oils. She is one of a group who quilt for world relief. They have donated more than 500 tied quilts over the past eight years to the Mennonite Central Committee to distribute. They have also donated ninety quilts of baby and youth sizes to Project Linus Quilts at Stonewall. These are for such local emergency vehicles as Royal Canadian Mounted Police and ambulances and also for grieving camps, where a child under stress is allowed to keep his quilt to take home.

Delphie was always interested in drawing and painting. Her mother would order "100 sheets" of drawing paper from Eaton's catalogue. When she and her two brothers and sister were young, they had a "quiet" time, which involved their sitting around the round oak table with the Aladdin lamp in the centre and draw. That was her beginning.

Years later while she and two neighbours were holidaying in Corpus Christi, Tex., they decided to go to a water colour workshop. They enjoyed the challenge and purchased the "red, yellow, and blue" paint tubes, bought some art paper, and had a most enjoyable winter. She loves the way in which water colours move—and dry much faster! Thus, she has been puttering for several years.

She is a member of the Stonewall Art Group, people of the fifty-five plus age. They have a session every Thursday morning, when they work with water colours, oils, and acrylics, according to each member's preference, which for Delphie include flowers, scenery, and seascapes. She has created many hand-printed cards.

The members take turns at bringing a "snack and coffee". They all display their works that they are doing or have done. A critique session is included. Among the group are very good painters, two of which have "art studies" backgrounds. Delphie enjoys this style more than structured classes where someone tells the group "what to paint and what colours to use!"

They work for eight weeks in October and November and then eight weeks in spring. In June, they usually have a show at the gallery. Delphie has sold a few paintings, given many away, and still has a stack. She has much fun in this activity. There is also a "South of the Lakes" show, usually early October, in which she has entered. She has sold many cards and even a few paintings. She does not expect to become famous—but it is a most relaxing hobby for her.

Delphie has been involved in several community groups. These include Meadows Community Club, Meadows Women's Auxiliary to the Community Club, Interlake Festival (music and speech) Committee, 4-H movement, and Women's Institute. She has been a member of the Meadows organizations for many years since moving to the farm.

To a class of kindergarten to grade four at Rosser School in the late 1990s, she and her mother gave a demonstration on carding sheep wool, spinning, knitting, rug braiding, and rag rugs. Her mother was over eighty-five years old then. As her mother demonstrated, Delphie told the story. The children were mesmerized! The early pioneer days took on a completely new meaning. In 2008, her mother was ninety-seven and still living independently in her own seniors' apartment at Stonewall, continuing to knit, sew, and read.

She and her husband Gunnar have taken many trips and seen many places: England, Scotland, Sweden (Gunnar has cousins here), Norway, Denmark, Hawaii, Tahiti, Fiji, New Zealand, and Australia. In addition, they have gone on two Caribbean cruises and visited the southern states from Florida to California, and, closer to home, northern Manitoba many times.

However, their most memorable trip was to Alaska and Yukon. They flew to Ketchikan, Alaska. From there, they toured the state and Yukon via various modes of transportation. They relished the museums which told about the gold rush days.

They rode on the White Pass and Yukon Railroad, which was completed in 1900, after the gold rush. They found this narrow gauge railroad to be awesome! They saw Dead Horse Gulch where the bones of 3,000 overloaded, sadly neglected packhorses now rest. They travelled along the Old Chilcoot Trail. They crossed over magnificent trestles and bridges and penetrated tunnels, amazed by how men with no modern machinery could construct them. It was very breathtaking. Delphie recommends that anyone who is interested in this railroad should go while it is still running.

They visited Rabbit Creek Bonanza, where they partook in the sport of panning for gold. No, they did not strike it rich! In the area, they saw the old dredges that were brought in piece by piece and assembled there. That was such a costly business.

They travelled the Yukon River by boat. Late one night, they read a newspaper on the longest day of the year—outside their hotel! They enjoyed the wildlife and scenery of Denali National Park, in Alaska. They rode the McKinley Express; but, when they approached the mountain, they were disappointed that its top was covered in cloud. At the other end of the line, they visited Anchorage. It was the year of the Valdez oil spill. When their tour arrived back in the Yukon, everyone (seventeen Canadians and seventeen Americans) stood up in the bus and sang "O Canada!" It had been a delightful trip under the supervision of a wonderful tour guide. When it was all over, a Dutch ship, SS *Rotterdam*, took them back south.

For a good Canadian place to visit, she would suggest a tour of the Maritime Provinces and Newfoundland. L'Anse aux Meadows, located on the most northerly tip of the island, is the site of the first settlement in Canada. Both the museum and the village are rewarding to visit.

Having teenagers as grandchildren and meeting their friends help to make her aware of the importance of education and in doing one's work. She has a few pieces of advice for those of that age. Always do as good a job as you are able. Treat your friends with respect, and always try to include any new classmates or those that seem to be left out of the circle. Take time to treat your parents and elders with love and care.

She has had an opportunity to discuss the merits of teaching with a neighbour's daughter. This girl has now graduated and is working for her second year and feels she is doing what she was destined to do. Delphie's advice is to enjoy the moments when a student really understands.

Pierre Elliot Trudeau had a zeal for life and seemed to inspire people to be prouder of Canada. She did not always agree with him, but she saw that he had a "spark" and perseverance that Canada needed in the time when he was prime minister.

Do unto others as you would have them do unto you. Take time to listen. Take time to smell the "roses" in our lives. These points describe her philosophy and she tries to live by them.

She enjoys painting cards and finding the perfect verse or "mini sermons" or sayings for special family and friends. She has learned to slow down in recent years as Gunnar has had lung surgery (successful cancer removal). Eight months later, he developed West Nile disease—the neurological type. He was so stricken with it that he did not know his family during the first week that he was in hospital. However, he has returned to golfing a bit again, and is enjoying his family and freedom of staying in the country where all their friends are. As a result of his sickness, the couple has not travelled as much. She does have hobby time, though, and realizes that life could be much worse.

48
Doreen (Olson) Lindquist

Cows can create adventures for anyone, often not pleasant ones. In Middlebro, there was a neighbour who lived in town but had a farm a few miles out. He would bring his cows into town for milking and a sleepover, milk them again in the morning, and then drive them out to his pasture.

One day, he developed a brilliant idea—at least for him. The school yard would be an ideal overnight resting corral. Because the yard had gates that could be closed, he would avoid having to round them up in the morning. However, cows have a habit of leaving their trademark.

The slipping and sliding began to wear on the teacher and the children as they used their playground. After a few weeks, Doreen could take no more of that nonsense. Early one morning, armed with a big whip and still clad in her night clothes, this brave young lady conducted her own kind of round-up. She put the run on about twenty of the herd. As cows will do, they decided to pass through the gate as one body. The fence was wrecked, but the cow problem was solved. Her school yard was now safe.

Doreen was born near Sprague. She attended a grade one to grade eight school about five miles (8 km) north of that community, a two-mile (3 km) hike from the farm where she was born. For grades nine to eleven, she attended a school in Sprague. It was necessary for her to attend Isaac Newton High School in Winnipeg in order to take grade twelve.

Her first experience in teaching took place in a two-room school, in Middlebro. This community is the most southeasterly town in Manitoba, a few miles from the U.S. border. She had about thirty-five students in grades five to nine. It was a wonderful community, in which the people were so hospitable and cooperative.

During the three years which she spent there, she learned much and made many life-long friends. She participated in many extra-curricular activities with the children—a few of which included square dancing, teen canteen, 4-H clubs, and baseball. Those were the days of an "official trustee" in Winnipeg instead of a local board of trustees. A feature of her time there was that she taught her first year with Ai Otsu, a Normalite of our year, and the next two with her sister Delphie.

During the third year of teaching, another interest entered her life. She became engaged to Axel Lindquist, from her home town of Sprague. They were married in July, after which Doreen took a break from teaching for a few years. The couple had three daughters in less than two years, Gaylene and twins Kristi and Karla. In 1957, the family decided to move to Atikokan, Ont., where Axel was hired by Steep Rock Iron Mines. However, this job turned out to be of short duration. They were in the process of building a house when Axel was laid off his job.

In 1961, when he was hired by INCO, a nickel mine in Thompson, they left their unfinished home and moved to northern Manitoba. At that time, Thompson had not yet appeared on the map. Axel and Doreen have enjoyed living there for the last forty-seven years. Both are now retired—she from teaching for twenty-nine years and he from the mine where he worked as a mechanic and planner. It has been fascinating to watch Thompson grow from an isolated community with no roads to a prosperous modern city of 15,000, mostly dependent on the mining industry.

Both have been active in the community. Doreen was on the first environment council and helped with Girl Guides as a Sparks and Pathfinder leader. Together, they have cross-country skied, bowled, canoed, built a cabin, played baseball, helped organize a museum, and been involved in volunteer work. She was honoured with a Queen's Jubilee medal in Queen Elizabeth's jubilee year.

She upgraded her education after they moved to Thompson, taking university courses through Inter-University North while teaching and raising a family, finally graduating with a Bachelor of Education degree. Probably one of the most enjoyable university courses was Outdoor Education—a fifty-mile (80 km) canoe trip—water survival, canoeing skills, food preparation, and other activities. It was a thrilling adventure.

Doreen conducted a private kindergarten—the first in Thompson—for six years. Then, when she entered the school system, she continued in kindergarten for another six years. After that, she taught grades six to eight, mostly English and mathematics.

The family has been able to take time for some travel. Two trips stand out in Doreen's memory. One was a cruise to Alaska. The other was a month-long trip to Sweden, where they visited with Axel's relatives, and to Norway and Denmark.

Where would be a wonderful place to visit? Doreen suggests that northern Manitoba would be a good choice. There are many lakes and immense forests. One of her favourite places is the family cottage at Paint Lake where they enjoy canoeing, fishing, and just basking.

Many people think that it is not possible to grow a garden in Thompson—not true. The summer days are long, with daylight from 4:00 a.m. until 11:00 p.m.

One of her favourite teachers was Marie Wilton, her grade one teacher, who was so kind and affectionate and always had time to listen.

At Normal School, Annie Bain supervised the housekeeping. Doreen worked for her in the linen room throughout the year. She was such a kind lady. The two remained friends for many years.

As a child, she loved *Anne of Green Gables* series, by Lucy Maud Montgomery. As an adult, she has read all of Elizabeth Berg's books, as well as many other authors.

She appreciated Pierre Trudeau for his stand on justice and acceptance when he was Prime Minister of Canada. She liked Pierre Berton's writings because he was a great Canadian whose love of our country was always evident.

Doreen enjoys music of all genres. She loves writing and trying her hand at poetry and at weaving, knitting, and quilting. Reading is also a favourite pastime. She likes writing and is working on stories of her early life and some of the adventures experienced by her and her family.

For young people interested in a teaching career, her advice is to prepare well. One of the shortcomings of our year at Normal School was the short time we actually had to practice teach. They should respect their students, especially since most problem children have underlying situations. They should set a good example and be open to new ideas but to be cautious about jumping on such "bandwagon" philosophies as open-area classrooms.

To young people in general, she advises that they not fry their brains with drugs or other addictive substances, that they be in control of their faculties, that they acquire a good education and lead a healthy lifestyle, and that they respect their elders and all with whom they come in contact.

Her own philosophy is fairness for all, care of our planet, and choice of a spouse whom one can love and respect. She feels that it is important for her to live modestly (a mansion being unnecessary), to go to a church of her choice, to keep up with the times, and to exercise her civic rights. She would recommend that everyone consider such a standard.

Class G

Dorothy Brownridge
Anne Bueckert
Nellie Enns
Pearl Fiterman
Betty Hughes
Joyce Lovell
Stan Petrowski
Eleanor Rankin
Shirley Ray
Tina Redekopp
Mary Regitnig
Joan Regner
Marguerite Reid
Margaret Relmer
Irene Ringland
Orest Roscoe
Vivian Roy
Harry Rudy
John Ryan
Bernice Rzasa
Verla Salmon
Flora Sampson
Fay Sandercock
Doris Saundry
Henry Schellenberg
Gladwyn Scott
Lois Scott
Michael Shewchuk
Marie-Ange Sicard
Viola Sigurdson
Janie Silverthorne
Yvonne Skagfeld
Melva Skeavington
Jenny Slawinsky
Elaine Slimmon
Aurise Smith
Helen Smith
Gladys Snyder
Mary Sobol
Wilfred Tomasson

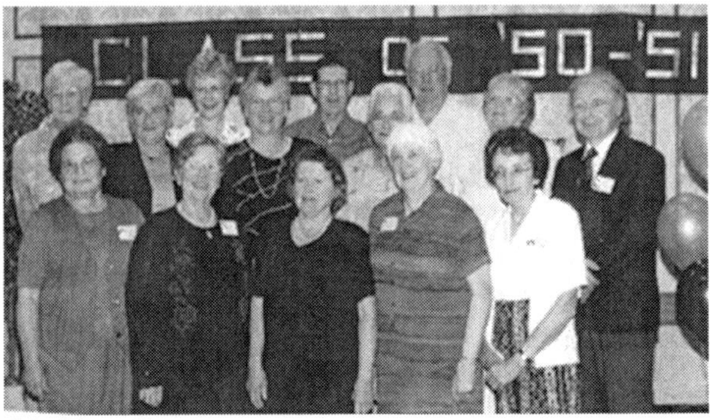

24. Class G

49
Dorothy (Brownridge) Haithwaite

What a memorable trip it was for a seventeen-year-old girl! She accompanied her aunt, her grandmother, and a friend visiting from England, setting out from Brandon during the first week in July by car to Long Beach, Calif. There were so many places of interest to explore along the way—such points as the Badlands, Grand Canyon, Hoover Dam, and others. What a thrill it was to see what she had only known from books! In California, the beach frequently beckoned and the popular points in Los Angeles had to be visited.

When the holiday was finished, she accompanied her uncle in driving back to Brandon in time for her to start school at the end of August. Since their route passed through Las Vegas, Nev., they decided to stop and discover what enticed people to come to this city. They chose the Golden Nugget, a popular hotel and casino. All progressed well until the security guard approached them and challenged the girl in regard to her age. Alas! Seventeen years of age was too young for a person to be in this setting. He advised her that she must leave. It was a good try, miss.

Dorothy was born in a farm home on 2-11-19, Elton Municipality. This farm is two miles (3 km) west of the intersection of Highway #1 and 18th Street, in Brandon, and then two miles (3 km) north. Brandon Airport was near the farm, creating an exciting place as a neighbour during World War II. A mile and one-quarter (2 km) from the farm was a small country school called Bloomsbury, where she attended for her grade one to grade eight. Then, she went to Earl Oxford School in Brandon for grade nine and Brandon Collegiate Institute for grade ten to grade twelve.

Since she had attended only a small country school with ten to fourteen students, she really enjoyed the schools in Brandon where there were so many other students with whom to interact. The class parties included such activities as hay rides and toboggan slides. In the music classes, the students learned songs which they sang at the city's Remembrance Day programmes. At Christmas, they sang carols in a live broadcast at local Radio Station CKX. In grade eleven, they performed *The Yeomen of the Guard*, by Gilbert and Sullivan, complete with costumes from Malibar, in Winnipeg.

One teacher at Normal School whom she remembers is Miss Pilling, our art teacher. Dorothy was astounded to encounter her there as she was one of the instructors at Brandon Normal School in the early 1920s when her mother was a Normal School student. Actually, the teacher whom she enjoyed in class most was Miss Douglas and the music which she taught.

Everything about Normal School life was wonderful. She lived in Mackenzie Hall in the main building. Her first learning experience was how to go from the third floor to the basement without becoming lost. She enjoyed the morning assemblies and the hymns we sang, many of which she still remembers.

Off-campus, she enjoyed learning how to travel in Winnipeg and which buses and streetcars to board. She was not involved in the social life much, which she feels

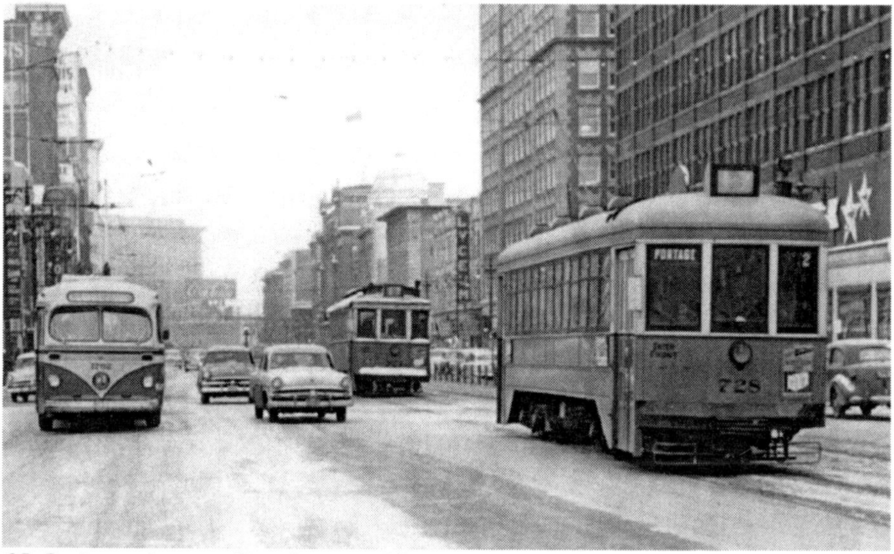

25. Portage Avenue Streetcar and Bus

may have been her loss. She did not enjoy the winter swimming lessons, but she did enjoy the walks to Assiniboine Park in the spring evenings.

She had not been a permit teacher, but she thought when she was at Normal School that she would have realized what she needed to learn if she had been one. For her first three years she taught grades one to nine at Rounthwaithe School. Then she moved to Brandon Hills for the next two years, where she had grades one to eight. By this time, she had married and was driving fifteen miles (24 km) twice a day. After that, she taught grades one to eight for two years at Stratherne, which was only an eight-mile (13 km) drive.

Then she ceased teaching, never to teach again—or so she thought. In 1968, an opportunity opened for her to teach kindergarten in Wawanesa School. This turned out so well that she taught at that level for the next twenty-six years, retiring in 1994. Kindergarten was one-half days at first, which worked out well for a farmer's wife. Then the policy changed to having classes all day every other day, one which had both good and bad points.

She cannot remember having had a favourite book as a child because she liked most books. She did like such fairy tales as *Cinderella* and *Sleeping Beauty*. She also liked to have the Thornton Burgess books read to her—*Peter Cottontail* and *Grandfather Frog*. In school, there was the *Highroads to Reading Series*, whose stories she enjoyed.

As an adult, Dorothy enjoys any book written by James Michener, but her all-time favourite was *The Covenant*, a book which she has read several times because of its appealing nature. Another author whom she particularly likes is Maeve Binchey.

Her hobbies include reading and knitting. Now that she is retired, she has more time to knit. Most of the mitts, scarves, and toques go to Samaritan House in Brandon, a ministry whose aim is to reach out and help those people in Brandon and its neighbouring communities who are in need.

She does not belong to any service clubs; but, when one lives in a small community, one automatically becomes involved in such community projects as being a volunteer worker, chairman, secretary, or treasurer. The local museum keeps her busy in July and August. Another group to which she belongs helps out with entertainment for the residents of the Personal Care Home. Also, she holds a number of executive positions in the United Church—which means endless meetings.

If someone from another country were to ask her somewhere to visit, she would suggest southwest Manitoba. Call into any of the small towns and check out their points of interest. Summer or early fall would be a good time to do this.

If Dorothy were addressing a group of teenagers, she would tell them to become involved in their community. They do not have to be the leaders, but if they start out as volunteers and help wherever they can, they will soon learn. They should watch the good things that are done, but also notice those that could be better. Eventually, they may feel comfortable to take on a larger task.

If you would like to enter the teaching profession, you must decide if you like children. You need to like being with them and not feel awkward around them. If you make friends easily and can strike up a conversation with anyone, you have a good start. Dorothy knew from the start that she would not be successful as a high school teacher, but she was quite comfortable as an elementary teacher.

A person who has had a positive influence on her life was a grade two teacher in Wawanesa. She was so organized and seemed self-assured and did everything well. She maintained a model classroom, which was neat and attractive, not messy like some classrooms.

A Canadian leader was Nellie McClung, who stood for women's rights and advocated that women must be allowed to vote. She was a delegate for Canada when the League of Nations met in Geneva and also served in the Alberta Legislature.

Her philosophy of life is to do the best that she can and to look to the future. She does not believe in looking at the past and regretting how badly that went.

Today, Dorothy lives on a farm two miles west (3 km) and two miles (3 km) north of Wawanesa. The farm is built on the site of the small town of Methven, which was thriving in the early 1900s, but soon died as the railway moved further west.

50 Betty (Hughes) Doroschuk

What a thrill it was to perform—not bit roles, but lead roles—in three Gilbert and Sullivan operettas: The *Mikado*, *The Yeomen of the Guard*, and *The Gondoliers*. In *The Yeomen of the Guard*, her favourite, she sang the role of Phoebe. She was in high school at Daniel McIntyre Collegiate, in Winnipeg. Later, she was a soloist at the graduation ceremonies for our 1950–51 Normal School class. She was on her way to a fulfilling career.

Betty was born in Winnipeg and obtained all of her education prior to university in that city.

As a non-resident of Normal School, she really does not have a stand-out memory of any event there. She is, however, appreciative of the fact that it was at Normal School that she met Yvonne (Skagfeld) Oliphant and formed a long friendship with her. Sadly, Yvonne passed away in 2006. She also must mention the fact that it was through the Normal School experience that she met and married Eugene Doroschuk. They were married in 1953 and have experienced a wonderful life together ever since.

She obtained a Bachelor of Music degree, a Licentiate in Voice Performance, and an Associate in Voice Performance degree from McGill University. She obtained another Associate in Voice Performance degree from University of Manitoba.

She taught in schools in St. James, Transcona, and Belmont. She also taught in Langley and Vancouver, B.C., and in Montreal, Que. Betty spent twenty years as a voice teacher in the Faculty of Music, at McGill University, nine years of which she was head of the Voice section.

Anne of Green Gables, by Lucy Maud Montgomery, was her childhood favourite book. In adult life, she enjoyed *Crime and Punishment*, by Fyodor Dostoevsky.

What a gratifying experience it was when one of her voice students won a Metropolitan Opera competition! Eugene and Betty were thrilled in attending a gala event at the "Met" to hear her perform.

When they lived in Montreal, they drove to New York about four times a year for various performances at the "Met". The building is fantastic inside. Very prominent over the seating area on the main floor are huge crystal chandeliers. Just prior to the commencing of a performance they slowly rise so that they do not block the view of the patrons. The theatre can host between 3,000 and 4,000 people.

Her favourite production was that of *Peter Grimes*, by Benjamin Britten. She particularly enjoyed listening to the renditions by Jon Vickers, a Canadian, who played the title role.

A trip to the USSR in 1980 was a learning experience. She found nothing unfavourable when they visited the country in a tour of fifteen people. At the time, that was the only way to go. The people were very friendly. They were able to go out alone at times because Eugene speaks Ukrainian and knows some Russian. Thus, they could communicate better with the local people.

During one visit to the subway system, they became lost. Happily, they met a student who kindly helped them find their way again. Although she liked the Montreal system, she found the Moscow one quite different. This system is very elaborate in structure, especially in the stations.

Another learning experience occurred when they visited Cuba. They saw no need to go to the beaches; but, instead, they preferred to go a small town a short distance from Havana. They wanted to see how the people lived. They were surprised to see that the clothes of the people are quite westernized. Many people speak English. When they visited a large mall, they noted that there was an armed guard at the doorway of each store.

They passed by a school during a recess break. Outside on the playground were happy children about twelve years old. A teacher was playing with them. All the children were in neat uniforms. While in Cuba, they drank bottled water to avoid sickness. However, after adding crushed ice to a beverage, not thinking about the fact that this was water, Betty became a bit ill. When she went to a clinic for treatment, she was treated royally.

She would urge teenagers to obtain as much education as possible and to pursue their dreams. Her advice to anyone considering the teaching profession is to go for it. Teaching is a wonderfully rewarding experience.

Glenn Pierce was her music teacher at Daniel McIntyre Collegiate. He was a wonderful musician who encouraged her to pursue a career in music. She has not regretted having followed his advice.

Doris Mills-Lewis, her first voice teacher, recognized Betty's talent and encouraged her to become what she could be. Betty also gives special recognition to her father. He, too, recognized her talent and sacrificed to give her voice lessons at a time when only the wealthy studied voice. He worked at the Canadian Pacific Railway shops and was a self-taught pianist and church organist.

Even as a hobby, Betty enjoys music. She works with young singers and she teaches piano to her two youngest grandchildren. For a change in venue, she enjoys solving New York *Times* Sunday crosswords and reading. In the community, she is active with Ballet Victoria and Northern Opera Theatre.

The Northern Opera Theatre was founded in Montreal in 1985 by Eugene Doroschuk, executive director; Betty Doroschuk, musical director; Colin Doroschuk, their son, stage director; and Jacqueline Sloan, their daughter-in-law, choreographer. Jacqueline was a former dancer with National Ballet of Canada. They produced operas in Montreal, Que., and Kingston, Ont., from 1985 to 1991.

Tommy Douglas was an unassuming person who believed in the rights of the common man. He would qualify as a great leader in Canada.

She suggests that a tourist should visit Montreal in the summer.

Her philosophy is, "Don't sweat the small stuff!" The older she becomes, the more that she finds this to be true.

Their three sons became an international pop-rock group—Men Without Hats—and were nominated for a Grammy. They were number one on charts all over the world and won many gold and platinum records. Now, granddaughter Sahara Sloan, at age eighteen, is pursuing a singing career at the Glenn Gould School in Toronto. She was awarded an $18,000 scholarship to attend. The music tradition continues, having been carried on by the last four generations.

Their married life has been fulfilling and filled with love. Betty has certainly been an exemplary model in the music profession for both her family and her students.

51
Orest Roscoe

What little boy has not in his imagination driven a race car, a steam locomotive, an airplane, or a pirate ship? Most young boys have enjoyed reading books about adventures in transportation.

One particular boy enjoyed reading the fifteen books in the *Dave Dawson* series, by R. Sidney Bowen. This series told of the adventures of Dave and his friends in the Royal Air Force during World War II, when they flew Spitfires and Hurricanes in defending their country. This reader was up there as his heroes flew over England, the Channel, and Western Europe as they fought their enemy—and returned safely to base. As he grew up, he broadened his reading and covered many types of books—so many that now no particular one stands out like *Dave Dawson* of his childhood days.

Orest was born in Selkirk and grew up in nearby Melrose, where he first attended school. He has no outstanding memories of his early school years as activities were normal and fairly routine, with an exception being a 28-day stint in isolation at the St. Boniface Hospital when he was in grade five because of a bout of scarlet fever. Isolation was the prescribed treatment at the time because this was before the days of modern antibiotics. Visitors were obliged to climb a ladder to the second storey level and to visit through an open window.

However, he does remember Dennis Nazeravich, his teacher in grades five and six and again in grades nine and ten. He was one who provided much encouragement to his students. Having been positively impacted by this man, Orest often speaks of him when working with others.

Except probably for Dennis, no one person has influenced him more than any other. It is difficult to name one because of his interacting over the years with many people who have left positive effects on him.

Regarding life at Normal School, he particularly remembers mealtimes in the dining hall because here he had the opportunity to associate with other students in residence. He made good friends and has kept in touch with several of them. As yearbook editor, he was very busy, especially in the last three to four months when he spent as much time in this activity as he did in attending classes. While his career path has taken him far away from Manitoba and from teaching, he often thinks of the friends whom he made at Normal School. He would love to hear from anyone from the Class of 1951!

Orest remembers Miss Douglas, our music teacher, mostly because he could not sing well. One day, Mr. Chidley, one of our mathematics teachers, called him to his office—a strange happening. When his student arrived, Mr. Chidley said to him, "Have you thought of going to university? You should go." Orest felt this was quite unusual because no one else did that for him. Nevertheless, he acted upon the advice two years later.

After teaching at age nineteen and facing forty-one students for one year in North Kildonan, a suburb of Winnipeg, he moved to Oakbank for one year. Then, he enrolled in electrical engineering at the University of

Manitoba, completing a Bachelor of Science degree in Electrical Engineering in 1957—the same year that Russia launched the first Sputnik satellite. He continued in graduate school, completing the academic portion of a master's degree in the same field one year later. He subsequently completed his thesis and received the degree in 1962.

He commenced his first full-time engineering position in 1958, at the Defence Research Board in Ottawa, researching the effects of the aurora on communications. In 1963, he became part of the Canadian pioneering team studying satellite communications and has worked in the satellite communications field ever since.

He held positions at the Defence Research Board, the Communications Research Centre, the Department of Communications, Telesat Canada, and Telesat Mobile Incorporated. At Telesat Mobile, he was Vice President, Engineering, responsible for MSAT, the satellite that provides mobile communications in Canada and the USA.

He has seen many changes in technology over the past fifty years, including such advances as laptops, cell phones, and the internet in the last fifteen to twenty years. Orest is still active in the field, currently working as a consultant.

As in his school years, his career mostly followed a normal, routine path, except for two opportunities. He spent two years in Oslo, Norway, on exchange, whereby he and a Norwegian engineer exchanged laboratories. As it occurred between 1967 and 1969, he considered this to be his centennial project during Canada's centennial year. This country was beautiful and clean and its people were friendly and had values similar to those of Canada. If he wanted to live anywhere outside Canada, he would choose Norway. He worked there before oil was discovered off her coast. Thus, the economy at the time was frugal, without any large revenue sources.

He also spent six months in Japan in 1978 to study the Japanese space program and to identify opportunities for Canadian/Japanese collaboration in space activities. This country was very crowded, but the people were very friendly. Like Norway, it is very mountainous; but here, minor earthquakes are felt monthly.

His chief problem was not being able to speak, read, or write in the Japanese language. At work, he was able to use English, since he worked with English-speaking colleagues. However, outside the workplace, he had to manage as best he could in everyday life activities. He soon managed this, and was able to travel extensively and to experience Japanese culture. It was very different from Canada; nevertheless, he fulfilled his reasons for going.

Orest feels that Japan is a successful nation because of her extensive rail transportation systems. It would be inconceivable to imagine the country being successful without them, especially in Tokyo where he worked and lived. His favourite city in Japan was Kyoto, with its wealth of beautiful and historic shrines and temples.

Orest travelled to various European countries on business and on vacation, but they were not as different from Canada as Japan was. He travelled to South America on business—to Brazil, Ecuador, Venezuela, Columbia, Uruguay, and Argentina. He also went to Mexico City five or six times, both on business and on vacation. He has also travelled extensively within the United States. However, the trips that stand out as being most different were those to Japan. He learned much in every country that he visited.

It is difficult to select one specific place in Canada, outside the usual tourist areas, to recommend to visitors to our country. However, he would mention Ottawa, our nation's capital, and Prince Edward Island as beautiful places.

His advice to young people is that they work hard, be innovative, be loyal, and do something besides their main line of work. For the last point, he recommends that they be involved in organizations where they can volunteer their services. A few examples would be Scouts, Guides, charitable agencies, children's sports coaching, and their church.

For those considering entering his career of engineering, he notes that there are many interesting developments on the horizon, especially in such areas as alternative energy sources and nanotechnology, probably within the next twenty years. They should not fear taking risks associated with creativity and innovation.

Lester B. Pearson stands out to him as a great Canadian leader because of his notion of peacekeeping, which he promoted sufficiently to have seen it become a reality in his time. Canada's role in Afghanistan today is somewhat different from Mr. Pearson's vision.

For hobbies, Orest enjoys such activities as curling, golfing, surfing the internet, woodworking projects, and gardening. His curling was best long ago. He took up golfing later in life and finds it great for exercise and socialization.

In community work, he has volunteered much in Ottawa. For example, he has led several building programmes in his church and has taken a major role in the development and residence construction programmes in seniors' organizations.

Orest and Joan were married in 1959. Joan has enjoyed careers as a teacher and as executive director of a social service agency providing services to seniors. They have three children and six grandchildren. Their daughter Robin is a Doctor of Veterinary Medicine, practising in

Ottawa; Stephen is a high school teacher in Mississauga, Ont.; and David has a Doctor of Philosophy degree in electrical engineering and is the engineering vice-president of a high tech company in Ottawa.

The family has lived in Ottawa since Orest arrived there in 1958, except for the two years when he worked in Norway from 1967 to 1969 and also when he worked in Japan in 1978.

52 Harry Rudy

Having the opportunity to gain useful skills in a school shop is a valuable experience for most students who are involved. However, for some, it poses a hazard which they might not recognize.

One day, a young shop teacher at Virden Vocational School was supervising a group of future carpenters busy with their woodworking projects. Wondering why a couple of boys seemed to be involved with a metalworking project that was not scheduled, he decided to investigate. What he saw horrified him!

One of his strays was in the process of clamping a .303 shell—a live one—into the vice. The next step was to apply a nearby hammer with force onto that shell. The boys were expecting the thrill of a detonation, little realizing what the consequences would be. The teacher promptly terminated the experiment and dispatched the instigator to an interview with the principal. The outraged teacher was adamant that anyone so unreliable and dangerous could not return to his shop. He gave a sigh of relief that a disaster had been averted.

Harry was born in Balmoral and took all of his schooling at Balmoral Consolidated School—from grade one until he had completed grade twelve.

He particularly remembers Alice Plante, his high school teacher who taught him from grade nine to grade twelve, mainly in such arts subjects as English, French, and history. She knew her subjects very well, and her preparation made them very interesting and appealing. She was a university graduate and would challenge her students to prepare to carry on their studies after high school, though it might take much work mentally and physically to reach this goal. The final result would be well worth the effort.

One spring day at Balmoral, a group of high school boys decided to play hookey from classes and to spend the afternoon in the local pool hall instead. A game of pool is much more thrilling than a boring class. Harry and his chum were matched against another couple of fellows on the first table. His buddy was preparing to sink a ball when he looked up and beheld in the doorway the presence of the principal of the school. The player froze in mid-shot! The match was abruptly terminated and the boys marched back to school under the watchful eye of the principal, after which they spent some time in detention. There must have been too many boys to punish by other means. The pool matches had to wait.

In 1949–50, Harry taught on permit in a one-room rural school at Prawda under the official trustee. Then in 1951–53, following Normal School, he taught a grade seven class and shop to grades seven to twelve at Virden Public School, in Virden.

Like most students, Harry had to work at Normal School to supplement his finances; and, upon applying for a job, he ended up on the potato-peeling brigade. His shift was during the noon hour. One day when he and his colleague had much to do and little time to do it, the boys let the machine remove the eyes as well as the peels. Of course, the spuds were really trimmed down. The next day, the chef was at the peeler to give his helpers a lecture on potato waste and to remove the eyes by hand.

George Chidley, one of our mathematics teachers, loved to challenge his students. He came to class well-prepared and able to keep the whole class busy throughout his teaching.

Harry obtained a Bachelor of Science (Honours) in Geology degree in 1957 from University of Manitoba and a Master of Science in Geology degree in 1958 from University of Alberta.

After graduating, he joined Gulf Oil in 1958 at Calgary, Alta. Two years later, he was transferred to Edmonton, Alta. Then in 1966, he left Gulf and joined Kewanee Oil Company in Calgary. He worked for several smaller oil companies in that city, progressing through a varied career as geologist, chief geologist, exploration manager, district manager, president, and consultant. In 1995, he retired from active employment, but remained in Calgary to be near family and friends.

During October and November of 2007, Harry and his wife Joan took a trip to China, starting at Beijing, on to Xian, Chungqing, Guilin, the Yangtze River, and finally Shanghai. China is a large, fascinating country with striking topographic variations and very friendly people.

Beijing harbours extremes in architecture from the original *hutongs* (walled courtyard houses) to extremely modern high-rises, in addition to the Forbidden City, the Harvest Temple, the Emperor's summer home, and the newest Olympic buildings for 2008.

The dense smog at Xian surpassed even that of Beijing, but it was worth the trip to view the Terra Cotta warriors. They were fortunate to have a side trip to a small village to see the works of the farmer artists, with a welcome by a Chinese band and dragon dancers. At a small elementary school, the children were so excited to see so many Caucasian tourists and were fascinated by the digital cameras and the ability to see themselves immediately on the camera. Like children all over the world, they were curious, happy, and mischievous.

Other memorable experiences on that trip included learning of the size of the old capital Chungqing (municipality population of 35,000,000 people), travelling on the Li River from Guilin through the famous karst topography mountains and cruising on the Yangtze through the Three Gorges, culminating at the huge dam. Again, the old and the new architecture at Shanghai were very impressive, and some of the modern buildings at Pudong were breathtaking.

For Harry, one of the most impressive places in Canada is Newfoundland. Although their bus trip was quite rapid, they relished the countryside, the geology, the scenery, the seaside, and the interesting people. September and October provide the best time for a visit to enjoy and appreciate the lovely autumn colours.

His advice to teenagers would be to pick a goal that interests and fascinates them and persevere in reaching it, no matter how difficult it may be. They should not be afraid to change or alter their goal if they feel what they have chosen is not right for them.

For someone considering geology, he would say that this is a very challenging and interesting profession, which has many different avenues available from a study of the earth, its make-up, and resources. This profession can open doors in the oil industry, mining metals and non-metals, teaching, and research.

Andy Baillie, of Gulf Oil, was the first geologist to hire Harry and give him challenging and exciting jobs in his chosen profession. Under Andy, he spent five years doing geological field work in the Rocky Mountains from junior geologist to party chief. The exposure to running field parties, handling assistants, and solving geological problems served him well later in his career.

Peter Lougheed, former premier of Alberta, was able to preserve the oil industry from collapse and build it up to become one of the main economic boosters for Canada. His vision and ideas for Albertans and Canadians has stood us all in good stead for the past twenty to twenty-five years.

Harry has been involved in community activities, serving with Boy Scouts of Canada for seven years, Little League Baseball for seven years, and Elks (BPOE) for sixteen years; and in his profession, as secretary with the Canadian Association of Petroleum Geologists for one year.

His hobbies are curling, skiing, golfing, travelling, and reading all types of books. His favourite books when young included *Tom Sawyer,* by Mark Twain; *Black Beauty,* by Anna Sewell; and *Wild Animals I Have Known,* by Ernest Thompson Seton. As an adult, he enjoyed reading: *Pillars of the Earth,* by Ken Follett.

Live your life to the fullest and practise this now! Do not procrastinate and wait until tomorrow as it is impossible to know what the future may bring. This is Harry's philosophy of life.

53
John Ryan

John, an author himself, wrote this account as a finished manuscript and requested that it not be edited. Therefore, I have left it in the first person unlike the other submissions.

I have lived most of my life in Winnipeg, with the exceptions being my early years, two years in Montreal, almost a year in Asia, and lengthy visits to Europe, Mexico and Guatemala, with shorter visits to Cuba and the USA. I was born near Hodgson, Manitoba—a little town adjacent to the Peguis First Nations Reserve. My father was a farmer and our home was almost four miles from the one-room school at Hodgson—so it was a long hike for a young duffer, especially in winter. Actually, I didn't start school until I was nine. It seems my father had some concerns about me walking along a winding dirt road through the bush and getting eaten by a wolf. What made him think wolves wouldn't eat a nine-year-old, I'm not sure. But it seems he was right—I survived those years.

Since this was a Grades 1 to 8 one-room school at Hodgson, I took my Grades 9, 10 and 11 at home by correspondence, and helped my father with all the usual work on a mixed farm—milking cows, looking after livestock, making hay, helping with the harvest, and so forth. In 1948 I left home to take my Grade 12 in Teulon and lived in a students' residence where I met Keith Huss, and for the next 60 years and counting we are still the very best of friends.

My first encounter with Normal School was a 6-week crash course during the summer of 1949 to prepare me for Permit Teaching at Hayek School, a little rural school ten miles north of Arborg—with an enrollment of 8 little kids, in Grades 1 to 8! From that 6-week training course, I can still recall Mr. Clarke extolling us "to teach faithfully and diligently"—in his colourful Irish accent.

And of course during 1950-51 I was at Normal School—rooming with Keith Huss and Harry Rudy in Frontenac Hall. Keith, Harry and I did our practice teaching at the Manitoba Home for Boys at Portage la Prairie, and the next year I wound up teaching at that institution for young juvenile delinquents. That's a bit of a story in itself . . .

From 1952 to 1955 I was at the University of Manitoba studying for my B.A.—with a double major in Philosophy and Sociology. I loved Philosophy but I hated Sociology because at that time the courses were little more than apologies for the capitalist system—and here I had grown up a Marxist and atheist at my father's knee. My B.A. became meaningful for me because of a filler course I took during a Summer School—a regional geography course on Canada and the USA. I discovered that through economic and cultural geography, and starting with a region's resource base, I could offer courses with a broad multidisciplinary approach. And hence my decision to take post-graduate work in economic and cultural geography.

During the summers while at the University of Manitoba I worked as a porter for CPR and at various types of construction work. Also during the months of May and June I taught at Balsam Bay and at Gladstone, 1954 and 1955, respectively. From 1955 to 1960 I taught at the Winnipeg School Division—Special Education classes at Mulvey, J.B. Mitchell, Kelvin, and Churchill.

During the summer of 1957 I travelled to Europe and spent two weeks in the USSR, where I attended the Sixth World Youth Festival in Moscow, and later travelled to Stalingrad. While on this trip I met Gale Clancy from Kenora, and the next year we got married. While Gale worked on her B.A. at the University of Manitoba, I continued to teach.

While teaching from 1956 to 1960, through night school classes and Summer Schools at the University of Manitoba, I obtained my B.Ed. and M.Ed.

From 1960 to 1962 I was at the University of Manitoba where I completed my M.A. in Geography. In the fall of 1962 Gale and I moved to Montreal where for the next two years I worked on my Ph.D. at McGill. I specialized in economic geography and the geography of the USSR. After my courses, Gale and I were to travel to the USSR where for my Ph.D. dissertation I was to make a study of state farms in Ukraine. Unfortunately, McGill was unable to establish an exchange agreement with a Soviet university, so I had to change my thesis topic—but it still had to be on socialist agriculture. In desperation, and to the relief of both me and McGill, we agreed that I could make a study of the agricultural economy of Manitoba Hutterite colonies.

I began my career as a geography professor in 1964 at United College, which in 1967 became the University of Winnipeg. I was there for the next 32 years, retiring in 1996.

I taught a wide range of courses which included: Introductory Geography, Canada, the USSR, Monsoon Asia, Economic Geography, Agricultural Geography, the Geography of Energy and Resources, and Economic Development.

I enjoyed my years as a professor enormously, and a number of my students still keep in touch with me. Because of the multidisciplinary nature of Geography, as events occurred in our country and the world at large, I was able to incorporate such issues in my courses, and I was able to do this from my perspective as a socialist geographer.

I always felt that professors in particular have a responsibility to be as objective as possible in whatever they teach. But try as we can, no one is truly objective, because we all perceive the world from our own perspective and life experiences. And because of this, students have a right to know where a professor stands on controversial issues, especially in matters that deal with economic or political policies. One thing I can say for sure, my students never had to guess where I stood. Right from my very first class in 1964, as a lowly lecturer, without a Ph.D., in the depths of the Cold War, I had the audacity to tell my students that I would not shy away from any controversial issues, but they ought to know that politically I was a socialist. However, they were not to get unduly upset because when dealing with capitalist issues I promised that I would be at least as objective as my capitalist colleagues would be when they dealt with socialism.

Oliver Wendell Holmes once said "Not to have participated in the passions and actions of one's time is to be at peril of being judged not to have lived." Fortunately for me, it's always been in my blood to get involved in matters of social justice and in the various important issues of our time—at all levels—from international affairs to University affairs—and I found it exhilarating and fun. In 1980 I was instrumental in unionizing the faculty at the University and served as the chair of the unionization committee. Later I served on the negotiation team and after 1½ years of bargaining we wound up with a contract that became a model for other universities. I also served as the president of the faculty association. I was promoted to Full Professor in 1978 and since my retirement I have the status of Retired Professor and Senior Scholar.

I had several sabbatical leaves, which included a memorable 8 months in Asia in 1978 during which time I completed 70 documentary case studies of farming in 12 countries—from Japan to Afghanistan. As for the Hutterite study, over a period of several years I made an intensive study of every single colony. No one had ever studied their agricultural practices before, so mine was a pioneer work, and remains so. It was published in 1977 by McClelland & Stewart as *The Agricultural Economy of Manitoba Hutterite Colonies.*

The arduous years of research on the Hutterite project got me my Ph.D., but indirectly this contributed to Gale's and my divorce. We parted on good terms in 1969 and have maintained a friendship ever since. Shortly after parting with Gale, I married one of my students, Marie Montsion. We had a tumultuous relationship—neither of us knowing why—and after five years we separated and divorced. We too have remained friends.

I spent the summer of 1976 in Mexico and the summers of 1977 and 1979 in Guatemala where I studied Spanish. I have also visited Cuba on five different occasions—once to cut sugar cane for Fidel in 1975.

During the provincial election of 1977 I worked for an NDP candidate and on the night of the election on October 11, I went to the campaign headquarters to view the results. On learning that the Schreyer government had been defeated, I happened to glance over my shoulder and suddenly saw a strikingly beautiful woman standing in the wide entryway. She wore a wide-brimmed red hat, a black bolero, and a white long-sleeved silk blouse—and looked Mexican. I immediately went to her and asked if she was from Mexico. She smiled and said she was from Indonesia. And here the night before I had decided I would spend some time in Indonesia during my sabbatical the next year! Amazingly, she too had plans to go back home the next year—to study batik. As we said afterwards, we knew instantly that we were destined for one another. At our fourth meeting we declared our love for one another, and for the next 19 years we revelled in a true fairy tale romance. And the year after we met we did go to Indonesia together.

Judith was a talented multimedia artist and called herself a "racial cocktail"—a true Eurasian—her origins being Indonesian, Dutch, English, French, Jewish, and Japanese. And she spoke five languages—Indonesian, Dutch, English, French and Spanish. We loved our time together and did a lot of travelling, including three months in a motor-home exploring Europe—East and West. Judith loved to drive so I navigated and took photos.

We bought a lovely big character home on Grosvenor—and spent 11 years renovating it! But in its way that was fun too, both of us being quite handy. We created a lovely big art studio for her and rebuilt the front which then provided me with a large study.

We thought our happiness and good fortune would never end, but then suddenly disaster and tragedy ensued. We had a lovely dinner the evening of May 10, 1996, and made a list of people to invite for a big party—to celebrate the recent completion of our renovations. The next morning she woke up with an excruciating headache—at the hospital they assured her it was only a migraine . . . later she went into a coma and the next day she died. An autopsy revealed that a blood vessel had weakened in the back of her head and that it hemorrhaged and bled into the cerebellum—killing her. I was devastated and I don't know how I managed to survive. And this happened two weeks after I retired.

Judith also had literary talents and I had urged her to write a book about her art and her life story, and that last winter she finally agreed and decided on a title, "*Where the wind carries me . . .*" Tragically, it was I who wound up writing her story. Writing it gave me a reason for living and helped me to deal with my grief. It's a 400-page art and biography coffee table book, with 250 colour plates of her art. It was launched at McNally Robinson on June 28, 1998—Judith's birthday. It became a best-seller and within four years all 2500 copies were sold out.

After its publication, *"Where the wind carries me . . ."* was submitted for the Benjamin Franklin Award for book design and book jacket design. It was also accepted by Germany's *Stiftung Buchkunst* for entry in the prestigious worldwide design competition at Leipzig. It was one of two books from Canada to enter the finals. I should add that it's in about two-thirds of Canada's public libraries and in most of our art galleries. Although the book is sold out, a lengthy description of it still remains at Amazon.com.

It took me about three years after Judith died to finally be able to live at peace with myself. We didn't have children . . . but had two lovely cats, Zephyr and Spice, who were with me until they both died last year. And strangely right at that time, through an unusual circumstance, I wound up with three lovely kittens . . . who have taken over my home and my heart. I have just completed a book about them, which is at the publishers: *The Saga of the Three Compañeros—Pantera, Leo and El Tigre.* It'll be about 150 pages, half text and half photos, and designed for both children and adults.

Gradually I resumed an interest in world affairs and have published a series of articles in journals and on highly regarded Internet sites. I have written on the events in Yugoslavia, Afghanistan, Iraq, Israel and Palestine, and of course on the situation in Canada. My most recent widely distributed article was on the advisability of a Liberal-NDP-Green coalition. And even more recently, Seymour Hersh, a journalist for the *New Yorker Magazine* and the writer who had exposed the My Lai massacre in Vietnam and the Abu Ghraib American torture scandal in Iraq, emailed and phoned me to talk about my 2006 article on Afghanistan. He is writing a book on Afghanistan and found my documentation of considerable interest, as well as my experiences in that country in 1978, six months after the indigenous Marxist revolution. For those who understand this early history, the belief is that if the American CIA had not created the mujahedeen and overthrown the progressive Marxist Taraki government in 1979, there would have been no army of foreign mujahedeen fanatics (including Osama bin Laden), no Soviet intervention, no war that destroyed the country, no Taliban, no 9/11 disaster in America, and no war there at present. There is no "winning" the war in Afghanistan, as the British and Russians found out, and as the Americans will discover. It will be up to the Afghanis to resolve their own affairs—after the tragic interference of foreigners for the past 30 years.

One would think that at my age and in comfortable retirement, I would hardly start off on a new career, but more than a year ago that's what happened. It started innocently enough as an academic exercise. In November of 2007 I discovered that an underwater electrical transmission cable (NorNed) had just been installed in the North Sea between Norway and the Netherlands—for a distance of 580 kilometres, going down to depths of 400 metres. In the meantime, in Manitoba a controversy was raging about the selection of a route for a new transmission line—to the east of Lake Winnipeg or to the west. Through Internet research, e-mails and phone calls to the Swedish company that built and installed the

NorNed cable—and a steep learning curve to almost become an engineer—I prepared a comprehensive, detailed proposal for such a cable to be installed in Lake Winnipeg—instead of an east or west land route. Of great help to me in this was my old buddy, Keith—it was fun to work together on this. I had a 3-part series on this proposal published in the *Winnipeg Free Press* in February of 2008. Shortly after, I had meetings with the Finance Minister, the President and CEO of Manitoba Hydro and other officials. Interestingly, Hydro had not done this research so they belatedly hired a consulting firm to follow up on my proposal and I was co-opted by the Hydro CEO to be his Special Advisor. So suddenly I once again had a job . . . with substantial remuneration!

For the past year I have been involved in meetings with the Hydro CEO and the president of the consulting firm. I wrote a number of reports based on my review and appraisal of the consultant's submissions. Even their recent third draft had major flaws and significant shortcomings. Because of some still unresolved problems with the transport of underwater cable by train in Canada, I did further research and presented Hydro with a different alternative—a combination of an overhead line, a short section of underground cable through the Grand Rapids area, followed by overhead line to the Conawapa power station on the Nelson. At the time of this writing, my proposal is still under consideration by Manitoba Hydro.

Because of my book on Judith and through serendipity, I came to know Helen Schreider, an artist in Santa Fe, New Mexico. She and her late husband had worked for *National Geographic*, had travelled the world over and had the most extraordinary adventures. They made a 20,000 mile journey in an amphibious jeep from the northern tip of Alaska to Tierra del Fuego, the southern most tip of South America. In a similar amphibious jeep they travelled the length of the Ganges, and afterwards spent 1½ years travelling from Sumatra to East Timor. Later during their travels they interviewed Chiang Kai-shek, the philosopher Lin Yutang, and Jordan's King Hussein. From Cairo they made their way through the Great Rift Valley to Mozambique, visiting the anthropologist Louis Leakey, and lion-man, George Adamson, who was behind the story of *Born Free*—Helen even played with Elsa's three cubs. In a land-rover they retraced the footsteps of Alexander the Great—24,000 miles—and almost lost their lives in the Baluchistan Desert where Alexander had lost a third of his army. And it was they who were given credit for discovering that the Amazon is longer than the Nile. They spent more than a year on the river, starting at its headwaters in Peru and after a perilous journey finally arrived at its mouth at the Atlantic Ocean. All this is recorded in many long articles in *National Geographic* and in their three books on these adventures.

Because of the complexity of life, Helen and I have a L.A.T. relationship—"Living Apart Together"—in the way that millions of loving couples have to do, the world over, because of certain circumstances. Although we have our homes 2,500 kilometres apart, we talk to one another every day by phone and enjoy lengthy visits several times a year, including ocean cruises and other vacations. We alternate our visits so the cats in each of our homes know us both. I recently wrote a book about her cats: *A Tale of Two Kitties—Taj and Bohdi.*

During my years as a professor I always tried to instill in my students a love for Canada and a sense of social responsibility. As for my philosophy of life, I suppose my guiding principle and objective in life, in my modest way, has been to try to change the world to be a somewhat better and happier place for humanity.

54
Gladwyn Scott

In 1954, Gladwyn was playing on a baseball team against Regina Royal Caps at a prestigious tournament in Indian Head, Sask., vying for first prize money of $1,000. Johnny Esaw, who became a well-known sports broadcaster and telecaster, was broadcasting the game to his Regina station. Johnny could not believe his eyes. Out there on the diamond, the veteran catcher, Jim Scott, had his two sons pitching to him. What a novel combination that was!

Although the Manitobans lost the game 6-4, Gladwyn was named a tournament all-star pitcher, which was quite an honour for the young man. Notre Dame Hounds—from Wilcox, Sask.—and Brandon Cloverleafs split top prize money after playing nine innings for a 2-2 deadlock. Eight thousand excited fans witnessed the tournament.

As brothers, Gladwyn and Glennis sometimes played together and occasionally competed against each other. They always had the greatest respect for their father, their mentor. Occasionally, he became a little annoyed with his sons when they did not do what he had taught them or when he thought that they were not working hard enough. As a catcher for them, he was a qualified critic. It was not until years later that the two brothers really appreciated the novelty of pitching to their Dad. What a phenomenal and memorable experience it had been for them!

Gladwyn was born at Hamiota. His wife, Marguerite, was born at Newdale. He had the unique experience of obtaining his first eleven years of education in a two-classroom school—one to six and seven to eleven—located in the small village of McConnell. He obtained his grade twelve at the high school in Strathclair. His principal for grade one and again in grade twelve was Walter Frederickson.

A favourite teacher was Charlie Miller, his principal in McConnell School for several years. His history classes came alive with his colourful stories. He had an enjoyable sense of humour and was always very encouraging and complimentary. He taught all subjects in grades seven to eleven, except French.

Gladwyn took his initial teacher training at Manitoba Provincial Normal School, in Winnipeg, in 1950–51. His athletic ability was apparent as he received a gold medal in physical education. After becoming a teacher, he continued his own education.

He obtained a Bachelor of Science degree, majoring in geology, zoology, and chemistry, at Brandon College in 1961. Next came a Bachelor of Education degree by summer schools from University of Manitoba in 1965. Finally, he obtained a Master of Education degree in Educational Administration from University of Manitoba in 1977.

His father farmed a half-section (130 ha) of land from 1928 to 1968. His mixed farming included raising cattle, horses, pigs, chickens, and turkeys and growing wheat, oats, barley, and flax. Gladwyn was the eldest of the children, who included one brother, Glennis, and four sisters.

On most days, the children played catch and hit grounders and fly balls to each other. Their dad, Jim, often batted balls to them and would catch for his two sons to give them practice in throwing accuracy and speed. He was a hard-working man and a wonderful role model. He exhibited a delightful sense of humour and was very encouraging. In addition, he was very musical and was involved in municipal affairs.

As a child, Gladwyn liked the book *The Three Bears*. He received it for being the most improved pupil in grade one. As an adult, he liked *Every Kid Can Win*, by Terry Orlick.

His principal vocation was educator—classroom teacher for 14 years, principal for 8 years, and superintendent for 21 years for an overall total of 43 years in his profession. A highlight of his career came in 1967, Confederation year, when he chaperoned a group of high school students from various Manitoba centres to Nanaimo, B.C., for a two-week exchange.

His involvement in sports has covered at least sixty years. During his teenage years, he was active in hockey, baseball, basketball, track and field, swimming, volleyball, fastball, and gymnastics—whether in school or in the community. At Strathclair, the high school had a very good Junior B (21 and under) hockey team which travelled to Birtle, Swan River, Crystal City, and Selkirk for play-off games. The team was provincial finalists with Selkirk Fishermen in 1950. Today, his favourite spectator sports are baseball and hockey.

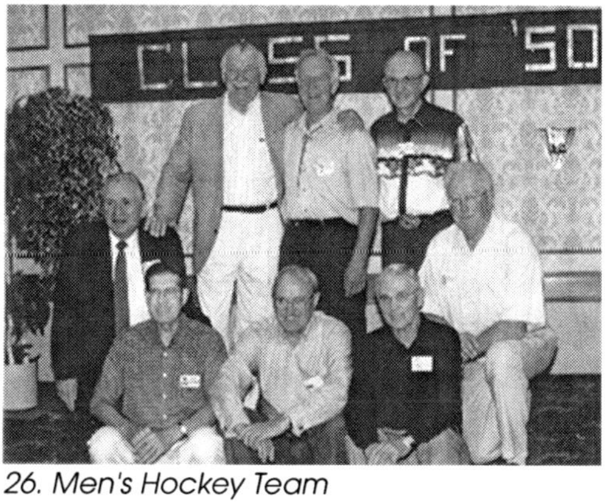

26. Men's Hockey Team

When Gladwyn taught in high school, he coached students in fastball, baseball, hockey, ringette, basketball, and track and field. Outside of school, he coached several teams. Some of them were: Hamiota Red Sox (baseball), Carman Goldeyes (baseball), Carman Beavers (hockey), Souris Elks (hockey), Souris and Warren minor hockey and baseball teams, and Westman Junior B All-Stars (hockey). The Westman team won the Manitoba title and placed fifth at the 1975 Canada Winter Games in Lethbridge, Alta. Hamiota minor baseball won seven provincial championships in five years. In 1957, the bantam, juvenile, and junior teams won Manitoba titles. The senior team, on which Gladwyn was playing coach, was provincial finalists.

As general manager of Canada's national youth baseball team, he travelled to Sydney, Australia, in November 1988 for the World Tournament for one month—Australia's bicentennial celebration. Australians are similar in many ways to Canadians except their vehicles are right-hand drive and they travel on the left side of the road.

He succeeded in reaching the professional level in baseball as a part-time associate scout for the Toronto Blue Jays from 1987 to 1993 and the Atlanta Braves from 1994 to 2001. The Blue Jays flew his wife Marguerite and him to Toronto to see the 1993 World Series between the Blue Jays and the Philadelphia Phillies. The Atlanta Braves enabled him to attend one-week spring training sessions at West Palm Beach, Fla., on two different occasions. Both were fantastic, memorable opportunities.

In 1996, he initiated and was the founding chairman of the Manitoba Baseball Hall of Fame and Museum. It was modeled after the Saskatchewan Hall. Because baseball had been an important part of his life, he gathered a group of other baseball people in January of that year. They set out to select individuals and teams who deserved special recognition for their involvement in the great sport of baseball.

They held their first induction banquet in 1997 at Brandon University, with twenty individuals and one team. Surprisingly, they drew 500 paying individuals. In 1998, they held the induction at Brandon's Keystone Centre; and, in 2001, they held it at Neepawa's Yellowhead Centre. Otherwise, the annual banquets are held at the Morden Recreational Centre. They have drawn from 600 to 740 people over the years.

The museum was officially opened at Morden in 1999, with Terry Hind cutting the ribbon and Frank McKinnon as master of ceremonies. This has been a fantastic success! Glennis and Gladwyn were inducted in 1998, while their father was inducted in the first class, in 1997.

Manitoba Baseball Hall of Fame induction is considered a great honour. There are many nominations of individuals and teams (three categories—major team, special team, and small community) for consideration by the selection committee. The museum outgrew its initial home and had to be expanded in 2008.

The Canadian Baseball Hall of Fame induction on June 28, 2008, was a fantastic and memorable experience. Meeting the other three inductees, Tony Fernandez, Billy Harris, and Peter Widdrington's wife and daughter was a supreme occasion. The four came from differing backgrounds, but all enjoyed such activities as attending a musical, "Cabaret", at Stratford, Ont., (fifteen minutes from St. Marys), signing autographs at the Super Golf Tournament on the 10th tee-off, and attending a game between Braves and Blue Jays at Rogers Centre in Toronto on June 29.

The entire Scott family (four children) and Gladwyn's brother and sister were all able to attend. At the conclusion of his acceptance speech, he became very emotional when he dedicated his award to his parents. Each inductee received a special black blazer and a beautiful plaque.

His advice for teenagers in regard to their future is to work hard and treat everyone with respect as they never know who might open a door in life for them. If the future includes a career in teaching, the student needs to want to help people develop whatever God-given abilities they may possess.

Gladwyn's own philosophy of life is to try to make this world a better place. Focus on the physical, mental, and spiritual growth of people in your jurisdiction.

He enjoys several hobbies. He writes for community newspapers—sports, recreation, and education articles in all communities, including Hamiota *Echo*, Dufferin *Leader*, Souris *Plain Dealer*, Stonewall *Argus* and Teulon *Times*, Interlake *Spectator*, Selkirk *Journal*, and Carberry *News Express*. He also interviews students of the month on local ACCESS television; supervises student teachers; and attends sporting events and concerts.

Gladwyn was always very active in communities where he and his family lived. These communities included Foxwarren (1 year), Cardale (1 year), Hamiota (5 years), Carman (7 years), Souris (13 years), Warren (14 years), Stonewall (6 years), and Carberry (8 years). He is —or has been—a member of the Masonic Lodge, Baseball Manitoba, and several recreation organizations.

On two occasions, he received Queen Elizabeth II gold medallions from MP Felix Holtman (Interlake, 1988) and Brian Palliser (Portage-Lisgar, 2002) for contributions to his community, his province, and his country. Recognition also includes Manitoba Sports Hall of Fame as an all-round builder in 1992; Manitoba Baseball Hall of Fame in 1998; Brandon University Hockey Hall of Fame in 2000; Manitoba Hockey Hall of Fame as a builder in 2003. However, he considers his Canadian Baseball Hall of Fame as "the icing on the cake".

Inspector John Menzie, with whom he worked at Gimli Summer School—1952 as a student and 1960 and 1961 as an instructor—had a positive effect on Gladwyn's life and work. He had a wonderful sense of humour, loved sports, and was a super human being, always positive with himself and others.

Two men stand out in Gladwyn's experience as making major contributions to Canada. They are Ed Schreyer and R. W. "Bobby" Bend.

Ed Schreyer was Premier of Manitoba from 1969 to 1977; Governor-General of Canada from 1979 to 1983; and Canadian High Commissioner to Australia, Papua New Guinea, the Solomon Islands, and Vanuatu from 1984 to 1988. Gladwyn met him at University of Manitoba Summer School in the 1950s. He was a caring human being who did what he thought best for all people.

R. W. "Bobby" Bend was another leader who made great contributions to Manitoba and education. Gladwyn succeeded him as superintendent of education in the Interlake School Division in August 1981. He, too, was a role model. In September 1981, Gladwyn initiated the renaming of the East School at Stonewall, a K-4 complex —R. W. "Bobby" Bend School.

He was a teacher, principal, and superintendent of schools at Transcona, Western (Morden), and Interlake School Divisions. He was an elected MLA who held Minister of Education and Minister of Health portfolios in the Manitoba Legislature. His oratory commanded the respect of his audiences. He was Manitoba Liberal leader and a great supporter of Jim Scott, who ran unsuccessfully in 1959 for his party. He was a highly respected and travelled baseball umpire throughout

Manitoba. Bobby was also a strong supporter of Gladwyn, who was highly honoured when his family invited him to give the eulogy at Bobby's funeral.

For a potential visitor to Canada, he suggests a visit to the Maritime Provinces in the fall to see the natural beauty, to meet the friendly people, and to experience the rich history.

He has enjoyed good health, but he did suffer a severe heart attack in November 1993. He is a bionic man now as he has two titanium hips—right on August 28, 2006, and left on April 18, 2007.

Gladwyn and Marguerite have four children—Michelle (1963), Rick (1970), Sharla (1972) are school teachers and Jeff (1966) works for Canada Post in Thunder Bay, Ont. Marguerite was a school teacher for three years before she and Gladwyn were married on July 29, 1961, at Hamiota United Church. They have always been very active in the church—attendance, and committees and she was also very involved in choirs, prayer groups, and Bible study.

The couple lives in Carberry. This town is the potato capital of Manitoba. McCain's operate a potato processing plant there which employs 300 workers. They provide McDonald's Restaurants with many of their French fries. Manitoba Starch Plant uses some of the potato by-products for starch.

Gladwyn feels that Manitoba Provincial Normal School, which he attended in 1950–51, was probably the best and biggest learning year of his life.

55
Viola (Sigurdson) Wild

Sharron Arksey, with the assistance of members of the family, provided her mother's story. Viola passed away on May 2, 2007, just five days after her seventy-fifth birthday.

What do you do if you are a young mother who must work and have no means of care for your pre-school daughter while you work? This was before the days of kindergarten. Some small communities found innovative ways to help its citizens in need. This rural one did find a way to help such a woman.

The local one-room school had a permit teacher of about sixteen or seventeen years of age, who taught grades one to eight with a few grades nine and ten students taking correspondence courses. To help the young mother, the school board agreed that, although the little girl was not of school age, she could go to school and be under the care of the teacher. The teacher developed an affection for the child, whose name was Sharron. When the young teacher gave birth to her own first daughter, what do suppose she named her? She was named Sharron—and the one who provided the information for this chapter.

Viola was born in Winnipeg and grew up in Oakview, a farming community near the Lake Manitoba Narrows. She took her grades one to eight at Darwin School, a one-room country school at Oakview, being able to pass grades one and two and then grades three and four in one year each. She took grades nine and ten by correspondence, with supervision provided by the Darwin School teacher. She attended Ashern High School for grade eleven, rooming with an aunt and uncle, and then Daniel McIntyre Collegiate in Winnipeg for grade twelve, rooming with family friends. As a result of her early acceleration, she finished grade twelve when she was only sixteen years old.

Following her high school graduation, Viola was a permit teacher for two years at Darwin School, the same school that she herself had attended. Upon leaving Normal School, she obtained a position at Lakeside School #225—also called South Lakeland School—and taught there from September 1951 to June 1953.

At that time, she married and, like many other women of this period, she put her career on hiatus. In the late 1960s and early 1970s, she taught health and spelling to grades seven and eight one afternoon a week at Langruth School. This gave the classroom teacher, Ray McNeill, who was also school principal, some weekly administration time.

Years after she received her teaching certificate, she obtained her Certificate in Municipal Administration through the University of Manitoba. In January 1974, Viola began a second career as a municipal administrator, working for the Rural Municipality of Lakeview. She held this position for almost twenty-four years, retiring in August 1997. As sidelines, she ran an Autopac (Manitoba provincial auto insurance) business out of the municipal building and was a Justice of the Peace.

A book which she enjoyed as a child was a teenage mystery published in 1929, *The Black Box*, by Thelma Lientz. She still had a copy of it in her personal library when she passed away. As a child, her daughter Sharron read the book after her mother told her how much she had loved it. Her other daughters read it, too. The love that her daughters have for mystery stories can be traced to this book. Where is the book now? It is affectionately a part of Sharron's own library.

Her interest in mysteries did not carry over into adulthood. She did not like the books that her daughters were reading; as she found them just a little too graphic and perhaps chilling. However, she was a fan of the author Maeve Binchy, whose books have been described as heartwarming.

Viola partook of several hobbies which interested her. She loved her vegetable and flower gardens and her houseful of indoor plants, which her family is trying to preserve. She also enjoyed reading, knitting, crocheting, and travelling. Since she was of Icelandic descent, she wanted to learn more of the language. As she attended classes, she discovered that she already knew much more than she gave herself credit. She attended baseball games in the summer—both league games in Winnipeg and games involving any of her grandchildren.

She also kept busy with community affairs. She was a member of the Langruth Community Club. For more than a decade, up to the time of her death, she was treasurer for Grace Lutheran Church. She was a member of the board of directors for Lakeview Children's Centre and she also volunteered on a weekly basis at the local child care programme after her retirement.

She served in all executive positions in the local branch of the Order of the Royal Purple. She attended TOPS (Take Off Pounds Sensibly) and was treasurer for one or two years. She was an active member of the Fifty and Over Club—the Langruth seniors' group. She was on the organizing committee of the Langruth Fall Fair. In her honour, one of the annual prizes is named after her.

Viola went on several trips outside Canada, most of them after her retirement. However, her trip of a lifetime occurred when she and her younger daughter Debbie visited Iceland in 2003. They were able to meet relatives on both her mother's side and her father's side of the family, and even some on her mother-in-law's family. Some of these relatives repaid the visit when they travelled to Canada in 2006. Apparently, her language ability was good enough for her to chat in Icelandic with those relatives as easily as if she had lived in Iceland.

She had been in the Maritimes in the autumn and loved the colours. She had been in Ottawa in the spring and loved the tulips. She might tell a person to go some place in Canada to enjoy an unobstructed view of the Northern Lights. Any of those places are well worth seeing.

Viola always said, "Just do your best." That probably sums up how she would have addressed young people on these topics of their present and their future. Her oldest granddaughter (Sharron's daughter) will graduate with her Bachelor of Education degree in the spring of 2009 and another granddaughter (Sharron's niece) will graduate with hers in 2010. It is not known who a favourite teacher at any level was.

Oli Eiriksson, her sister's father-in-law, was reeve of the Rural Municipality of Lakeview in 1974 when Viola was hired in the office. She took on the municipal position with no experience and no training, just a willingness to learn what needed to be learned and with the support of people like Oli Eiriksson. It opened up an entirely new career for her. She was grateful to him for hiring her and for supporting her in those first few years as she learned the job and completed the training.

Viola and her husband Don raised six children, four girls and two boys. The youngest son died in a car-pedestrian accident in 1984 at the age of twenty-one. This was without a doubt the hardest experience in her life. Losing a child is unthinkable.

All four daughters went on to further education with her influence being seen in this as she valued education. The oldest son took over the family farm. There are eleven grandchildren.

Don was diagnosed with cancer in 1987 and died in 1990 after a series of treatments and a brief remission. Viola became a nurse in addition to being a spouse in his last months.

The family has amusing pictures of their mother. One is of her going on a Seadoo ride with one of her sons when she was seventy-three years old. Another presents her shaking hands with a wax figure of Mel Gibson in Las Vegas, Nev. She said to the figure, “Mel, it’s so nice to finally meet you.” Throughout her life, she was always willing to try anything new.

Until her death, Viola lived on the family farm thirteen miles (21 km) south of Langruth.

56
Elaine (Slimmon) Dale

"That's my mom up there receiving her diploma!" This is what one of her sons said to the person sitting next to him. He thought that this was, in his words, "Pretty neat!"

It was the 1993 convocation at the University of Manitoba. His mom was receiving her Bachelor of Education degree! She was no ordinary mom. She had four grown children, and three grandsons. Her youngest son—who expressed the sentiment—was so proud of her. She was humbled and pleased with the comment.

It took her ten long years to accomplish the feat, all the while being a teacher, a student, and a domestic engineer. Many mothers have graduated, but she was a grandmother who was near the retirement age.

Elaine was born in Shoal Lake. Her first educational experience was in two one-room schools—Reidville and Raven Lake. Her high school was Shoal Lake Collegiate. She obtained a Bachelor of Education degree from University of Manitoba. Nothing really memorable happened for her in school. However, she accomplished a feat within her family, being the only one of seven children to complete high school.

Elaine admired Mr. Lightly, our vice-principal and social studies teacher, for his sincerity and his ability to remember people. He was an inspector in her area when she was in elementary school. At Normal School, he remembered her and others from the Shoal Lake District.

Attending Normal School was her first experience in living in residence. She enjoyed the get-togethers in students' rooms—Rupert 1. The girls were especially happy when someone had been home and had brought back goodies (even roast chicken) from their mothers' pantries. The treats were appreciated and, as a result, did not last long.

She taught in the one-room school district of Huntley, in the Belmont-Neelin area; in the St. James School District, in suburban Winnipeg; and in Winnipeg School District 1.

Teaching ESL (English as a Second Language) can be educational, not only for the students who struggle to learn our language, but also for the teachers as they listen to stories from the immigrants. Having taught ESL for nearly twenty years in the 1980s and the 1990s, Elaine has heard some very dramatic stories. She provides the reader with two examples.

In one class, she asked her students to tell the class how they reached Canada. After the coffee break, several urged her to ask David about his experience. David lived in Romania under the regime of Nicolae Ceauşescu and served in his country's Merchant Marine.

One night, off the coast of Turkey, he decided that this was his opportunity to gain his freedom. When it appeared to be clear, he dived off the ship and swam toward shore. Local fishermen rescued him from the water and, since he was a foreigner, turned him over to the authorities. He was placed into a refugee camp; and, from there, he eventually arrived in Canada.

Someone asked him, "Why would you risk your life in such a manner?"

Dramatically, he replied, “I had nothing to lose. There was nothing to live for in my country.”

On another occasion, there was John, a young fellow with a good sense of humour who liked to tease and expected teasing in return. He worked during the day and attended classes in the evening. Sometimes, he would doze off during the lesson.

One evening, when he dozed, Elaine said to him, “I guess you were out too late with your girlfriend last night.” This time, he made no reply. At coffee break, he apologized and said that he was not sleeping very well. She realized that something was bothering him. Therefore, she asked if she could help. He then told his story.

In escaping from Romania, he had hidden in a truckload of exports, driven by a friend. He was very careful not to divulge any information that might lead to his friend because of the dire consequences. His elderly parents lived just outside Bucharest, the capital city. He had not heard from them and could not contact them. Mail was being intercepted. He was worried that the regime had harmed them in some way.

Elaine suggested that he contact the International Red Cross to see if they could help. They were able to contact his parents and acted as a go-between for him and his family. Shortly thereafter, he accepted a job in the Yukon, after which she lost track of him.

As a child, Elaine enjoyed reading *The Yearling*, by Marjorie Kinnan Rawlings. As an adult, she enjoyed *Exodus*, by Leon Uris.

In the 1970s, she visited Lucerne and Berne, Switzerland, and saw places, architecture, and the Alps, about which she had only read. It was so exhilarating!

Elaine’s husband and his business partner operated a refrigeration and air-conditioning business and sold

General Electric equipment. Instead of giving bonuses, GE took their sales representatives on trips, one of them being to Lucerne, Switzerland. Her husband and his partner earned the trip for them and their wives through their sales. There were probably about fifty representatives and their wives, plus GE officials and their wives who went. This was one of several trips the partners and their wives took together.

One evening, their tour group had dinner accompanied by Swiss entertainment. The emcee asked people to try the instruments—one being the long Swiss horn. Two Canadian tourists from Saskatchewan were contestants. At the end of the evening, they were going out the door at the same time as these girls. Elaine and her husband chatted with them and their escort, a Swiss gentleman who had lived in Canada and made a point of entertaining Canadians. He had met the girls at the railway station earlier when he was picking up his daughter. After the chat, he took them back to the railway station where they caught a train for Italy.

He offered to take the two sales representatives and their wives for a drive the next afternoon. They accepted the invitation, thinking that he meant within Lucerne. He picked them up at one o'clock and brought them back to their hotel at seven o'clock!

He took them through the mountains, even to the town in the Canton of Uri where William Tell was born. Being typical tourists, they were photographed in front of his statue. Then, they visited what seemed to be a diner and meeting hall in the middle of a huge meadow in a valley. Here the local farmers and mountain dwellers met for cards games, conversation, and food on Sundays. Since this was Sunday, they met and talked with some locals. They also saw a unique cemetery on the mountainside. The graves were in tiers, with photographs of the deceased on the tombstones.

The buildings in the area were very old and very well preserved. The year in which they were built was carved into the wall beneath the eaves. It was an amazing experience.

Elaine suggests that tourists in Canada visit anywhere in the Canadian Shield—especially in the Manitoba-Ontario border area—away from the tourist spots. Each season has its own special beauty.

For pastimes, she likes gardening, reading, cottage life (experiencing nature), curling, and golfing.

She has been quite involved in community activities. These include the following: Local Community Club (Westridge), United Church of Canada, Pembina Business Girls Curling Club, Pembina Ladies Curling Club, Manitoba Ladies Curling Past Presidents' Association, and Rotary Auxiliary. With Rotary Auxiliary, she attended conferences in such places as Regina, Sask.; Kenora, Ont.; and Thief River Falls, Minn. However, she did not have the opportunity to attend any overseas.

During her curling days, she did not win any memorable trophies, only those within her local club. Her rink represented their district in the Senior Women's playdowns one year, but they did not win. Also, they have represented their district in the Golden Gals; but again, they were not winners.

Over the years, she has participated in many bonspiels, both ladies and mixed, at various towns in the province, and also in North Dakota and Minnesota. Sometimes, her rink won prizes. However, whether they won or did not win, it was always fun. In the process, they always met interesting and friendly people.

Do not become a slave to technology—use it to expand your knowledge. Learn to converse intelligently.

Be physically active. These pieces of advice she would present to young people.

For those aspiring to be teachers, she has this advice. Develop your social and inter-personal skills. Be respectful of others, whether they be your superiors, your workmates, or your students.

There are many persons who have had a positive influence on her life, but one stands out—her neighbour and friend, who has always been ready when needed. Elaine knows that she can count on her friend, even if it is only for a sounding-board for her ideas or frustrations.

Duff Roblin was the former premier of Manitoba who was instrumental in building the floodway around Winnipeg, between 1962 and 1968. It has saved the province and the country untold dollars in flood damages. Anyone who remembers the disastrous flood that inundated some parts of Winnipeg in 1950 will appreciate the importance of that floodway.

Her philosophy of life is to live for today as the past cannot be changed and no one knows what the future has in store.

CLASS H

Irene Branconier
Harry Craig
George Krahn
John Lord
Lyall Simms
Geoffrey Smith
Shevaun Smith
Shirley Solar
Donna Sproat
Verna Spurr
Jean Stadnyk
Marian Staple
Joan Stanbridge
Joyce Stanbridge
Steve Stasiuk
Garnet Stevens
Shirley Stevens
Audrey Stevenson
Margaret Stewart
Leon Stocki
Joyce Stroud
Vicki Styba
Valerie Swiderski
Alice Sydor
Emily Szarkowicz
Eva Tabalotny
Alice Tanchak
Olive Tarbath
Gwen Thera
Tina Thiessen
Theresa Tkachuk
Verna Toews
Victor Toews
Lucille Tougas
Carmella Trudeau
Helen Unruh
Bessie Vatcher
Blanche Vercaigne
Roy White

57
George Krahn

Winnipeg was celebrating her 100th anniversary of incorporation. The guests of honour were HRH Princess Margaret and her husband, Lord Snowdon. The city sponsored a luncheon for them. One boy and one girl from each school in the city were invited to attend. How thrilling this must have been for those children!

George, who was employed in Sturgeon Creek Regional School at the time, had the honour of sitting at the head table next to Lord Snowdon. He reported having had a very pleasant conversation with the prince. He, too, seemed to relish the opportunity. Other adults not at the head table were in the gymnasium and watched the event on closed circuit television.

George was born in Winkler. He attended grades one to ten in rural one-classroom school districts in which his father was his teacher. He took grades nine and ten by correspondence. The schools were Edenthal, Burwalde, Rosenort, Altbergthal, and Sommerfeld. He took grades eleven and twelve at the Mennonite Collegiate Institute, a private school in Gretna.

When he was in grade three, a very traumatic event occurred. The mother and baby sister of one of his classmates died in a horse-drawn vehicle during a blizzard. For George, the funeral was very dramatic.

He lived in the Bible brimstone belt of southern Manitoba, in which he learned that a person goes either to heaven or to hell on death. That belief was stressed in the preaching on that day. He lived in a home that did not have the media facilities that are common today. Thus, he was unaware of other beliefs. In later years, he saw in the opera *The Damnation of Faust*, written by Hector Berlioz, a good portrayal of heaven and hell, similar to what he had been taught as a child.

Although he felt that his dad was a good teacher, he particularly remembers his high school principal, Mr. Schaefer. This man made Mennonite history come alive. That was important as George had a Mennonite background.

He earned a Bachelor of Arts degree and a Bachelor of Education degree from the University of Manitoba. He earned his CFP designation from the Canadian Financial Planning Institute.

George was in the field of education for twenty-nine years. On permit, he taught a class of forty-one students in grades one to three in the rural school district of Chortitz. Eighteen students in grade one spoke only German, but this was no problem since George also spoke German. He taught grade six for two years in Morris and for three years each in Birkenhead School District and Winkler. He spent twenty years in education in the St. James School District. This included three years of teaching junior high at Golden Gate School and seventeen years of administration.

His administrative posts were Assiniboine School, Britannia Junior High School, Bannatyne School, Bruce Junior High School, and Sturgeon Creek Regional Secondary School. His final year in St. James School District was as an assistant school superintendent.

In 1979, he retired from teaching and took a correspondence course from the Financial Planning

Institute, a Canadian facility. When he entered his second career, Jim Lawton was his friend and mentor. Jim showed him how to be successful in the field of financial planning. With this kind of support, George enjoyed the work very much.

As a child, he enjoyed reading books in the *Hardy Boys* series, by Franklin W. Dixon. After he became an adult, he read a book which he had missed when he was a young boy—*Call of the Wild*, by Jack London.

Past community service includes Kinsmen, Rotary, community clubs, and singing in church choirs. His hobbies in order of involvement are golf, fishing, opera and ballet music, and online poker. He played squash and tennis when he was younger.

A memorable trip for George and his family was to Expo 67, held in Montreal, Que. Two things stood out. A telephone company presented a movie showing a 360° documentary about Canada and her people. The other one was impressive in a negative way. They were in a campground in which there was a ditch for the sewage. In an effort to keep it somewhat sanitary, workers treated it with lime.

He would suggest that one should visit Massacre Island on the Ontario side in Lake of the Woods and Fort St. Charles on the Northwest Angle on the Minnesota side. In June 1736, La Vérendrye and twenty other men in his expedition were beheaded and scalped by unfriendly natives. They were later buried at Fort St. Charles. The fort has been rebuilt and is now a refuge and sanctuary for Catholic priests. Another place to visit in the area is the beautiful Rushing River Provincial Park on the east side of the lake.

He admonishes youth to plan to make a difference in their lives. They should see the movie *Lions and Lambs*, which is set in the Afghan War. The person whom Robert

Redford portrays challenges a young, rich, spoiled, college student to make a difference in his life.

For a person who insists on a teaching career, one should teach in a good private school, a French immersion school, or a similar type of school as the public educational system today is like a zoo. Since he knows families who are homeschooled, he feels that this is a good alternative.

Lester Pearson stands out as a great Canadian. First, he excelled in his peace efforts, for which he won a Nobel Prize. Then, when he became Prime Minister, he had to lead minority governments. In this difficult task, he again performed well.

Mr. Lightly, our vice-principal and social studies teacher, really impressed George when he was in Normal School. He was tall and he exuded confidence, calmness, and power. Normal School was like play-school. George was involved in sports. However, what he really liked was the night life in the canteen. There were "canned" music and dancing, among other social activities. He noted that the female students outnumbered the male students by about ten to one.

It has been incredible to have lived in Canada all of his life, even though he now spends part of each year in California. He is most thankful that his parents emigrated from Russia in 1928 and settled in Canada. After forty-four years, his mother flew to Siberia to visit her sisters. The Soviet system had made it so different from what she had experienced before leaving there earlier. George also notes that after World War II, there was an era of opportunity for young people in Canada, even if they had little education.

He maintains that he is totally responsible for his life. No one else is responsible for the fortunes—good or bad—in his life, except himself. What he is to be is up to him.

58
Shirley (Solar) Maurice

When little children are involved, expect the unexpected. It was in an "open area" school. As she taught a lesson or read a book, she would sit on a small chair and the children would sit in a circle or group at her feet. One day, a little boy seemed to be more interested in her than in his lesson. Gently, he ran his hand on her ankle. What was his interest? Was it her nylons? After the lesson, all the children except this little boy returned to their table and chairs. When everyone was out of earshot, he approached his teacher and whispered quietly into her ear, "You need a shave!"

Shirley was born in the St. Boniface Hospital, in Winnipeg. Her first school years were spent at Cromwell School, near Beausejour, where her father taught in a one-room school with eight grades. When she was three years old, she was allowed to go to school if she "sat quietly" in one of the smaller desks near the front of the room. At five years old when she was in grade one (at last!), her dad "used" her talents of being unafraid and of being able to carry a tune to help him teach songs to his students. She would sing the whole song through, then one line, with the other children repeating. Then she would do the same with two lines, and then three lines until the classes had learned the song—all by rote.

By the time that she was seven, her dad took her and her brother with him to Lac du Bonnet, leaving her mother in Rembrandt School to teach eight grades plus correspondence. The marriage was in trouble and the school inspector—the only "counsellor" who was neutral—suggested this arrangement would give her mom a rest and maybe the marriage would survive. Shirley was to "mind" her brother; but, by Christmas as they were boarding with a family near the school, her dad decided that the children would be better with their mother. That turned out to be a good decision.

When her mother had to go to Winnipeg by bus for a Friday appointment (offices not being open on Saturday), Shirley was assigned to supervise the whole school while she was gone. There were *no* "subs" to take over. All the work was on the blackboard and she knew how to dictate spelling, to correct mathematics, and to collect answers from the questions on the board. Good behaviour was expected! Older sisters in upper grades took care of dressing the younger children in winter, of leading playground games, and of supervising lunchroom. These were assets!

Shirley finished grade ten at Rembrandt and then went to Winnipeg to complete grades eleven and twelve at Isaac Newton High School. There, she found three very good friends, despite boarding with her mother's friends, baby-sitting, and trying to understand high school.

For the school year 1949–50 after Gimli Summer School, she taught grades one to eight in Fryer School, at Silver, on a permit. She had twenty-seven students and earned $1,000 a year, a figure set by the Department of Education.

From 1951 to 1954, after attending Tuxedo Normal School, she taught kindergarten to grade six in Ridgeville. This was a two-room school, with the principal having grades seven to ten and correspondence. From 1954 to 1956, she taught grades three to five in Snow Lake. A Normal School colleague, Nora (Kabernick) Perry, was also on staff.

Between 1964 and 1966, after several years away from teaching, she substituted in the Protestant and Catholic schools in Elliot Lake, Ont., for teachers on maternity leave and for principals. Her assignments included grade eight classes—shudder!

From 1966 to 1972, she taught third classroom of year one in Allard School in St. James, a part of Winnipeg. As Shirley described it, the school was brand spanking new! She went from that school to another new one in 1972. She had the third class of year one children at Ryerson School in Fort Garry. She stayed here until 1990 when she retired to enjoy the three grandchildren. Her husband Gerry was already enjoying them, having retired early.

Shirley and Gerry Maurice were married in December 1956. From July to December of that year, she worked for the Toronto-Dominion Bank. Thus, she became a teller. Gerry was in the Air Force flying T-33s and Sabre jets. As a result, they lived in Trenton, Ont., and Chatham, N.B.

When there was a change in the federal government, they soon learned that they were *not* going to Europe, but returning to Manitoba—with Shirley pregnant and both jobless! Gerry went into recreation and made a successful career. With a baby girl, they moved to Elliot Lake, Ont., where Gerry was Collins Hall manager and in charge of all the recreational programmes for the town and the five mines surrounding the town. A son arrived in 1960. When uranium became not as viable as it had been, they moved back to Winnipeg.

During her first year of teaching at Ryerson School in Fort Garry School Division, the board informed their teachers that they would not have their contracts renewed unless they held a degree. Therefore, about 1982, Shirley began a crash study programme with university courses, summer school, and intercessions. By 1986, she had earned her Bachelor of Education degree, majoring in history and minoring in English, with as many primary courses as she could find.

The division kept up with the changes by offering non-credit courses in the "new" mathematics, the whole language idea in creative writing (she continued phonics!), the "new" social studies and science curricula. She even worked on a committee with Peter Luba from the Department of Education, writing a "problem-solving handbook" for years one to three. These courses were scattered through her final eighteen years of teaching.

Besides being a teller in the Toronto-Dominion Bank, she had three other jobs outside the home. One summer, she was as an aide in a nursing home. During another summer, she was a waitress in the Idylwylde Tea Room at Clear Lake, in Riding Mountain National Park. She also had a volunteer position ushering at the matinée at the Manitoba Theatre Centre.

As a child, she read every library book that came to Rembrandt School before her mother had put the "sticker" in the front of each book. She particularly enjoyed *Five Little Peppers*, by Margaret Sidney, and *Love You Forever*, by Robert Munsch. The *Pooh* books, by A. A. Milne, were read over and over in her teaching of primary children. Now, she enjoys reading the short stories and novels by Winnipeg native Linda Holeman and mysteries by Mary Higgins Clark.

She has knitted a blanket for the bed of each of her six grandchildren. She has printed signs for curling rinks, the Manitoba Curling Association, and her church. Miss Pilling, our art teacher, performed her job well and Shirley has made good use of her felts.

She served in the UNICEF store when there was a branch in Winnipeg. Twice a month, she volunteered at the food bank at her church in Fort Richmond. She has participated in her church choir—sometimes as lead—and in her church library. In addition, she has been coordinator for funeral luncheons, and, after nineteen years, has just resigned from the fall supper committee.

Most of her work involved teaching her own music, gym, and even French before specialists were trained. She felt that she needed to improve her French for her classes. Also, Gerry's family was fluent in the language. With those two incentives, she had an urge to travel to Jonquiere, Que., for a 6-week immersion course in French. Her dream was fulfilled. She thoroughly enjoyed stepping into this culture and participating in it. She ate, slept, and thought in French. What a memorable experience it was! It was a trip which she will never forget.

For an experience in culture, a visitor to Canada should consider going to Winnipeg in August. That is when Folklorama is in session. It is a time to meet the different nationalities as they stage two weeks of food, fun, dance, and culture for the public. The performances are definitely exquisite.

For advice to teenagers, she offers an oxymoron: Respect yourself. Give yourself a good trial at a career you think you want. Weigh the pros and cons and change course before life becomes complicated with "stuff". Do not allow others to be affected negatively by your choices.

She has met students who had been in her classes and now are at the University of Manitoba specializing in primary education. Her advice by example is to love what you do. Shirley had set the example for her students.

Her inspiration, her guide, and her role model were provided by one of her teachers, Mrs. Mary Solar, her mother—all 5' 2" (157 cm) of her. When Shirley was a permit teacher, she was close enough to walk home the five and one-half miles (9 km) carrying her book bag every weekend. She would sit at the kitchen table, plan the month, plot the week, and follow the plan for eight grades.

Each of her principals was a positive influence in her teaching career. A vice-principal, Mrs. Jan Lowe, had a special talent to accentuate the positive when she did her yearly visits in Shirley's classroom at Ryerson. She and Bryant Hasker were, without a doubt, the best team for whom she worked in her thirty-four years in the profession.

Pierre Elliot Trudeau made an impression on both Gerry and Shirley. They felt that he believed English and French could coexist without breaking away—and "Fuddle Duddle" lives on.

She has had a career which she loved, a family of whom she is proud, and a dearly loved husband for almost fifty years. His family is still part of her life. They have been able to surmount many problems. Thus, she feels that when you come to the end of your rope (or think you have), tie another knot and hang on! In brief, do not give up.

When she arrived at Normal School, she discovered that every teacher on staff was special—unlike high school, which she found very difficult. Every teacher was speaking her language. She mentions some of them.

There were our principal, Mr. Moorhead; our vice-principal and social studies teacher, Mr. Lightly; and the Turners. She, like others, remembers Miss Norton and her rendition of the "great, grey-green Limpopo River". Shirley always read aloud to her classes with the voice of

Miss Norton in her head. She wanted to coordinate her clothes and jewellery just like Miss Smith did! She learned from Miss Douglas and is still in a choir. Who else but someone with the name Mr. Herron would there be to teach science? She seemed to know what Mr. Clarke was going to say before he said it.

She particularly remembered Miss Ring when she was in a country school one Friday afternoon in October. She was catching in the "gym" baseball game with no glove. A grade four boy fired a blistering pitch over the plate and caught her right ring finger, breaking it. Ow! All she had was a box of band-aids!! What would her teacher have thought if she knew that there was a pail of water from which the students drank and saved the excess in a basin for hand washing, and that no well existed on the property? She learned from each of the teachers and loved them all!

She was a resident at Normal School and considered herself lucky because, after study hour, there was a choir practice or speech choir, or something new to learn in the gym (volleyball and basketball), helping Johnny in the canteen, playing baseball or hockey (in figure skates), or visiting in other rooms in the "hut". Her permit year was exciting, successful, and memorable; but her Normal School year proved that teaching was the only life for her. She travelled home by bus when she could afford it and told her mother about Normal School *all* weekend. She had made the right choice of a career.

59

Verna (Spurr) Lavergne

Do you know young people who are anticipating a career in teaching? Have they talked to a teacher—or several—about the pros and cons of this profession as a life work? One former teacher has some thoughts on this. She would like to encourage young people who are considering teaching as a profession.

To her, it is the most important and rewarding career there is. It is a joy to see children learn. It is the skill, knowledge, encouragement, patience, and love of the teacher that is successful in developing and nurturing young minds. What vocation would bring more satisfaction than the success of children learning? Be confident and positive. Never give up! They should think about this former teacher and what others have advised.

Verna was born in Rocanville, Sask., where she took her first three years of schooling. Her family then moved to Bredenbury, Sask., where she completed grade eight. Then, they moved to Sinclair where she finished grade eleven.

That summer, she attended summer classes at Provincial Normal School in Winnipeg and received her Letter of Standing to teach on permit for one year. However, that fall, she attended grade twelve in Welwyn, Sask. In the following September, she taught one year on permit at Elim South District, a rural one-room school near Welwyn. That was an exciting year and a tremendous learning experience!

The staff at Normal School was truly outstanding, particularly Miss Ring, our health teacher, who was an inspiration to the young female students. Verna vividly recalls how she encouraged them to become "proper ladies" as they would be models for young people at the schools in which they would be teaching.

Verna was one of the residents of Mackenzie Hall in the main building. After Christmas, because this hall was to be redecorated, about twenty girls, with their beds, desks, and personal belongings, were moved to the big dormitory in the Bell Tower. Everyone was aware that "Boris" the ghost lived in the Bell Tower and that there was tremendous apprehension about his dwelling there! What if he should appear?

He did materialize one night after midnight—being impersonated by a group of girls who had remained in Mackenzie Hall. What was that noise? The would-be ghosts, enrobed in white sheets and, with noise makers, raided the Bell Tower dormitory. Boris escorted his friends to the room and rudely awakened the sleeping beauties with their eerie noises. What panic broke out—no lights and frantic girls dashing everywhere! The ruse was successful and kept everyone from enjoying a good night's sleep. There must have been some sheepish expressions on the faces of the victims when the truth about the ghostly horde was revealed.

Upon graduation, Verna was a classroom teacher in Lenore and Carberry, following which she transferred to Kenora, Ont., where she taught until she was married. After her two daughters were born, the family moved to Burlington, Ont., where she taught until her retirement.

Early in her teaching career, the music supervisor in Kenora, Mr. Swanson, had a profound influence on

Verna's ability to succeed in teaching music. He taught the music lesson in each classroom once a week. He was her mentor, who greatly influenced her ability to make instruction interesting, varied, and functional, encouraging her to participate in music festivals and to teach music in other classes within the school. He was a person who could sense a hidden talent and who would help to develop it in order to share the skill of teaching music to others. What an opportunity that was for her!

During her thirty-two years of teaching, she took numerous university courses, received diplomas from professional courses, and attained her Specialist in Special Education and Primary Specialist Certificates. She directed school choirs and played a leadership role in presenting workshops in English, environmental studies, and music for teachers on professional development days. She also worked on various curriculum workshops. At this time, her daughter, who was completing her Bachelor of Education degree, took her special education and, thus, mother and daughter together completed these courses. What a joy that was for both!

As a child, Verna's favourite reading was a collection of poems by Robert Louis Stevenson and his book *Treasure Island*. Recently, she enjoyed reading *Chalk, Challenge, and Change: Stories from Women Teachers in Ontario, 1920–1979*, by Retired Women Teachers of Ontario.

In her earlier days of teaching, she was active as a CGIT leader, a choir director, and in curling. As her husband Bill was a Kinsman, she became a member of the Kinette Club, served on the executive, and eventually became president. They have been members of the Roseland Golf and Country Club for many years and Verna was an executive member and served as president of the women's section. Bill is a bridge life master and an accredited bride instructor, and she is his assistant in the latter endeavour. They play bridge as a social pastime. With all their activities, their days are always full.

When she moved to Kenora, Ont., to teach, she soon realized that this area is a must-be-seen part of our country. The amazing Lake of the Woods with its ten thousand islands, nestled in the rocky terrain with stately evergreens, is a wonderful spot to absorb the magnificence of nature. It is a refreshing, relaxing place to spend holidays and to enjoy!

One of the most enjoyable trips that she and Bill experienced was their Royal Caribbean cruise on the ship *Song of America*. Accompanying them were five other couples, most of whom had been former school chums of Bill. The camaraderie and frivolity day by day enhanced the marvelous surroundings on this trip of a lifetime!

There are many people who have made a great contribution to Canada. One outstanding Canadian was Lester B. Pearson, who was awarded the Nobel Peace Prize in 1957 and was prime minister from 1963 to 1968. His administration created the Canada Pension Plan, universal medicare, and the new flag, all of which have remained supreme through the years.

Many teachers have provided great contributions to Canadian children. One of Verna's favourites was Annie B. Fraser, a mature lady with great dedication and respect for her grade eight students. Her ability to make learning fun and to display love for and to reach out to all children in her class was a true inspiration. Her success stories have been the subject of conversations for many years.

As of 2009, Bill and Verna have been married for forty-eight years. They have two daughters, Debbie and Nancy. Debbie, their teacher daughter, is married to Martin Rauch. They have one daughter, Shannon, who is the only grandchild of Bill and Verna. Nancy is an esthetician and has her own esthetics studio in Burlington.

60
Steve Stasiuk

Strike! Strike! It happened when he was in grade eight. No, it was not a labour strike, but a student strike—in a small Manitoba town in the 1940s. The Dauphin-Ochre River School District was in the process of being formed. One of the proposed casualties was the teacher of grades nine, ten, and eleven in Sifton.

The powers-that-be gave notice that they were going to move him—Mr. Stanko—and these grades. How dare they do this dastardly deed! Although this teacher had his faults according to the students, they recognized that he was a high-quality teacher and wanted to keep in their community both him and the grades which he taught.

The students of those grades decided to act. After organizing a plan, they invited the students of grade eight, of which Steve was a member, to join as they would be in that class group in the next school year. After consolidating their plan, they marched through the streets with their placards and chanted that they wanted Mr. Stanko to stay.

The event drew the attention of CBC radio. Therefore, on the nine o'clock news that evening, the word spread across the province. This was considered an unusual occurrence. The school district authorities decided to soften their stance a bit. The teacher and the three grades remained for two or three years, after which, they succumbed to the "progress" of the time.

Steve was born in Sifton. All of his schooling before Normal School was obtained in the same town.

From Normal School, he remembers Miss Pilling, our art teacher, for her counsel on how we should dress. He particularly enjoyed the sports which were held after classes and participated in mainly fastball, and continued playing in this sport until 1965. He umpired in both baseball and fastball over the years.

After Normal School, he obtained a Bachelor of Teaching degree from Brandon University. Steve taught in rural schools in Sifton, Ochre River, and Gilbert Plains. Then, he moved to the positions of classroom teacher and principal in Dauphin.

His first school was in the Dauphin-Ochre River School District. It was a rural one-room school with eight students in grades from one to eight, with some grades vacant. The school was heated by a wood-burning pot-bellied stove. The students drank from a crock water fountain and paper cups. However, a few students brought their own cups. The school was closed after Steve's first year there.

Everyone moved to an older school for the following year. In this school, where he was for one year, there were fifteen students. Then, he moved to a junior high school in which he had thirty-two students. In his next school, he had average enrolments in the upper thirties.

Steve and his wife Lillian embarked on a memorable trip to the Baden-Soellingen, Germany, Canadian Army base where Lillian's brother was stationed. Among other sights, they enjoyed seeing the Black Forest and made a short visit to Strasbourg, a border city in France. They joined a tour with the Canadian soldiers to Italy.

After driving through Switzerland, which was very tidy and clean, they found a great difference on crossing the border into Italy. The places seemed so ramshackle and dirty. They visited such cities as Florence, Rome, and Pisa and also made a few side trips. The trip involved mainly the looking at buildings and statues.

When in Pisa, Steve gazed at the tower. No, he was not going to climb that structure. What if it would fall over at this time? It appeared that it would. Lillian was brave because she wanted to see what it is like up there. Thus, Steve watched at a safe distance.

From their hotel room window in Rome, he noted the small, poor homes in the vicinity. Sanitary conditions were bad. They could not drink the water in either country; however, there was better water on the base.

In his school years, he enjoyed *The Tragedy of Hamlet*, by William Shakespeare. Later, it was basically education books at the university level which he read.

For hobbies now, he enjoys wood working, puzzles, and dancing. His woodworking projects are mainly constructing lawn ornaments. He does the cutting and applying the undercoating. Then, Lillian does the actual painting of them as she has a particular skill in how she does it. They have not sold the ornaments, but have made them for themselves and their children. Some of these are now returning when a family moves and does not have the room for them any more.

He also enjoys an art known as pretty tunching. In the process, he uses a needle and tunches yarn on the underside of a piece of material. It comes out as a picture on the upper side with the use of different colours of yarn.

In his community, he is a member of the Knights of Columbus and the Ukrainian Catholic Parish. The Knights give bursaries to local high school students and sponsor the local Christmas parade. Steve and Lillian miss the parade because of their going to Texas for the winter. The organization also donates to charities in the community.

For an enjoyable Canadian trip, Steve recommends being in northern Manitoba in the summer.

He admonishes young people to work hard and be true to themselves. For those desiring to be a teacher, he exhorts that they be sure that that is really what they want.

Mr. James Stanko was a teacher whom Steve respected. He was very knowledgeable and strict. This student was willing to go on strike for him. Dorothy Brummitt was a principal under whom Steve worked. Through her example and advice, she made him a better teacher.

When he retired, he enjoyed not having to go back to work. He did miss it on the first day as he saw neighbourhood children going to school. He decided to go to Brandon on that day, just to be away. After that, he did not miss it. For a few years, he was kept very busy with volunteer work as he was yet unable to say, “No.”

Each winter, he and Lillian go to southern Texas. They travel within a radius of one hundred miles (161 km) of Weslaco. They usually visit Mexican border towns during this time. However, they have not eaten food or drunk water on any visit across the Rio Grande in the twenty years that they have been going to Texas.

This area in the lower Rio Grande Valley has a semi-tropical climate. There is a rainy season and a dry season. Most of the rain comes from hurricanes. Palm trees are a common sight. Grapefruit farming is an important industry.

Steve’s philosophy of life is to be the best person that one can be.

61
Emily (Szarkowicz) Hilhorst

Information for this chapter was submitted by Emily's children, who provided what they could recall about their mother. Emily passed away in August, 2006.

She loved the companionship of her friends at Normal School, not only on campus but also when they went shopping and went on picnics. In the fall, she needed a coat for winter as that season in Winnipeg can be very cold. She shopped in various stores, and after careful consideration, she selected one that she found in The Bay, a favourite store for many students. Although she spent an entire year paying for that coat by instalments of $15 per month, she was happy with her purchase.

She frequently talked about Grant Avenue, which, at the time, was a dirt road that ran by the Normal School, upon which one took one's chances in not becoming stuck in mud or snow! Those were the good old days.

Emily was born in Ituna, Sask. She attended Sponden School, a one-room school within walking distance of the farm where she lived, until grade ten. For grade eleven, she attended Goodeve High School, and lived with her older sister. After that, she attended Ituna School, where she graduated from grade twelve.

In 1949, following summer classes at Normal School, she obtained a Letter of Authority to teach on permit.

Thus, it appears that she knew from high school that she wanted to be a teacher and immediately went after that goal.

For the year 1949–50, she taught at Oak Hill School as a permit teacher. While she taught there, she met the man who later became her husband. Bert Hilhorst attended Oak Hill School as a student, and then was the one responsible to go to the school every morning and start the fire in the wood stove. It is thought that he may have continued doing this chore when Emily taught there.

For the summer of 1950, she persuaded her sister Stella to go work with her at the Sanatorium at Neelin, south of Brandon; and Stella left the farm to join her sister there. Following that, Emily attended Normal School for the 1950–51 year, and Stella took a job as a nanny and attended a business college in Winnipeg. The two sisters met frequently, and spent time together—shopping, at movies, at the park, and on picnics.

For the year 1951–52, Emily taught at Richmond Hill School, a position that she loved. She did have to haul armloads of firewood to feed the fire in the school's stove. Then, in October, 1952, Emily and Bert were married. After her marriage, she remained on the farm to work alongside her husband and to raise their four children.

It is not known if she had a favourite book when she was a child. However, when she was an adult, she was an incredible reader of many and varied books.

She was a wonderful homemaker and excelled in baking, cooking, preserving, knitting, and gardening. Anyone who arrived at the home to visit for a while was always welcomed, and before leaving, was invited to the table. Emily provided a sumptuous meal of homemade bread or buns, sliced home-cooked roast and chicken, home-cured and smoked ham and sausage, pickles, and vegetables from the garden, finishing off with a freshly baked cake or cookies. If anyone came from a distance which necessitated spending the night, there was for breakfast in the morning a royal spread of bacon, eggs, and milk from the farm, and the latest homemade jam or jelly that one absolutely must try. Her hospitality was truly second to none. What a wonderful home it must have been to visit!

In the community, she volunteered with the Holland Hospital Guild and the Bruxelles Women's Group.

She and Bert took a trip to Toronto, Ont., where, along with her sister and brother-in-law, they visited many churches, shrines, and grottos. It was an experience which she really loved at the time and about which she enjoyed to relate afterwards.

Emily and Bert loved to spend time with their son, daughter-in-law, and their children who live in High Level, Alta., about an hour drive from the Northwest Territories border. They would go fishing in the Peace River and the Hay River. They went north to the town of Hay River, N.W.T., on the shore of Great Slave Lake, and on to Yellowknife, N.W.T., and explored Wood Buffalo National Park and such northern Alberta communities as Rainbow Lake, Fort Vermillion, and Zama Lake.

Since they also had family in the Interlake Region of Manitoba, they visited back and forth. Emily had a brother who lived for many years in Dryden, Ont., and another in Thunder Bay, Ont. They would frequently visit them and the brother from Dryden would take them fishing on the lakes from Dryden to Thunder Bay. Those are deep and very beautiful lakes. She enjoyed these trips so much that she would recommend to everyone a trip to the North Country wilderness of Canada.

Emily had very specific advice for young people. Dress appropriately, sit up straight, listen to your parents, do as you are told, do not backtalk, go to church, pray to God for guidance, be of service to others—especially the disadvantaged—drink sparingly and avoid becoming drunk, do not smoke, avoid drugs, do not sleep with someone you do not intend to marry, do not sleep with him/her before you are married, do not gamble all your money away, work before playing, and watch television only after the work is finished. She may have had further advice, but these points provide a general idea of the example which she expected of young people.

Emily has stated that milking cows and farming make a hard life. She probably would not recommend the teaching profession to a young person these days, given the challenges before them. However, if a young person in the community had decided to go to university to major in Education, she very much respected and supported that person. Emily's philosophy would coincide with her advice to young people—and would include an emphasis on prayer.

It is not known if she had a favourite teacher at any level of her schooling. Mother Theresa provided a good model and influence for Emily. She considered former Prime Minister John Diefenbaker to have made a great contribution to Canada.

Until her passing, she resided in their retirement home on the farm, south of Holland.

62

Olive (Tarbath) Johnson

How would you like a slice of freshly roasted muskrat? The potential existed in one rural Manitoba school as a result of a discussion in class concerning the use of wild birds and animals for human consumption. It was common in the area to eat wild game since much trapping was performed. The boys were quite adept at catching such animals as rabbits, which provided numerous meat dishes. The class saw the merit of this activity.

On the following day, one of the older students brought his teacher a neatly "dressed" muskrat for her to cook for her evening meal. The boy was actually trying to be helpful, although he may have also been testing her since muskrats were not used for food. She was a bit surprised, but not horrified, when she received the donation. She graciously accepted it and took it home to her landlady, who decided that it might be better not to prepare it for their supper. Instead, she suggested that it would be more useful as dog food—which it became. It is amazing what can result from a simple lesson in class.

Olive was born on a farm near Rathwell and Treherne, and began her schooling in East Treherne.

One day when she was riding her horse to school, a flock of birds suddenly flew close by, startling her horse so much that Olive lost her balance and fell off. Away galloped her mount until he reached the safety of the neighbour's pasture. What would she do? The neighbour, who was not far away at the time, came to her rescue. Soon, the horse had settled down and allowed the man to lead him back to rejoin his rider. What a very embarrassed ten-year-old girl she was! Now, she could continue on to school as she was not hurt when she fell. Possibly, the neighbour told his family about the incident, but there was no teasing her for having fallen as it was not uncommon for a child to fall from a horse.

Olive remembers Mr. Lightly, our vice-principal and social studies teacher at Normal School. She appreciated his confidence-building remarks and his ability to gain respect without being forceful.

The girls in Thompson Hall were a very friendly “sensible” group, who were under the guidance of Pat Williams as house captain. Much giggling from the girls would occur at night, especially in the room next to that of the captain. Eventually, she would have enough and would tap on the wall and tell the girls to simmer down. Olive was innocent, being at the other end of the hall; but someone told her about the antics in this particular room.

After graduating from Normal School, Olive taught at Glencove, a rural school near Glenboro. Then, she taught at Bru, a rural school near Cypress River.

At Glencove School, the facilities were quite modest. The children obtained their drinking water from a well on the grounds and kept it in an insulated jug in the classroom. There was a very small library, possibly average for the time; but it did not compare with a school library of today. The basement was a heated area, the same size as the classroom above, less the space taken by the oil furnace and the toilet. The children were able to play games here, especially during cold weather.

After she married, she assisted with farm work and raised a family of two boys and two girls.

In her childhood, one of her favourite books was *Shepherd of the Hills*, by Harold Bell Wright. As an adult, she liked *Pearls: Philosophies for Living*, by Greg Tange.

Her hobbies today include gardening, reading, card-playing, travelling, and sight-seeing. In her community, she has served on the Board of Directors for Cypress River Credit Union, Cypress River Seniors' Lodge, and Cypress River Activity Centre. The activity centre is for the seniors, where one meal a day for five days of the week is provided. Such facilities as shuffleboard and a pool table are also available here.

Olive found a trip to Alaska and the Yukon both beautiful and informative. The lakes, trees, mountains, and glaciers were gorgeous to behold. She learned about the hardships of building roads and railways when the area was being developed. She became more informed on the "gold rush days" and the local industries of today.

As she rode on the White Horse and Yukon Railway, she was amazed with the spectacular scenery seen from the train. However, the train ran quite slowly because of the track being rough. At first, Olive wondered if this were a dangerous adventure as it appeared that the train might jump the tracks at any moment and plummet into the deep chasm below. The anxiety of all the passengers gradually subsided and it became a beautiful, scenic ride.

She recommends the Tiger Hills area southeast of Brandon, as a beautiful Canadian place to visit—especially when the flax and canola crops are in bloom.

Her advice to young people is that they be kind and honest with others and with themselves. They should try to maintain their own self-esteem despite difficulties that they might face in life.

If one is considering the teaching profession as a career, one should prepare by obtaining experience in dealing with young people. Babysitting, volunteering in a day-care centre, and assisting with organizing young people's activities are some ways of finding out about working with children. If such provide satisfaction and success, one may continue with the formal training for becoming a teacher.

Susan McKee was Olive's grade eight mathematics teacher. She helped her student develop a new understanding of many methods which became useful later in her teaching career.

Emma Hallgrimson is someone with whom Olive can discuss personal negative or positive issues which confront her. Her friend can make helpful suggestions without causing her to feel foolish or self-conscious.

Olive considers Tommy Douglas, "Father of Medicare", to have been a great Canadian. He made an outstanding contribution to the health care of lower income families in Canada.

Her philosophy of life is to live by the "Golden Rule". Live every day as though it were your last one on earth.

63
Tina (Thiessen) Hildebrandt

Her lecture was interrupted when several students in the back of the classroom were distracted by something on the floor. Before she knew it, the entire class surged out through the windows, leaving their teacher in the lurch in front of her desk. Much to her relief, a brave young man came to the rescue to save his teacher from any danger. With a hue and cry, he exterminated the culprit in record time. It was a short pencil-thin viper. Quite a diversion from teaching primary reading techniques!

Tina was born in Winkler and began her schooling in the same town. Her primary teacher, Ella Adrian, impressed her young student so much with her stunning appearance. She was so dressed up! In grade three, Tina would receive 93⅓%, her friend would receive 100%. Tina did not like this at all!

Although in 1950, her first choice was to go permit teaching, she accepted the modest Manitoba scholarship to attend Normal School instead. The fact that she developed a case of shingles was positive proof that she possessed an inordinate fear of teaching—practice teaching, in particular. If the course had lasted five years, she probably would have dropped out.

At Normal School, she served tables, mainly at breakfast. Before she had this work, she had never met guys of different ethnic backgrounds; but, now, she had a table of them in her charge. Oh, how those hungry boys devoured all the food that she placed before them!

For herself, she felt that the food was good. As soon as everyone left the dining hall, she and the other girls scrambled to reset the tables as classes would soon commence. If there were a table without a waitress, Mrs. Savage would look for someone waiting in the entrance for her meal. Her sweet request for a waitress for the meal at hand was difficult to decline. Like so many students, it was necessary for Tina to work to earn money as she even could not afford to go to swimming lessons.

She particularly remembers Mr, Lightly, our vice-principal and social studies teacher, who was such a gentleman and who had the skill of assessing the ability of students, even the quiet ones. Regretfully, he succumbed to Alzheimer's disease.

Tina taught in schools in Winkler and Altona, and in a school in Nigeria. What a pleasant surprise it was when the board of a two-room rural school near her home town hired her. She was on her way to be a workaholic, but her principal tried to prevent that scenario by frequently allowing double and triple recess times, giving her time to orient herself. Each year she was blessed with a different inspector whose encouragement was invaluable.

Moving to a town school in Altona was another challenge that turned out to be most positive. As her university credits increased, it was gratifying to be promoted to junior high. In those days, discipline was not the problem it seems to be today.

In 1970, she married Jakob Hildebrandt, an experienced teacher whose résumé ranged from Shamatawa to Zaria (Nigeria). Three years later, the couple signed up to teach under Mennonite Central Committee's Teachers Abroad Program, which assigned both to schools in Nigeria.

Tina's school lacked much—particularly books. She was unable to add to the few books in the library. There were very few supplies; and, when she opened a package of paper, students wanted even the covering paper. The buildings, a former Catholic seminary, were actually good, despite some windows lacking. This was a teachers' college, where she taught her students how to teach remedial reading and mathematics. One of her classes consisted of good teachers who were returning to upgrade their qualifications. In spite of its shortcomings, the school was still considered one of the best in Nigeria. Unlike his wife, Jakob, who taught in a government high school for boys, was able to obtain books.

During the tenure of their assignments, "universal primary education" was introduced and teachers' salaries —abysmally low until then—were doubled. Since Tina and Jakob were under a monthly MCC allowance, this did not affect them. They lived on a reserve of residences for teachers, creating a village outside of a town of 3,000, which had few stores. When they walked to the top of a nearby hill in the evening, they could see smoke rising from the homes in the town. The people of this very rural community were not well-to-do. The students brought their own knives and forks to use in the dining hall, and they purchased their own compulsory uniforms.

It is always gratifying to hear of the success of one's former students. Tina is happy to include a church bishop, a doctor, an industrialist, a naturalist, and many public-spirited citizens as her former students. Despite duty days, recess patrols, and nightly homework, it has been fulfilling. To God be glory for health and strength.

In 1996, Jakob and Tina flew to Omsk, Siberia, where they were picked up by someone in a small, rickety car which had been imported from Germany and which two families owned. Their destination was the comfortable home of her aunt, who lived in Sonsofka, a town with a population of 3,000. The residents of this town were not well-to-do. Tina admired how self-sufficient each family appeared to be, depending on its own gardens and livestock. She has a vivid memory of a vast expanse of golden grain being harvested by five combines.

Stories of the repressive days of the Communist system were related mostly with a sense of humour in the days of *glasnost* and *perestroika*. Jakob's aunt had to work hard in previous Communist times at a commune, leaving her two little sons uncared for. One day, she went on strike, feeling that she should look after her household no matter what happened to her. This good worker could have been fined by the authorities, but she escaped any penalty. The people would say that their employers pretended to pay their workers and the workers pretended to work. During their visit of three weeks, Jacob and Tina did not have the opportunity to ride on the Trans-Siberian Railway; but were aware of its presence.

Tina recommends that visitors go to the southern Manitoba city of Winkler and the surrounding Mennonite villages in summer. Altona's Schwarz House has a gallery in the park featuring prize-winning sculptures and art by internationally renowned painters, both indoors and out.

Tina would advise a young person that the teaching profession is rewarding; but is also quite strenuous, especially today. During her 32 years in the profession, she never entertained the idea of changing her career.

As a teacher, she enjoyed sharing *The Boxcar Children*, by Gertrude Chandler Warner, with primary children. Her community activities today involve working in the Mennonite Central Committee thrift store; but, in the past, she has served on the board of the Seniors Centre. For pastimes, she likes to read, to sew, and to travel.

64

Roy White

One day when he was in high school, he decided to play Tarzan. It was not a scorching day, but a day in winter. There was a rope hanging from a tree branch. There was a frozen ditch that begged to be crossed. Now was a good time to test that rope and his agility. Crash!

As the rope gave way, Roy felt the ice shatter under his weight. The water was so very cold! Unceremoniously, the defeated aerialist crawled out of the ditch as rapidly as possible. He scurried to his boarding place to change clothes and to dry off. His pockets were still full of ice as he removed his cold trousers.

He was a celebrity for the next week. Children and adults would point him out, "He's the one." At the 50th reunion of his high school, what do you think they remembered after all those years? Tarzan had landed upon the ice.

Roy was born in Hartney. He commenced his education at Whitewater S. D. 336 Hartney, a one-room school with thirteen students, grades one to nine.

After attending Normal School, he obtained a Bachelor of Arts degree and a Bachelor of Education degree.

In schools at High Plains, Cameron, Warren, and Hartney, he was both a classroom teacher and the principal. From 1964 to 1966, he taught at Wudil Teacher Training College, in Nigeria. When he returned to Canada, he became Midland Division superintendent at Carman.

Wudil is a small village in Nigeria. While there, Roy taught Principles of Education and various academic subjects as the need arose.

For two years, Roy, Edith, and their three children lived in a comfortable house on the southern edge of the Sahara Desert. The camel caravans went right past their gate. The authorities provided the family with three servants—a garden boy, a steward, and a cook. The steward provided the children with very good care. The two older boys obtained their education via official correspondence courses from Manitoba.

The local people had sufficient food and good housing. They showed much friendship toward the White family. Overall, the family was quite satisfied with living there. However, despite that, there was a concern about what was happening in Nigeria at the time. The Biafran War was being fought. Roy prefers not to go into detail about some aspects of life there. Matters changed greatly for the native people, depending on which tribe they were members. He felt that one would not want to be a Nigerian then. It was so dangerous and uncertain for them.

After his time in Africa, Roy was Director of Communications and Education, Manitoba Association of School Trustees, in Winnipeg, for fifteen years. This was followed by ten years as a self-employed consultant in education, working out of Winnipeg.

He retired from this organization at age 58. Then, he became a consultant on the operation of boards—any kind of board, even corporate. This work took him across Canada, but he performed much work in the Arctic, particularly in the Northwest Territories. This continued until 2005.

You have never really experienced a blizzard unless you have encountered one like the one that caught Roy during his time in the North. For ten days, he was stranded in Baker Lake Hotel. Each morning, the school superintendent would arrive with an extra pair of coveralls to protect Roy from the frigid wind and then lead him to the board office through the ferocious blizzard. It was a blind excursion as they groped their way from hydro post to hydro post, guided only by the sound of humming and snapping wires above them.

If he were young and just beginning his profession, he would heed the call of the North without hesitation. His favourite community was Fort Good Hope along the east bank of the Mackenzie River, almost to the Arctic Circle. This community originated as a fur-trading post of the Northwest Company in 1805.

As a child, Roy enjoyed reading *Wahb: The Biography of a Grizzly*, by Ernest Thompson Seton. There were only about six readable books in the one-room school library. Another book which he read was an engineer's story of his part in the building of the Canadian Pacific Railway. Every time he drives through Saskatchewan on Highway #1, he looks for the village of Secretan, which was named after that engineer. Recently, he finished reading the book *A Short History of Everything*, by Bill Bryson.

For hobbies, Roy enjoys wood carving, tennis (which he learned in Africa), golf, pool, and cooking. With all of these activities, he does not have time to be bored.

He has been involved in too many service clubs or community organizations to recall all of them. A few of the positions which he has held include the following: president of the Manitoba Education Research Council, chairman of the Teachers' Certification Board, chairman of the School Act review, life member of the Manitoba Superintendents' Association, and honorary life member of the Manitoba Trustees' Association. Since retirement, he has resolved never to go to another meeting. He has not been entirely successful, but he goes to very few now. He says that life is great for him.

When Roy was teaching in Hartney, two of his students from his school in Africa visited him and his family. He arranged to take them by train from Winnpeg to Kitimat, B.C. He was so impressed with the sight of the majestic Mt. Robson, the highest peak in British Columbia, as the train passed by. It was such a wonderful trip, one which he would recommend to anyone.

He advises teenagers to follow their dream, but not to become mired in a life which they do not like. They should have the courage to move on. When considering teaching as a career, young people should be aware that this is not for everyone, but it is wonderful for those who succeed.

Mr. Lightly, our vice-principal and social studies teacher, stands out for him. This man was sincere, straight-forward, and normal. He remembers his fellow students, his roommates, and other residents of Frontenac Hall, most of whom are still in touch with him, even though they are spread across Canada. Fellow Normalites honoured him by electing him Student Body President for the second term.

Roy feels that his wife Edith had more positive effect on him than anyone else. She was always supportive of her husband when she felt what he was doing was correct. On the other hand, she did not hesitate to tell him when she thought differently. He gives her credit for being correct most of the time.

Roy has much respect for Ab Richardson, one of his high school teachers. This man recognized that his students had much value in them. Prime Minister Pierre Elliot Trudeau was an outstanding leader because he caused the people of this country to feel proud to be Canadian.

For Roy, life just seemed to unfold, each new step being better than the previous one. He thinks that our age group is a part of a blessed generation. We missed the dirty thirties through which our parents had to live—and most never got over them. We missed the war that took the lives of many who were just a few years older, including many of our older siblings. We have enjoyed the security of the growth that followed the war. We did not have to worry about employment as there was always a job somewhere, unlike our baby boomer children who always had to compete. He could go on, but we all have experienced many positives in our lifetime. So, be thankful. Enjoy retirement.

"There is a destiny that shapes our ends. Rough hew them as we may." This summarizes Roy's philosophy of life.

TIME

A suitable topic for an octogenarian

When I was young time was infinite
Christmas was always years away
Summer holidays went on forever
Growing up was an eternity
Learning was every day all day
Everything was exciting
The future was tomorrow.

Now at eighty.

A day becomes a week
A week a month
A month a year
A year a decade
The future is yesterday
Old is a jet plane speeding to eternity.

I am not complaining. We were a blessed generation.

The thirties built our character
We were too young to go to war
We had the privilege of university
We never had to worry about making a living
Times were good
Life was good.

Life is still good it is just going by too fast.

Roy White, recent octogenarian

CLASS J

Carl Braun
Etta Craig
Belva Hassett
Peter Hiebert
Peter Klassen
Lorene Lyle
Michael Maksymets
John Pauls
Mary Produnuik
Anne Pronchuk
Sylvia Syrnyk
Yvonne Ver Wilgen
Elaine Vincent
Elaine Wall
Erica Wall
George Ward
Anita Wenden
Florence Westfall
Edna White
Shirley White
Marlyne Whyte
Mary Williams
Patricia Williams
Helen Wilms
Olga Wingarek
Jeneva Wood
Edna Woods
Natalie Woods
Isabel Woods
Michael Yarmie
Pearl Young
Pauline Yourkin
Harry Yoshida
Mary Yule
Bertha Zacharias
Sylvia Zadorozny
Bernard Zakaluk
May Zook

65
Carl Braun

It's January 21, 1937:
Blasts of ice crystals,
Billows of white from chimney
Straight to heaven in a Manitoba January kind of way.
Squeaks from snow that tingle the ear—
Otherwise, ominous silence
All the way to school—
On a particular January morning—

While we are quietly finishing our breakfast, and before we get into our winter togs, the radio man announces, "... bitterly cold today ... BRRRR." And bitterly cold it was. The sleigh is parked by the kitchen door ready to deliver five bleary-eyed children to school. Even the barn, perhaps 20 metres back, is all but shrouded in ice crystals. BRRR, indeed! The long wash line with long johns, yesterday's laundry that hasn't yet dried, stark reminders of cold, bitter cold—ghastly frosted phantoms suspended from small to larger, to ever larger, stiff robots dizzily dancing in crazy rhythms in the Arctic breeze! BRRR! One can sense Jess and Bell's reluctance to embark on the two-mile trek they know so well. Very quickly they are encased in ice crystals, jetting clouds of steam from nostrils, rime-flecked manes, each snort amplified like an exclamation point to highlight "bitter cold!" Apart from this, the only sound, amplified clinks and clanks of harness steel, and the ominous squeals and squeaks of steel runners on the hard, packed snow trails. The signature CHK CHK CHK's of Pappi's tongue urges Jess and Bell to trot just a little faster. (I will always carry the image of us huddled together like five fluffed and puffed up Hungarian partridges to ease the snap of the prairie winter blast. And through the ice fog, I see Pappi, his back to us, a massive statue draped in heavy buffalo fur, motionless—like an ice-age prairie sasquatch. That's January in Burwalde, a Manitoba January). I'm so glad that Peter and I are sitting close to the back of the room, all but over the heat register which this morning bathes our back sides with blasts of hot air.

The bell rings. O Canada and the Lord's Prayer quickly follow, and the usual singing of choruses. Then roll call. (I was puzzled for months about that word, "present" since it was never followed with a present.) Miss Suderman asks us to take out our readers ... everyone settled in for another day, another week of school, the usual. And then without warning, fire! Flaming tongues—brilliant orange, yellow, red—lashing from the register, which in my super-powered imagination would later evoke images of a hundred thousand dragons spewing fire at unsuspecting little victims.

I believe in the miracle of a child's memory to all but filter out whatever transcends the bearable, though not always. All I remember after our rush to the frigid outdoors is being back on the straw-lined sleigh to escape from the scene of this horrendous unfolding drama, the odd "booh whooh's" of ones as terrified as I am, juxtaposed against the unbelievable exclamations of bravado, "School's out! Whoopee!" "How lucky for us!" (To this day, I marvel that I recognized the voices.) As for me, I bemoan the fact that I haven't had time to grab my brand new Christmas scribbler and pencil from Grossmammi Braun.

> Weeks, even months pass and the image of flames reaching out at me, especially in my dreams, is an on-going occurrence, and my refusal to go to school is seen as no more it seemed at least, as a brand of typical Carl-type sissy behaviour. I call out in my dreams, and nobody comes. Some mornings I get dressed for school, go toward the sleigh and then dash back into the house. The dead silence of my brothers and sister and Pappi leaves no doubt as to their feelings. I remember Mammi begging one morning for me to go because that was the day Miss Suderman was going to decide who could proceed from the Primer into the Reader. Even her coaxing didn't work. Ernie was the only one happy about my resistance to go. We'd spend the day playing at home." (Carl would learn later that he had missed forty-five days of school.)

These are the words of Carl Braun as he remembers his horrendous experience with the burning of his school.

Carl was born on a farm near Winkler. He started school at Burwalde #529, a two-room school, grades one to ten. After completing the grades offered there, he took his grade eleven, partly by correspondence, and partly at Winkler Collegiate Institute. He completed his grade twelve at WCI.

He had a major choice to make when he graduated from Burwalde School. Where would he obtain his grades eleven and twelve in order to graduate from high school? He could obtain them by correspondence or attend a Mennonite private school. The curriculum at the latter had a significant German component and the discipline was reportedly very harsh. Thus, this seventeen-year-old youth chose the correspondence route.

Since he did not have adequate space at home for studying, he went to the school despite its meagre science supplies. He bluffed his way on reports or did not submit them regularly. It was not long before his tutor realized what his student was doing and expressed concern. The situation went from bad to worse. At last, he was given an ultimatum. He must submit his missing assignments or withdraw. He selected withdrawal. Thus, except for some music study, he enjoyed a relaxing winter.

Shortly before Easter, his father made a comment completely out of the blue, "Maybe you could go to Winkler after Easter and try to salvage part of the grade." Carl seized upon the opportunity. The high school there had a high passing rate record on the provincial departmental examinations, and most of the courses by this time were in the review stage for the June examinations. How could he review the courses if he had not "viewed" them in the first place?

The ancient "twin desks" would turn out to have redeeming qualities for Carl. He was alone for the first week. His seatmate was missing because of surgery. He eventually met this seatmate—Jerry Hildebrand. The young man was an angel for this new student! Jerry's notes were a life saver—so organized, so clear, and so complete. He turned out to be one of the absolutely kindest, most selfless people whom Carl was ever to meet. The boys became friends quickly. Carl salvaged his year through what he considers nothing short of a miracle. He did have an ability to compose essay-type answers. He considers himself to have been what David Cork, in *The Pig and the Python*, calls an "articulate incompetent."

He began his post-secondary education at Manitoba Provincial Normal School. After that, he obtained a Bachelor of Arts degree, a Bachelor of Education degree, and a Master of Education degree at University of Manitoba through years of evening and summer classes. Concurrently, he specialized in music, obtaining piano teacher certification (A.M.M.) from University of Manitoba and piano performer certification (A.R.C.T.) from Royal Conservatory of Music. He then obtained a Doctor of Philosophy degree from the University of Minnesota and an honorary Doctor of Laws degree from University of Manitoba.

In addition to English, Carl speaks Low German (Plattdeutsch) and German (language of the church, and second school language).

He shared somewhat cramped quarters in Strathcona Hall with Victor Toews, who also came from a Mennonite community. They had become acquainted when they attended a previous six-week permit teacher's course. Carl was a member of Class J because he and his brother Ernie, in Class B, had decided not to be in the same class.

While he became acquainted with many students, he remembers special times with Victor Toews, Orest Roscoe, Ed Maza, Pete Fast, Jerry Hildebrand, Merv Farough, and Ernie—all Strathcona dudes. When any of them received care packages from home, they freely shared the contents.

He particularly remembers one fellow who was unfamiliar with proper laundry skills. While performing his weekly laundry, he provided his heavy woollen sweater with a steaming, soapy bath. Anyone but a novice could predict the result. What went into the machine as a hefty size 42 emerged minutes later just large enough to fit the average size doll.

The meals, on the whole, were passable. Some of the desserts were quite good. As for shepherd's pie, he has not sampled it since. In addition, he does not expect that he will look for a piece any time soon. He assumes that we all withstood the saltpetre that was added to the food.

He still feels that some of the teachers demonstrated very effective practice and an abundance of patience and care. It must have been a challenge for them, considering the somewhat "rough edges" that some of the students had on entering into a setting quite alien to previous experience.

He remembers with great fondness so many classmates from Class J and beyond. He agrees with a comment made by Shirley (Solar) Maurice at the June 2007 luncheon that we had always been "a caring group and still cared about each other." He considers it very special that we continue to belong to a "community" so many years later.

He has fond memories of the class projects. Class J opted for a "Selkirk Settlers" theme. He does not state it specifically, but the class earned the best marks in the interclass competition. What a beautiful way this was of involving all members of a class in incorporating music, art, movement, and drama into one production! The Class choir under John Pauls' direction did quite a remarkable rendition of the 23rd Psalm, a version that was new to Carl, and one which he still loves. His class had some excellent singers in the group, and Shirley White did a professional take on the Highland fling.

There certainly was much learning—plenty of organization, planning, and working together, which, at times, was a challenge. He thought that the instructors executed a marvellous job of emphasizing the positive in their evaluations. Throughout his long career, Carl would see many reincarnations of integrating the arts with other aspects of the curriculum, always with a splash, always with banners proclaiming the "new and innovative"—just one instance of educational amnesia, the endemic malaise of many educational bureaucrats.

He has positive memories of both Mr. Moorhead, our principal, and Mr. Lightly,our vice-principal. Although so different in personality and approach, in many ways the two complemented each other. He thinks many of us remember Mr. Moorhead for some of his favourite hymns which he would volunteer during morning chapel. Two notables were “From Every Stormy Wind that Blows,” and “Where Cross the Crowded Ways of Life.” Healthwise, “the stormy winds” would soon take over in Mr. Moorhead’s life, more than Carl had realized.

Carl, his brother Ernie, Duane Duff, and Ed Maza went to visit him at his house in July following our year. All had been working at the school during the summer. He was a very mellow man, obviously weakened, and physically in stress. What struck Carl was the warmth he exuded as he received his four students. He demonstrated so clearly that we were one of his!

Through the years, Carl has been proud to have been associated with these folks at Normal School, many of whom have served the children of Manitoba so well—high-class teachers, consultants, a Minister of Education, superintendents, principals, professors, pastors, and missionaries. There have been many footprints of expertise, love, and compassion, far beyond what anyone could ever trace.

Carl spent his first thirteen teaching years in Manitoba schools, including an eight-grade rural school, and elementary, junior high and senior high schools in the towns of Winkler and Fort Garry. He held full-time professorships at University of Manitoba and University of Calgary. In addition, he held short-term visiting professorships at University of Regina, University of British Columbia, University of Minnesota, Western Washington State University, and Mount St. Vincent University (Halifax, N.S.). For many years, he was involved in piano tutorials as a member of the Greater Winnipeg Music Teachers’ Association.

The summer following their first year of teaching, Carl and Ernie decided that they would need more education and enrolled in American history and German at University of Manitoba. After only a few days, disaster struck! Carl received word that one of his grade two pupils had contracted polio and passed away the next day. How emotional this experience was! He immediately went home. With the help of members of the school board, a student choir was quickly organized to sing a couple of hymns at the funeral. He chose one of the hymns which had been used at another funeral, despite the emotional effect that it had on him.

On his way to the funeral service, he had left an older brother, Ted, in the Winkler clinic waiting to be seen by one of the physicians. When he returned, his brother was lying on one of the clinic benches obviously in agony. Carl knew that Ted, a strong, dignified, self-assured person would only in the most dire circumstances expose himself publicly to what could have been construed as weakness. Something was wrong, very wrong. The result was that Ted would spend the next thirty-six years in the polio ward of the King George Hospital in Winnipeg. Carl and Ernie dropped their classes and returned home where their family had need for them. It was a summer of very dark clouds!

He wants to make it clear that he was never a particularly brilliant student. However, he did have the ability to know when to leap onto the backs of giants and hitch some quite significant rides. When he had completed his candidacy examinations at the University of Minnesota, he shopped for a supervisor to walk him through a dissertation, hopefully quickly and painlessly. He tried two or three before he settled on co-advisors—one, a well-seasoned research psychologist and the other, an internationally known language educator. It turned out that he had chosen wisely, and he managed to obtain his “ticket” in close to record time.

What was significant and very surprising to him was that he received an International Outstanding Dissertation Award, which would have ripple effects throughout the balance of his career. The results showed first with a number of lucrative writing contracts, invitations to write for some of the publications with wide international distribution, and more speaking engagements than interested him.

Ultimately, the visibility would lead to his nomination and consequent election to the board of the International Reading Association for a three-year term. The organization, often known as "IRA", had more than 90,000 members in over 100 countries at the time.

Subsequent to his term on the board, he was elected to the presidency of the organization, the first non-U.S. president. Since it was International Literacy Year, the spin-offs were quite incredible—membership on the International Task Force on Literacy, delegate to various world education conferences, an invitation to UN headquarters to consult on matters dealing with the "Conventions of the Rights of the Child", a number of UNESCO meetings, and speaking gigs in Thailand, New Zealand, and Australia. The culminating tasks of the president were hosting one North American Convention, his being in Las Vegas, Nev., for 13,000 delegates.

A more significant event was a World Congress on Literacy in Stockholm, Sweden. The Congress culminated in a reception at Town Hall. Carl was the host, and what an experience that was! The ambience, the history, and—more important for him—the expectations, were thrilling. He was seldom really overwhelmed during the years in executive office. This was a notable exception. He put all of his resources to work in mustering feigned confidence and a measure of panache. All of this was an experience, but oh, it was so far from "the farm" in Manitoba which he had long left behind—and no Nobel Prize for the boy!

In May 2007, he was awarded two honours in Toronto for his contributions to world literacy. He still enjoys attention, but he was frankly embarrassed by such tributes as, "We honour your exemplary leadership and your commitment to world literacy, and especially your unwavering commitment to improve the role of women and children in developing nations."

He doubts that any ripples from that doctoral tome have sent significant vibrations to many in developing countries. He also doubts that anyone has ever marked his footprints in those faraway villages of poverty and disease. However, he does believe that his significant place in life has been with children and teachers. That is where he began—in the one-room school. He still has some opportunities—and the nerve—to work with children as together they enjoy working through a piece of rousing reader's theatre. That is where he feels the tingle of accomplishment, so satisfying, even exhilarating—56 years later.

It is touching the individuals, or small groups of individuals, with whom we live and work daily that has the potential for difference. He thinks about Margaret Mead's comment, "Never doubt that a small group of thoughtful, committed citizens (or individuals) can change the world; indeed, it's the only thing that ever has." He has always believed that idea.

There have been numerous persons who have influenced him during his lifetime—former students, colleagues, teachers, and musicians. Choosing one person has been virtually impossible.

He thinks of Alan, who was referred to the University of Calgary Language/Reading Clinic. Alan, an eight-year-old, had been a battered baby, but was adopted into a wonderful family. His brain was clearly damaged and his speech was halting, arrhythmic, even robotic. He was in grade three—a non-reader. His response to the regimen prescribed by Carl and his student clinician was a combination of movement, kinaesthetic involvement, music, and more. This experience taught Carl more than he could ever describe. Alan, two years later, won the academic award in his class and a significant Science Fair award, by now a completely fluent speaker, an avid reader, self-assured, and happy.

He also thinks of Ruth Neill, nee Hoehn, teacher par excellence on the Sandy Bay reserve in the Manitoba Interlake district. Ruth, one of his former students, demonstrated almost every human and professional quality that would define his notion of the model teacher. When some of the classes in Sandy Bay had few, even no students on Friday afternoons, Ruth had the full complement. Her students would not dare to be absent for fear that they would miss something "special." Something special might have been learning a new song, listening to an extra story, or going out on a nature walk.

However, probably the person who had the most effect on Carl was one who had taught him. She was Miss Norton, our literature instructor at Normal School. There were at least two other instructors who would influence him as much as Miss Norton. He feels that some of the things Ruth may have learned from him, and some of the ways in which he and his colleagues worked with Alan in the clinic, in indirect ways at least, did indeed bear some of the footprints of Miss Norton.

Like Miss Baker (Psychology), Miss Smith (Basic English Composition and Grammar), and Miss Douglas (Music), Miss Norton was one the planters of ideas and notions which would grow into quite unrecognizable fruits in years to come. He cannot say that Miss Norton really stood out in any way until she produced Kipling's "The Naughty Elephant's Child." For Carl, that was a gift that has given many times through the years. The story was good, but the production was outstanding!

The use of language, the demonstration to reflect nuance, the expert phrasing, the timing and the placement of pause, and all those facial contortions—the winkles, wrinkles, and crinkles punctuating, and generally, embellishing the performance—were something to behold. It was a masterful performance! He will always carry in his "echo chamber" the sound of "*... the banks of the grey-green, greasy Limpopo River, all set about with fever trees, to borrow new noses from the Crocodile.*"

It taught him more about language and language instruction than any series of lectures on language that he has endured through the years. It also taught him much about the elements that make language memorable, the elements that are likely to draw attention, and even more important, that language in "wholes" is the only way in which sense is created and communicated effectively.

Perhaps more than anything, Miss Norton demonstrated the place of literature in the curriculum—which language is taken in like our mother's milk, defying the need for endless skill, drill, and kill exercises. Her production has figured in no small way in Carl's interest in the cross-over between music and oral language. He has felt some of the ripples even in his more recent work with his daughter, Winn, as they continue to explore learning possibilities through reader's theatre. He would love to have a video of Miss Norton and compare it with the ongoing replays in his personal eidetic cinema, and just "drink it in" once more.

He had the pleasure of meeting Miriam Norton years later. As president of the Winnipeg Chapter of the International Reading Association, she hosted a reception at her home. What a gracious hostess she was! Carl had always considered her quite old, not necessarily ancient, just old. Thus, when she introduced him to her mother, his jaw all but dislodged. His teacher was really younger than he thought when he was a Normal School student.

Carl has always been a dreamer, from childhood to senior. He still remembers a poem learned many years ago.

If I were Lord of Tartary
Myself and me alone,
My bed should be of ivory,
Of beads and gold my throne.

He has had such dreams. However, on a more realistic note, he always hoped that his personal and professional resources would result in the enhanced welfare of students, particularly many of the children—and some adults—whom he and his colleagues used to serve in language clinics, recognizing fully that literacy carries the potential to change lives, and in later life, the lives of their families.

Music has always ranked high in his interests and aspirations. In his mind, he would love, at least once, to have performed a piano concerto—a Tchaikovsky, a Beethoven, a Rachmaninoff (especially #3), a Prokofiev, or even a Mozart or Haydn. Yet, in his imagination, he does conduct musical performances, sometimes even when he is out for a jog. Little ability is required, and lack of discipline never gets in the way. He is firmly resolved to sublimate and to work a little harder at a couple of Chopin Études which are within reach—even as he lowers his personal expectations.

Musical activities of various sorts would best characterize his principal hobby, even if during many times of his life music as a hobby and music as vocation intersected inextricably. This is not surprising as, even during his doctoral studies, he was considering a music major. He has directed school and church choirs (children's)—including high school operettas. Over the years, he has accompanied choirs, vocal and instrumental soloists, and played at many weddings. He continues to do some playing as a therapeutic diversion.

His fascination with language and writing is vying for front row status. It seems as though there is a tension between his two "principal loves" as they are competing for time and energy.

For him, defining his philosophy is like attempting to define a rainbow, a smile, a kiss, or the taste of good chocolate. You begin to define what you have experienced, and suddenly the words render the beautiful mundane, even dull. He is reminded of Keats who claimed that "philosophy can unweave the rainbow; it can clip the angel's wings." He believes that Keats was alluding to a preoccupation with analysis.

He states a few of the core beliefs which he has come to cherish, and for the most part, to live by. Love and compassion, he believes, are at the centre of a life worth living, and he always hopes that his expression of these virtues defines who he is. He believes that the Golden Rule has a greater place in the world today than ever before. He was touched deeply by the reaction of the Amish community in Pennsylvania in the way in which they dealt with the horrendous losses in the wake of the sniper "hit" on their school children in 2006. They demonstrated true Christ-like living. It was a demonstration of forgiveness and love unparalleled in our daily news reports.

He and his wife Evelyn spend many hours volunteering in a Salvation Army Hospice, and now more than ever before, he has come to grapple with the notion of compassion. There are many times when he questions the extent to which he is able to demonstrate compassion, especially in the presence of some of the residents. He is bothered at such times. He wonders if he might be too wrapped up with his own needs.

As for a philosophy, he is led to believe that he must shed some of the personal baggage in order to open space for the baggage of others. As much as he likes to fight it, the challenge clearly lies in becoming less self-centred.

He likes to believe that his actions are guided by a desire to leave the planet just a little better than it is. That is inclusive, and as he understands things, it means that he take into account not only how he treats his neighbour, but also how he treats God's creation. As he strives to fulfill his purpose on this planet, he realizes more and more the need to remain connected with God, the creator, and his son, the Master Teacher.

Being an educator, he states a few ways in which his philosophy plays out in his life from a learning and instructional standpoint. He believes that truth is communicated through action, good literature, and striking metaphor. What he reads into the actions or words of another is coloured by his beliefs and his experience. He was a high school English teacher for several years; but he had taken only one university English course, completely turned off by demands to regurgitate the interpretation of a professor of Chaucer, Shakespeare, or any other author. Years later he would resonate with Margaret Atwood's salty quip, "squeezing the last pimple of significance from a piece of literature."

The biggest problem that he would ever have with graduate students was being faced always with the question, "I'm not sure what you want." Carl's response would be, "I can't possibly know what I want since I don't know what you're capable of giving me. Your response to what you consider a 'wishy-washy' demand will offer me some insight into your personal crucible of knowledge."

Students came with an expectation that they could find "the answer" by reading the text. He wanted their reaction to, even anger at, what others thought. This caused them to explore creatively. In his last two clinic courses, he simply announced on the first days of seminar, "You'll all get at least a B unless you hear from me early enough in the programme to pull up your boot straps." How he wishes that he had thought of that earlier in his career!

His students were free to explore their potential, free to risk being wrong, and free to become truly professional. He believes that this is a reflection of his philosophy. He also believes that, in both school and university classrooms, much potential is laid waste through the fear of failure of the course grade.

He has always believed that his job in the classroom was to create an environment in which learning would thrive. Eventually, he invited students to challenge not only what they read, but also what they heard from him. Eleanor Boyce, who taught at the Normal School a few years after our year, and later at the University of Manitoba, in concluding a course she taught in Winkler, challenged her audience, "If you forget everything I've said, remember to teach your students that paper never refuses ink." What good advice that was! He senses a message there for us all—students, teachers, parents, pastors, rabbis, priests, and the electorate!

Finally, he believes Marguerite Somerville, prominent Canadian ethicist, strikes an important note for all, certainly for him, "Hope is the oxygen of the spirit." He wants to remember that always!

The main residence for Carl and his wife Evelyn is in Calgary, Alta. Then, for three months of the year, they live near the town of Kenora, Ont.

66

Elaine (Wall) Rex

Play ball! That call created many memorable experiences for a young girl who participated on a girls' baseball team. This capable player and her team won many games. She even practised with the boys' team during school noon hours.

One particular game stands out in her memory. She had been hurling to her male battery partner when, suddenly, she stopped and called him to the mound. What strategy did she want to discuss with him in regard to the next batter? This is a normal practice between catcher and pitcher, although it is usually the catcher who initiates such a conference.

Out strode the catcher to the mound, approaching her closely so that the opposing team could not hear the conversation. Pop! Down the front of his shirt fell a frog that his female pitcher had found in the grass. Girls! How deceptive and unexpecting they can be in a time of serious business! Years later, this incident was recalled by her friends.

Elaine was born on a farm located at 30-2-12, near Clearwater. She attended Clearwater Public School for grades one to eleven and rode the train to attend the high school in Crystal City for grade twelve. She also took university classes after attending Normal School.

Her favourite teacher prior to Normal School was her principal, Joe McCracken, who taught all subjects in grades nine to eleven. She attributes to him the qualities of being interesting, knowledgeable, compassionate, and fair. He expected all of his students to work to the best of their abilities, to respect each other, and to play fairly.

As a teenager, Elaine was a member of 4-H, where there was a good teaching programme, including the learning of crafts, the conducting of meetings, the interacting in the community, and speaking at rallies. For a time, she served as president of the club.

Elaine has fond memories of Room 1 in Thompson Hall, which she shared with Elaine Vincent, Sylvia Lee, and Ivy Douglas. It was a double room at the end of the hall, large enough for late night birthday parties, discussions, and mentoring each other, or even responding to knocks on the window after hours to let someone in through it. Here they laughed, cried, and became friends for life.

Miss Ring, our health teacher, is the staff member whom she particularly remembers. She taught us basic health and so much more. Her methods expanded beyond the classroom and into every aspect of the community life which she knew that we would experience.

Elaine's first experience in teaching was at Dunallen School District, located about ten miles (16 km) north of Boissevain. She left there on November 10, 1951, following a tragedy that befell her sister. Thus, she stayed at home until Christmas, after which she taught grades one and two at Darlingford, where she remained for two and one-half years.

When she was teaching at Dunallen, she had a most embarrassing experience. One cold November morning when she and three children from the farm where she boarded were riding to school a bit late in a horse-drawn buggy, she urged the children to have the horse pick up the pace. The horse, with the encouragement, set off at a gallop toward the school yard. When the children managed to bring the horse to a halt, the seat lurched, snapping the bolt which was anchoring it. Suddenly, everyone and everything—teacher, students, blankets, books, and lunch pails—tumbled unceremoniously to the ground. How hilarious that was for the children peering out the windows in the school! Elaine and her fellow riders picked themselves up amid the laughter of the spectators.

From 1979 to 2008, Elaine operated a small business as the owner-manager of a dental supply company, selling directly to dental offices and laboratories. Being a people person, her work was based on service, by which she knew her customers very well. She found this was more rewarding than the money which she earned. Most of her business was carried on outside Winnipeg, but in the later years, she operated in the city.

Elaine would tell teenagers that our destiny is shaped by the choices which we make each day and that everything becomes history which cannot be erased. Teenagers, especially, are influenced by their peers. At this age, it is difficult to imagine that our association with our classmates, many of whom we shall never see again, lasts such a brief time. However, their influence, good or bad, may stay with us. She encourages young people to focus on being role models rather than looking for one to follow.

A school superintendent once told Elaine that teachers are born, not made, and that he "can stand a great teacher on his/her head in a corner and he/she can still teach". She believes that one's intention should be passion for the work before the paycheque. A teacher should love students first and think of them as stars entrusted to him/her to develop and polish. The teacher should help them to believe in themselves and that encouraging words from the teacher may be the only ones that the students may receive.

As a child, she enjoyed reading *Heidi*, by Johanna Spyri; and, as an adult, it was *Gone with the Wind*, by Margaret Mitchell. Today, her hobbies consist of reading, sewing, playing cards, and learning how to use a computer.

For many years, she was a member of the United Church Women and has led women's ministries and Bible study within the church. Other church activities were organist in a small congregation for thirteen years and teaching Sunday school. She attended Bible School at Springs Church in Winnipeg. She and her husband Alf became involved in community associations wherever they lived. She has served for twelve years with the residents' association in the building where she lives.

She and her family travelled to Fort McMurray, Alta., many times to visit relatives, with Elaine, herself, having made the trip at least forty times. They participated in many tours of the oil fields, becoming quite familiar with the process of extracting at the surface. Because of the method used, it was easy to experience the entire process. Although this type of procuring oil takes a toll environmentally, she wonders how many of the thousands of petroleum-based products would consumers be willing to forfeit.

Rachael Skilleter is a dear friend and mentor who has had a positive influence on Elaine's life. The two friends are in constant communication even though more than 1,000 miles (1,600 km) separate them. Rachael is a woman of great wisdom and faith, who is firmly grounded to the plumb line of life. Everyone needs a mentor who is able to share the joys and challenges of life together. She can rely on Rachael to give advice that Elaine needs to hear, not what she wants to hear.

For a visitor to Canada, she would recommend Tofino, on Vancouver Island, where she has fond memories. Elaine and Jean McClelland (chapter 36) married Agriculture Faculty roommates—Alf Rex and Ken Tully, respectively. Together, the two couples have visited the area numerous times. They would rent a cabin on the beach to watch monstrous tidal waves crash on rocks in pre-dawn hours. Such a mystical aura and breath-taking event this was! She informs us that storm-watch vacation special offers are available and highly recommends them. During visits of ten days at a time, they would see many wonderful places in the area.

Two weeks before Alf died, Ken phoned Elaine to check on his friend and learned that he was not doing well. On the same evening, Ken phoned back to say that he would go to see Alf for a few days because he preferred doing this rather than receiving word to come to the funeral. It was a wonderful visit in which both men were uplifted.

During many class reunions and luncheons, a comment made regularly was that the class of 1950–51 was unique. We bonded then and the bond remains strong today. Carl Braun told Elaine that, years after graduation, Miss Baker, our childhood development teacher, commented to him about this uniqueness. The staff realized that they had never had a class like ours. Elaine would like to think that we collectively have made a great contribution to the shaping of our nation of Canada.

She believes that her philosophy of life is fairly simple. Everyone is born with a purpose that our Creator has for us. Strive to discover that purpose and fulfill it and take time to develop relationships. Love people for who they are, not what they have done. Life is one of choices and each day will be what one makes of it.

We are in our twilight years with many more behind us than ahead. It is not too late for new dreams and goals as we can still make a difference in the lives of those around us. In the words of songwriter Lee Anne Womack: "Whenever one door closes, I hope one more opens. Promise me you'll give faith a fighting chance, and when you get the chance to sit it out or dance, I hope you dance."

67
Pearl (Young) Langille

She always had a "too-good" appetite, especially for sweets. A Valentine party in the country school house was an ideal place for food—sweet food. The best part of any party was the food. On this occasion, someone had brought a jelly roll. On seeing it, her mouth began to water. At last, it was time to sample it. How good that tasted! Would there be enough left over for her to have a second slice?

After a time, she noticed that there was just one slice that no one seemed to want. That must be just for her. Happily, she picked it up and took a big bite. Ugh! How awful it tasted! Her mouth was full of not only jelly roll, but also dirt. Unknown to her, it had fallen on the floor and then had been put back onto the plate, dirty side down, just to fool someone like her. She was the victim. Everyone had a hearty laugh at her expense. What did she learn from this experience? Do not be so greedy!

Pearl was born in Weyburn, Sask., and began her schooling in that town.

Her favourite teacher was Jean Kettles, her grade eight teacher in a one-room rural school in the 1940s. She taught every grade from one to eight, having a total of over forty students, including four of her cousins. The youngest of those cousins was extremely unruly, requiring the patience of Job. However, this teacher was equal to the task, even though it was her first year of teaching. She was fair and patient with all of the students. Pearl is privileged to be able to phone her occasionally now.

She feels that this same Jean Kettles had the most influence on her life and work. She was a role model of what a teacher should be. If it had not been for her, Pearl would not have been able to continue school after grade eight. Jean and the school inspector persuaded her father to allow her to complete high school. This took some doing as she was the only one of a family of twelve whom her dad allowed to continue schooling. His stipulation was that she would stand first in the class. You are assured that she kept her nose in the books for the following four years!

She admits that she does not remember the names of most of the teachers at Normal School. She has difficulty in remembering names—a real negative in teaching. However, she does remember Miss Ring and was impressed by her quiet manner and her control of the class. When one of the students suffered a seizure, Miss Ring calmly utilized the opportunity to practise what she had taught her classes about such an occurrence, using the proper procedure to help the student recover.

Since Pearl was an introvert, she was not often involved in activities outside the classroom at Normal School. One memory she has is the "torture" of gym classes, becoming unconscious on one occasion. She was paired for the Indian wrestle with a larger and heavier student than she. Since she knew that she could never fling her opponent up and over without straining her muscles, she offered little resistance. Consequently, she was literally banged onto the mat and "knocked out" for the remainder of the class.

Another impossible gym experience was trying to leap frog over a six-foot (183 cm) plus fellow, ending up riding on his back instead of landing on the floor. How she did dread gym classes!

She did make a few friends at Normal School, one with whom, Emily James, she has kept in touch over the years, although they have not seen each other much since the 1950s. She knew Dorothy Keffen, her roommate in the main building, from high school days. Later on, Pearl enjoyed a visit in her home. All things considered, she found Normal School an interesting, helpful, and positive experience.

As a permit teacher, Pearl taught at Moline, near Rivers. After graduating from Normal School, she taught at Boss Hill, near Virden; at Kelowna, B.C.; and at Winnipegosis. She was a substitute teacher at several locations.

When she was attending rural one-room schools as a student, she had a fear of the school inspector, who visited twice a year. What if he would ask her a question that she could not answer? She was terrified of the possibility.

This fear was still apparent when she was teaching, making her feel very nervous. The school where she was teaching was situated beside a field where the grain had been threshed, leaving much straw in which the students liked to play. They had actually piled straw over the top of some low bushes, making a straw house.

One day at noon hour, teacher and students were inside their straw house, eating their lunches, when someone arrived. The inevitable happened. Here was the school inspector! Pearl gingerly crawled out, full of straw —in her hair, down her neck, and all over her clothes. What a spectacle she must have been! What did the inspector think? He made no comment, for which she was thankful. However, she was never so embarrassed in her life—before or after!

In 1973–74, she took a secretarial course. Following graduation, she worked in a newspaper office in Amherst, N.S., for one year. She held several temporary typing jobs in Halifax, N.S. Then she worked as an executive secretary for the Non-Academic Staff Association, a trade union at the University of Alberta, in Edmonton, Alta., for four years.

Pearl was not thinking about learning on a trip that she and her niece took to the United States in 1953. First, they visited her sister and family in Colorado Springs, Col., and then they continued to Nashville, Tenn., to attend the Grand Ole Oprey.

While in Colorado, which is semi-desert, they visited the Garden of the Gods and underground caves at Colorado Springs. In this "garden", huge, tall, reddish spires scattered all over a valley. What a really spectacular sight this was!

On a tour of the underground caves, they viewed stalactites and stalagmites—huge icicle-like formations composed of dripping water containing minerals that had frozen. The former hung from the roof of the cave while the latter stood on the floor. Within these formations was a "bridal" chamber where some couples chose to be married. Another oddity was the "fat ladies entrance", a very narrow passage through which a few tourists were not able to pass. These people had to return to the surface. In today's "obesity epidemic", there would be many more people unable to navigate this entrance.

Another point of interest was a vertical rock wall where climbers could practise their skill, or lack thereof. Her sister told them that several times a year a novice climber would suffer severe injuries or even death from falling. Yet, that did not deter others from climbing.

When she was a child, Pearl enjoyed reading *Anne of Green Gables*, by Lucy Maud Montgomery. Later, as an adult, she enjoyed *Who Has Seen the Wind?* by W. O. Mitchell.

She still enjoys playing her Gibson guitar (antique 1951), singing, and "jamming" with her grandson. She likes to work with jig-saw puzzles having 1,000 pieces. After completing the pictures, she frames them for wall pictures, particularly those from paintings by Thomas Kincade. She likes to read, but she is doing less because of her "old" eyes.

In the community, she has worked with Autumn House. Locally, this is the Cumberland County Transition House Association for abused women and children.

A place in Canada that she feels is well worth visiting is the area between Amherst and Parrsboro, N.S. It resembles the Cabot Trail in Cape Breton, although it is not quite as spectacular. The view overlooks the Bay of Fundy with its tides, which reportedly will be a great source of electricity in the future. The autumn season is the most colourful time of the year in this area.

There is much advice that Pearl could give a group of teenagers, although most of it would be too old fashioned to be heeded. She would advise them to take life seriously and always strive to give their best. She would also inform them that morality, honesty, and dependability will bring them the best in life—a clear conscience, peace of mind, and satisfaction. To be able to look back on their lives when they are old, knowing that they had accomplished something worthwhile is worth much.

To young persons considering teaching as a profession, she would point out the need for a love of children, firmness accompanied with kindness, patience, and praise for a child's best efforts. Also, they should be prepared for a job which, at times can be difficult, though overall most satisfying.

As a great Canadian, she would name a modern day leader, Bill Casey, who has made, and continues to make, a great contribution to Canada because of his honesty. He is the Member of Parliament for Cumberland County, where she lives. She is aware that his courage in standing up for his beliefs made news across Canada. At present, he is attempting to bring order and cooperation among the members of parliament. If all leaders and politicians were as honest as he is, Canada and the world would be entirely different.

Her philosophy of life is that we are born for the purpose of serving our Creator and living our lives according to his commandments. While not popular today, it is the way that gives us the best in this life and also a hope for eternity. This is also an anchor in times of distress and provides comfort and fulfillment that cannot be found any other way.

Appendix

Place of Birth

California
Dunsmuir: Isabelle (Neeley) Dowling

Manitoba
Argyle (RM): Evelyn (Graham) Jones
Arnaud: Mary (Dishnick) Chubey
Balmoral: Harry Rudy
Binscarth: Aileen (Harbottle) Huss-Seidel
Broomhill: Helen (Finlay) Morrow
Chater: Isla (Gliddon) Lawrie
Clearwater: Elaine (Wall) Rex
Cypress River: Dorothy (Carnegie) Blakeman
Darlingford: Bernice (Morrow) Lewis
Dauphin: Jack Morton
Elm Creek: Wilma (Miller) Furniss
Elton (RM): Dorothy (Brownridge) Haithwaite
Gilbert Plains: Ethel (Galloway) Currie
Gladstone: Rose (McColl) McIver
Glenboro: Vera (Jones) Skayman
Hamiota: Wilma (Hedley) Treloar, Gladwyn Scott
Hartney: Roy White
Hodgson: John Ryan
Horndean: Peggy (Friesen) Lawrence
Killarney: Peter Peters
MacGregor: Winnie (Cathcart) Wolfe
McCreary: Emily James
Manitou: Cecile (Droux) Fisher
Medora: Frances (Burnett) Dickinson, *Lois (Leigh) Moore
Minnedosa: Shirley (Bold) Fairbairn
Oakburn: Harry Backlin

Plum Coulee: Abe Friesen
Portage la Prairie: Ruth Armson
Pulp River: Eugene Doroschuk
Rosebank: Jean (McClelland) Tully
Rosendale: Ena (Kandall) Sparrow
St. Boniface: Joyce (Griffith) Garner, Keith Huss-Seidell, Shirley (Solar) Maurice
St. Claude: Henrietta (Heiget) Leduc
Selkirk: Marie Brownlees, Orest Roscoe
Shoal Lake: Elaine (Slimmon) Dale
Sifton: Steve Stasiuk
Sprague: Delphie (Olson) Norberg, Doreen (Olson) Lindquist
Swan River: Dorothy (Twilley) Shewfelt
The Pas: Joan (Barr) Allison
Tilston: Virginia (Eilers) Lyons
Treherne: Audrey (Donald) Henitiuk, Olive (Tarbath) Johnson
Virden: Betty (Forsyth) Sumner
Winkler: Carl Braun, Jerry Hildebrand, George Krahn, Tina (Thiessen) Hildebrandt
Winnipeg: Edna (Brown) Dreger, Betty (Hughes) Doroschuk, Irene (McFee) Coleman, Sarah "Eva" Muir, *Viola (Sigurdson) Wild

Ontario
Corinth: Duane Duff

Saskatchewan
Edgeworth: Shirley (Fulmore) McCracken
Carnduff: Jacob Enns
Ituna: *Emily (Szarkowicz) Hilhorst
Rocanville: Verna (Spurr) Lavergne
Swift Current: Sylvia (Lee) Haverstick
Weyburn: Pearl (Young) Langille
Young: Henry Dick

* deceased

Place of Residence

Alberta
Calgary: Carl Braun, Henry Dick, Harry Rudy
Delburne: Wilma (Hedley) Treloar
Stony Plain: Audrey (Donald) Henitiuk

British Columbia
Abbotsford: Abe Friesen
Ladner: Isla (Gliddon) Lawrie
Nanaimo: Jean (McClelland) Tully
North Vancouver: Jack Morton
Pitt Meadows: Marie Brownlees
Prince George: Harry Backlin
Surrey: Duane Duff
Victoria: Betty (Hughes) Doroschuk, Eugene Doroschuk, Shirley (Bold) Fairbairn

Manitoba
Alexander: Winni (Cathcart) Wolfe
Brandon: Vera (Jones) Skayman, Ena (Kendall) Sparrow, Betty (Forsyth) Sumner
Carberry: Gladwyn Scott
Carlowrie: Mary (Dishnick) Chubey
Cypress River: Olive (Tarbath) Johnson, Evelyn (Graham) Jones
Dauphin: Steve Stasiuk
Elkhorn: Cecile (Droux) Fisher
Headingly: Bernice (Morrow) Lewis
Holland: *Emily (Szarkowicz) Hilhorst
Langruth: *Viola (Sigurdson) Wild
Manitou: Irene (McFee) Coleman, Wilma (Miller) Furniss, Dorothy (Twilley) Shewfelt
Meadows: Delphi (Olson) Norberg
Morris: Edna (Brown) Dreger
Stonewall: Emily James
Thompson: Doreen (Olson) Lindquist
Virden: Virginia (Eilers) Lyons
Waskada: Frances (Burnett) Dickinson
Wawanesa: Dorothy (Brownridge) Haithwaite, *Lois (Leigh) Moore

Winkler: Jerry Hildebrand, Tina (Thiessen) Hildebrandt
Winnipeg: Ethel (Galloway) Currie, Elaine (Slimmon) Dale, Jake Enns, Sylvia (Lee) Haverstick, Keith Huss-Seidel, Aileen (Harbottle) Huss-Seidel, Peggy (Friesen) Lawrence, Henriette (Heiget) Leduc, Shirley (Solar) Maurice, Helen (Finlay) Morrow, Peter Peters, Elaine (Wall) Rex, John Ryan, Roy White

New Jersey
Haworth: Dorothy (Carnegie) Blakeman

Nova Scotia
Amherst: Pearl (Young) Langille

Ontario
Burlington: Joyce (Griffith) Garner, Verna (Spurr) Lavergne
Clearwater Bay: George Krahn
Fort Frances: Joan (Barr) Allison
Kanata: Orest Roscoe

Saskatchewan
Carnduff: Sarah "Eva" Muir
Moose Jaw: Rose (McColl) McIver
Ogema: Shirley (Fulmore) McCracken

Washington
Seattle: Isabelle (Neeley) Dowling

Yukon
Whitehorse: Ruth Armson

* deceased

LaVergne, TN USA
28 September 2009
159085LV00001B/1/P

9 780981 078441